I0044488

Veterinary Medicine: Research and Practice

Veterinary Medicine: Research and Practice

Editor: Shawn Kiser

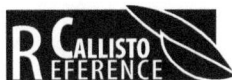

R CALLISTO REFERENCE

www.callistoreference.com

Callisto Reference,
118-35 Queens Blvd., Suite 400,
Forest Hills, NY 11375, USA

Visit us on the World Wide Web at:
www.callistoreference.com

© Callisto Reference, 2019

This book contains information obtained from authentic and highly regarded sources. Copyright for all individual chapters remain with the respective authors as indicated. All chapters are published with permission under the Creative Commons Attribution License or equivalent. A wide variety of references are listed. Permission and sources are indicated; for detailed attributions, please refer to the permissions page and list of contributors. Reasonable efforts have been made to publish reliable data and information, but the authors, editors and publisher cannot assume any responsibility for the validity of all materials or the consequences of their use.

ISBN: 978-1-64116-120-6 (Hardback)

Trademark Notice: Registered trademark of products or corporate names are used only for explanation and identification without intent to infringe.

Cataloging-in-Publication Data

Veterinary medicine : research and practice / edited by Shawn Kiser.
     p. cm.
Includes bibliographical references and index.
ISBN 978-1-64116-120-6
1. Veterinary medicine. 2. Animal health. 3. Animals--Diseases. I. Kiser, Shawn.
SF745 .V48 2019
636.089--dc23

Table of Contents

Preface

I am honored to present to you this unique book which encompasses the most up-to-date data in the field. I was extremely pleased to get this opportunity of editing the work of experts from across the globe. I have also written papers in this field and researched the various aspects revolving around the progress of the discipline. I have tried to unify my knowledge along with that of stalwarts from every corner of the world, to produce a text which not only benefits the readers but also facilitates the growth of the field.

Veterinary science is the branch of medicine that is concerned with animal health. It involves the analysis, treatment, diagnosis and prevention of animal diseases. Veterinary science covers the treatment of all domesticated and wild species of animals. It also furthers human health and well-being by monitoring and controlling zoonotic diseases in animals. Research in veterinary science explores the prevention and control of diseases in animals. This book presents the significant veterinary science concepts and theories and explores the interrelation and incorporation of these methods in the field of livestock management. There has been rapid progress in this field and its applications are finding their way across multiple industries. This book is designed to serve a broad spectrum of readers from experts to students who want to gain a better understanding of the subject.

Finally, I would like to thank all the contributing authors for their valuable time and contributions. This book would not have been possible without their efforts. I would also like to thank my friends and family for their constant support.

Editor

Congenital infection with atypical porcine pestivirus (APPV) is associated with disease and viral persistence

Lukas Schwarz[1†], Christiane Riedel[2†], Sandra Högler[3], Leonie J. Sinn[2], Thomas Voglmayr[4], Bettina Wöchtl[1], Nora Dinhopl[3], Barbara Rebel-Bauder[3], Herbert Weissenböck[3], Andrea Ladinig[1], Till Rümenapf[2] and Benjamin Lamp[2*]

Abstract

In 2013, several Austrian piglet-producing farms recorded outbreaks of action-related repetitive myoclonia in newborn piglets ("shaking piglets"). Malnutrition was seen in numerous piglets as a complication of this tremor syndrome. Overall piglet mortality was increased and the number of weaned piglets per sow decreased by more than 10% due to this outbreak. Histological examination of the CNS of affected piglets revealed moderate hypomyelination of the white substance in cerebellum and spinal cord. We detected a recently discovered pestivirus, termed atypical porcine pestivirus (APPV) in all these cases by RT-PCR. A genomic sequence and seven partial sequences were determined and revealed a 90% identity to the US APPV sequences and 92% identity to German sequences. In confirmation with previous reports, APPV genomes were identified in different body fluids and tissues including the CNS of diseased piglets. APPV could be isolated from a "shaking piglet", which was incapable of consuming colostrum, and passaged on different porcine cells at very low titers. To assess the antibody response a blocking ELISA was developed targeting NS3. APPV specific antibodies were identified in sows and in PCR positive piglets affected by congenital tremor (CT). APPV genomes were detected continuously in piglets that gradually recovered from CT, while the antibody titers decreased over a 12-week interval, pointing towards maternally transmitted antibodies. High viral loads were detectable by qRT-PCR in saliva and semen of infected young adults indicating a persistent infection.

Introduction

Congenital tremor (CT) of piglets is a common phenomenon characterized by a generalized shaking involving the whole musculoskeletal apparatus. CT is generally classified in two types of disease. While histopathological lesions are missing in type B, the type A is associated with variable hypomyelination of brain and spinal cord. These histological lesions are found as inherited genetic defects in male Landrace pigs in type A-III [1] and in Saddleback pigs in type A-IV [2]. Other causes of CT occurrence are infections with viral agents like Classical swine fever virus (CSFV), responsible for type A-I [3]. CT of type A-II is prevalent in piglets worldwide, occurs as a sporadic disease affecting single litters, as an outbreak over several weeks affecting a high proportion of farrowing's or as an ongoing problem frequently affecting gilt litters [4]. Viral agents responsible for CT A-II were sought for decades. In 2015, the novel divergent porcine pestivirus strain "atypical porcine pestivirus (APPV)" was identified in North America and subsequently also detected in Europe [5–7]. Other closely related strains were termed congenital tremor virus (CTV), because they were detected in piglets clinically affected by CT, creating a synonymous name for the same viruses. Serum of affected piglets was used to inoculate pregnant sows to establish the link between APPV and congenital disease. This infection study could reproduce congenital disorders in the offspring [8]. However, Koch's postulates

*Correspondence: benjamin.lamp@vetmeduni.ac.at
†Lukas Schwarz and Christiane Riedel contributed equally to this work
2 Department of Pathobiology, Institute of Virology, University of Veterinary Medicine Vienna, Veterinaerplatz 1, 1210 Vienna, Austria
Full list of author information is available at the end of the article

remain to be proven for APPV. Recently, a first successful cell culture isolation of APPV was reported [5], which might be the key for infection experiments with a defined inoculum.

It is known that pestiviruses may induce various clinical symptoms depending on virus species and strain, as well as on age and immune status of the respective hosts. Beside acute hemorrhagic disease, as documented for CSFV or highly virulent strains of Bovine viral diarrhea virus II (BVDV-II), an infection with most pestiviruses yields mild or subclinical disease in the immune-competent host [9]. Pestiviral infections during gestation may have a detrimental effect on the embryo or fetus, causing stillbirth, neurological defects or malformations [10]. Dysmyelination or hypomyelinogenesis is a characteristic neural lesion in ovine fetuses infected with Border disease virus (BDV) in the late gestation period [11] and such lesions are frequently associated with CT [12]. The clinical signs and histopathological lesions of the so-called "hairy shaker" lambs substantially improve in a few weeks [13, 14], but the exact mechanisms responsible for congenital hypomyelination after in utero infection have not been discovered to date. Historically, CSFV was the only pestivirus known to cause natural infections with clinical significance in swine [15] usually resulting in different clinical symptoms with high morbidity and mortality. CT is a frequent symptom of congenital CSFV infections of piglets. A first novel "atypical pestivirus" (Bungowannah virus) was found in Australian pigs in 2003 but no link to CT was given. Instead, Bungowannah virus caused stillbirth and sudden death of young piglets [16]. The Bungowannah virus is still circulating at the site of initial discovery, but this virus or relatives were never found at other locations [17].

Here we report on the identification and characterization of atypical porcine pestiviruses in seven Austrian farms affected by CT. Clinical symptoms and the course of disease in single litters were followed up over several parities. Histopathological examination showed that clinical symptoms were linked to characteristic hypomyelination in the CNS. APPV could be isolated and propagated on porcine cell lines and the infection was visualized by immunofluorescence. Prevalence of APPV was analyzed by RT-PCR and APPV specific antibodies were determined with a novel NS3 based blocking ELISA to get insights into APPV epidemiology. Monitoring naturally APPV infected and CT affected piglets over a period of 24 weeks gives evidence for a persistent infection. The first documentation of virus shedding via semen in a meanwhile clinically unsuspicious boar, which had been a shaking piglet before, is of special importance with regard to the epidemiology of APPV in the field.

Materials and methods
Sample collection

All animal use protocols employed in this study are approved by the institutional ethics and animal welfare committee and the national authority according to §§26ff (Animal Experiments Act from 2012; BMWF-68.205/0188-WF/V/3b/2015). All APPV strains and sequences analyzed in this study originate from these Austrian field cases. In 2015 and 2016, we investigated the pathogens in five Austrian piglet-producing farms, which were experiencing problems with CT and subsequent growth retardation in rearing piglets (Table 1). These cases of CT were brought to our attention by the responsible veterinarians, which reported on several additional cases distributed all over Austria. None of the farms had used vaccines against CSFV according to the Austrian legislation. Veterinarians of the University Clinic for Swine in Vienna conducted the clinical examination and collected samples for diagnostic evaluation. Furthermore, we included a retrospective evaluation of clinical samples from two previous outbreaks, which occurred in 2013 in farms in lower and upper Austria. The clinical examinations in the affected farms only gave a snap shot of the signs and course of disease in some farms. A continuous monitoring of production performance, mortality and pathogen prevalence was not possible in all farms, since the cases occurred in regular commercial breeding farms. To present a typical example, we investigated the outbreak in farm A in detail regarding production losses, clinical symptoms and pathological findings over a 6 month period. Available data about piglet production before and during the occurrence of clinical signs of CT in the other farms is summarized in Table 2.

Farm A

Farm A is a piglet production site located in the northwestern part of Upper Austria. 105 Large-white × Landrace crossbred sows are managed in a 3-week batch-farrowing interval in seven groups consisting of 15 sows each. Gilts are obtained from a gilt producer. Two teaser boars are kept on site for sow stimulation during artificial insemination. Before entering the production cycle, gilts are housed in a separately managed isolation unit for three to nine weeks, which is managed separately. Here, all gilts are vaccinated against parvovirosis and erysipelas (Parvoruvac®, Merial SAS, Lyon, France) and treated alternately with fenbendazole (Panacur 4%, Intervet, Vienna) and ivermectine (Ivomec, Merial SAS) to prevent introduction of sarcoptic mange and round worms. Serum samples of all gilts are screened for PRRSV antibodies before integration into the sow herd. This herd was free of PRRSV before and after occurrence

Table 1 Synopsis of farms participating in the study

Farm	Year of CT outbreak	Location	# of piglets in pathological examinations	Data generated in the respective farm
A	2015	Upper Austria	10	Exemplary description and prevalence studies
B	2016	Upper Austria		
C	2016	Upper Austria	3	Genomic APPV sequence and long-term monitoring
D	2016	Upper Austria		
E	2016	Upper Austria		
F	2013 and 2016	Lower Austria	2 (in 2013)	Virus isolation
G	2013	Upper Austria	2 (in 2013)	

Table 2 Impact of CT occurrence on piglet production, piglet mortality and the splay legs syndrome

Farm	WP/S/Y before OCT	WP/S/Y during OCT	Mortality of CT-affected piglets	Splay legs observed in CT-affected piglets
A	25.5–26.5	23.57	Up to 30%	Yes
B	24.5	17.2–19.6	i.d.	No
C	25.6	22.8–24.0	i.d.	Yes
D	26.2	26.0	0.6%	No
E	26.5	23.45–23.86	Up to 25%	Yes
F 2013[a] (2016)	i.d. (24.1)	i.d. (24.0–24.05)	i.d. (<0.6)	i.d. (no)
G	i.d.	i.d.	i.d.	i.d.

WP/S/Y: weaned piglets per sow and year; OCT: occurrence of congenital tremor; CT: congenital tremor; i.d.: indeterminate, due to inexistent or inconsistent records.

[a] Material was investigated retrospectively and therefor no accompanying data available.

of CT. An average of 26.0 piglets was weaned per sow and year in farm A before CT symptoms occurred.

Pathology

A complete necropsy was performed on ten piglets of farm A and seven affected piglets from the other farms. Here, we describe the findings from five clinically affected piglets from farm A and five littermates without symptoms. The piglets were euthanized, a gross pathological examination was performed and samples were taken. For histological examination brain, spinal cord, and organ samples of all piglets of farm A and a healthy control animal from a farm without CT problems were fixed in 10% neutral buffered formalin. Formalin fixed brains were cut into coronary sections of 2–3 mm thickness and embedded in paraffin wax. Organ samples and coronary and longitudinal sections of cervical, thoracic and lumbar spinal cord were cut and embedded in paraffin wax, too. Of all embedded organs 1.5 μm thick sections were cut and stained with hematoxylin and eosin (HE). Furthermore, brain and spinal cord samples were stained with a combination of luxol fast blue and HE (LFB-HE) to determine the extent of myelination. Immunohistochemical investigations using a primary antibody (ab109186, dilution 1:1000; Abcam, Cambridge, UK) for determination of olig-2, a marker for oligodendroglial cells, were performed automatically on an autostainer (Lab Vision AS

360, Thermo Fisher Scientific, Waltham, USA). Briefly, 2 μm paraffin-embedded sections of the piglets' brains and spinal cords were placed on coated slides and dried to enhance tissue adherence. Antigen retrieval was performed on deparaffinized and rehydrated sections by heating in citrate buffer (pH 6). Endogenous peroxidase activity was blocked by incubation in H_2O_2. After application of the primary antibody a polymer detection system (UltraVision LP Large Volume Detection System; Thermo Fisher Scientific), consisting of a universal secondary antibody formulation conjugated to an enzyme-labeled polymer was used. The polymer complex was then visualized with an appropriate substrate/chromogen (diaminobenzidine [DAB]; Labvision/Thermo Fisher Scientific). Subsequently, all sections were counterstained with hematoxylin, dehydrated and mounted.

For transmission electron microscopy, samples of cerebellar white matter, cerebellar peduncles, and medulla oblongata of one clinically affected piglet and one piglet without symptoms from farm A were cut in 1 mm^3 cubes and fixed in 2.5% neutral buffered formalin and 2.5% glutaraldehyde (Merck, Darmstadt, Germany) in 0.1 M phosphate buffer (Sigma-Aldrich, Vienna, Austria), pH 7.2, at 4 °C for 3 h. Afterwards samples were post-fixed in 1% osmium tetroxide (Merck) in the same buffer at 4 °C for 2 h. After dehydration in an alcohol gradient series and propylene oxide (Merck), the tissue samples were embedded in glycid ether 100 (Serva, Heidelberg, Germany). The ultrathin sections were cut on a Leica Ultramicrotome (Leica Ultracut S, Vienna, Austria) and stained with uranyl acetate (Sigma-Aldrich) and lead citrate (Merck). Ultrathin sections were examined with a Zeiss TEM 900 electron microscope (Carl Zeiss, Oberkochen, Germany) operated at 50 kV.

Detection of APPV genomes and sequence analysis

Total RNA was extracted from field serum samples, semen, saliva or tissue samples using the QIAamp Viral RNA Mini Kit (Qiagen, Hilden, Germany) according to the manufacturer's instructions. RNA was eluted in 60 µL RNase free distilled water and directly used for RT-PCR or stored at −80 °C for subsequent analysis. RT-PCR was carried out using the OneTaq One-Step RT-PCR Kit (NEB, Ipswich, USA) or the One Step RT-PCR Kit (Qiagen) according to the manufacturer's instructions. Several primer pairs (available upon request) that were hybridizing with highly conserved regions in different pestivirus species (BVDV, BDV, CSFV, Bungowannah, and APPV) were designed according to published sequences available in NCBI GenBank. Resulting PCR amplicons with suitable length were subjected to gel electrophoresis, purified by the peqGOLD Gel Extraction Kit (Peqlab, Erlangen, Germany), and sequenced by a commercial provider (Eurofins Genomics, Ebersberg, Germany) using the PCR primers. DNA fragments belonging to APPV were sub-cloned in the pGEM-T easy vector (Promega, Madison, USA).

Sequences of Austrian APPV strains were submitted to GenBank with the provisional entries KX778725 (AUT-2015_A), KX778726 (AUT-2016_B), KX778724 (AUT-2016_C), KX778727 (AUT-2016_D), KX778728 (AUT-2016_E), KX778729 (AUT-2013_F), KX778730 (AUT-2016_F), KX778731 (AUT-2013_G). First analyses were carried out using NCBI's Basic Local Alignment Search Tool for nucleotides (BLASTn). Phylogenetic pairwise comparison and identity calculations were carried out with CLC Main Workbench 7.6 (CLCBIO, Aarhus, Denmark). Alignments and phylogenetic trees were generated with the software CLC Sequence Viewer 7.6 (CLCBIO) with bootstrap values based on 1000 replicates. For construction of the phylogenetic trees, homologous sequences of APPV and other pestivirus species deposited in GenBank were used as indicated.

Quantitative reverse transcription-PCR (qRT-PCR)

For the quantification of viremia and virus burden, viral RNA was also extracted with QIAamp Viral RNA Kit (Qiagen) according to the manufacturer's instructions. RNA was eluted in 60 µL distilled water and 1.25 µL was directly used for amplification with the Invitrogen One-Step qRT-PCR Kit (Thermo Fisher Scientific) on an ABI 7500 cycler (Applied Biosystems, Foster City, USA). The APPV specific primers P1 (5′-AGTTCAGAAAT CCGGTAGCTG-3′) and P2 (5′-CTACCAGCCTGA GGTCTTC-3′) were used for amplification and the probe P3 (5′-FAM-GTTTCGACACCAAAGCTTGGG ACACTCA-TAMRA-3′) was used for detection. A recombinant bacterial plasmid harboring the sequence encoding the NS5B gene of APPV strain AUT 2016 Farm A was purified using the QIAGEN Plasmid Midi Kit (Qiagen) and spectrophotometrically quantified. The copy number of recombinant plasmids was calculated following the formula: N (molecules per µL) = (C (DNA concentration in µg/µL)/K (fragment size in bp)) × 185.5 × 10^{13} (factors derived from DNA weight, volume and the Avogadro constant). In order to obtain a standard curve, a tenfold dilution series of cDNA was included in the qRT-PCR setup. Cycling conditions were 42 °C 15:00, 95 °C 5:00 and 45 cycles of 95 °C 0:05, 60 °C 0:33 (amplification and fluorescence detection step). Genome copies were calculated by 7500 System SDS Software (Applied Biosystems) based on the standard curve. The genome equivalents from 1.25 µL of the purified RNA were projected to copies per 1 mL serum using the multiplication factor 342.9. Sample concentration during RNA preparation (140/60 µL = 2.3) reduced the volume projection factor (1000/1.25 µL = 800) yielding this factor. The copy number per swab was calculated by multiplying with factor 171.4, because the swab was washed out in 500 µL of buffer (500/1.25 µL = 400, concentration factor 2.3).

Determination of the genomic sequence of an Austrian APPV strain

The genomic sequence of APPV isolate AUT 2016 Farm C (GenBank KX778724) was determined employing primers designed based on an available APPV genome sequence in GenBank (KU194229.1, primer sequences available upon request) [8]. Resulting PCR products were purified, cloned with the help of T-vectors and sequenced as described in sub-section "Detection of APPV genomes and sequence analysis". RACE-PCRs were not employed to determine the ultimate 5′- and 3′-termini.

Recombinant antigens

For expression in *E. coli* the coding sequence of the NS3 helicase of APPV AUT 2016 Farm C (AA1513-2006) was amplified by RT-PCR and inserted into a modified pet11a vector (Novagen) with a C-terminal polyhistidine tag (petNS3H-APPV). After expression via a T7 RNA polymerase promoter in *E. coli* strain Rosetta 2™ (Novagen) the protein was purified by ion metal affinity chromatography (IMAC) using Ni^{2+} Sepharose (HisTrap™; GE

Healthcare). Amount and purity of APPV-NS3H was accessed by sodium dodecyl sulphate polyacrylamide gel electrophoresis (SDS PAGE), and identity was confirmed by immunoblot analysis with an anti-His antibody. Purified proteins were further purified by size exclusion chromatography (Superdex 200 10/300, GE) and served as antigen source for ELISA studies. The APPV NS3 helicase sequence was sub-cloned in a pcDNA3.1 vector for eukaryotic expression and immunofluorescence tests (pcDNAGFP-NS3H).

Monoclonal antibodies against pestiviral proteins

As reported earlier, we generated a panel of monoclonal antibodies against the nonstructural proteins of CSFV using heterologous protein expression in the E. coli and standard technics [18]. Over the last years this panel was extended to antibodies against the nonstructural proteins of BVDV [19] and Bungowannah virus (unpublished). In addition, we generated monoclonal antibodies against the structural proteins of CSFV [20] and BVDV [21, 22]. Briefly, BALB/c mice were immunized with recombinant proteins until seroconversion was observed. Spleen cells were prepared and fused with sp2/0-AG14 myeloma cells to generate monoclonal antibody producing hybridomas. Finally, secreted mAbs were evaluated using ELISA, immunoblot and immunofluorescence assays as needed. Each of these fusion experiments yielded up to 100 different reactive monoclonal antibodies. This extensive collection of antibodies against all pestiviral proteins is screened for APPV cross-reactive antibodies using different assays in an on-going project. Until now, we successfully screened different anti-NS3-helicase panels and found two APPV cross-reactive antibodies. Both antibodies were generated by simultaneous immunization with CSFV and BVDV NS3H.

Serological reagents and ELISA studies

ELISA screening of different hybridoma cell culture supernatants from our library of cross-reactive monoclonal antibodies (mAbs) against pestiviral NS3H was performed as described previously [23]. Briefly, purified recombinant APPV-NS3H was dissolved in ELISA coating buffer (0.1 M sodium carbonate, pH 9.5) and diluted to a final concentration of 10 μg/mL. 96-well ELISA plates (Maxisorb™; Nunc) were coated with 0.5 μg of the APPV-NS3 and blocked with phosphate buffered saline containing 0.01% Tween 20 and 10% fetal calf serum (FCS Gold Plus, Bio&Sell, Feucht, Germany). After incubation with hybridoma cell culture supernatant, specific binding of mAbs was detected with horseradish peroxidase (HRP)-conjugated goat anti-mouse immunoglobulin (Dianova, Hamburg, Germany) and 3,3′,5,5′-tetramethylbenzidine (TMB; Sigma) substrate. The specificity of

mAbs was further analyzed in immunoblots and immunofluorescence using the recombinant protein.

The presented indirect ELISA system was modified to analyze the ELISA blocking activity of serum samples from APPV infected pigs. After coating with APPV-NS3 the ELISA wells were blocked either with FCS as a mock control or with the swine sera to be tested. The Cut-off value at a relative signal intensity of 0.5 was determined empirically using defined positive and negative sera. APPV antibody negative sera were obtained from sows and piglets of unsuspicious farms that never experienced problems with CT and were tested negative for APPV by RT-PCR. Defined positive sera originate from sows and piglets from affected farms with high indirect ELISA titers. APPV-NS3H specific antibodies from reactive sera were further characterized in immunofluorescence assays using BHK cells transient transfected with a pcDNA3.1 vector encoding green fluorescent protein fused to the NS3 helicase domain of APPV (pcDNAGFP-NS3H). Reagents suitable for immunofluorescence detection of APPV infected cultured cells were prepared by affinity purification of the porcine APPV NS3H specific antibodies from sera. One milligram of recombinant APPV NS3H was coupled to a NHS-column (HiTrap NHS-activated HP; GE Healthcare, Chalfont St Giles, UK) according to the manufacturer's recommendations. Ten milliliter of an APPV positive porcine serum was diluted 1:5 in Tris buffer (100 mM, pH: 8.0) and passed over the APPV NS3H-coated matrix. Unbound antibodies were removed and the bound antibody fraction was eluted using a glycine buffer (50 mM, pH: 3.0) and concentrated by ultrafiltration.

Virus isolation

For virus isolation, 50 μL serum of diseased piglets from different Austrian farms were used to inoculate 5×10^6 SK-6 or PK-15 cells in a six-well format. After 3 days, the infected cells were passaged and a tenth of the cell culture supernatant was further passaged on the same cell line. All cells were grown in Dulbecco's modified Eagle's medium (DMEM) supplemented with 10% fetal calf serum (FCS Gold Plus, Bio&Sell) and maintained at 37 °C and 5% CO_2. Virus infections and passages were analyzed by immunofluorescence and qRT-PCR.

Results
Exemplary description of the CT outbreak in farm A
In farm A, the occurrence of CT was first observed in July 2015 in suckling piglets. About 70% of all newborn piglets showed various degrees of trembling or shaking, with 80% of the litters being affected (Table 3). The only symptom visible in most piglets was head shaking, while trembling of the whole body was noticed in severely affected

Table 3 Course of reproductive performance of sows (mean weaned piglets per sow and year) of farm A and the percentage of CT affected piglets in each farrowing batch

Farrowing group	Date of parturition	% of piglets affected by CT	Mean # of weaned piglets per sow
2	16.07.2015	70	11.43
3	07.08.2015	80	10.73
4	28.08.2015	20	9.07
5	18.09.2015	80	8.33
6	10.10.2015	30	9.92
7	29.10.2015	25	10.93
1	21.11.2015	30	11.00
2	09.12.2015	0.8	9.13
3	01.01.2016	30	9.71
4	22.01.2016	0	11.20
5	11.02.2016	0	11.64
6	03.02.2016	7	10.64

animals (Additional file 1). Stress factors induced or increased shaking symptoms significantly, while no shaking or solely minor tremor was observed during relaxation or sleep. Severely affected newborn piglets were incapable of sucking milk resulting in mortalities of up to 30%. In single piglets a fatal combination of CT and splay legs was observed. During the outbreak of CT between July 2015 and January 2016 productivity dropped from 25.5–26.5 to 23.57 weaned piglets per sow and year. After the outbreak had ceased, productivity levels returned to 25.5–26.5 weaned piglets per sow and year.

Pathology

Ten animals of farm A, five clinically affected and five clinically healthy littermates, were examined and compared to a healthy control animal from a farm without CT problems. On gross examination the piglets showed no severe lesions. Excoriations of the legs, alveolar lung edema and emphysema were present frequently. Four animals out of ten—two affected, two not affected—showed scattered petechiae in the renal cortex. In all animals, brain and spinal cord showed no obvious lesions on gross examination. In the majority of clinically affected animals ($n = 4/5$) few vacuoles were present in the white matter of the cerebellum in LFB-HE-staining, while in the unaffected littermates vacuoles were extremely rare or absent (Figures 1A and B). In the healthy control animal no vacuoles were found (Figure 1C). There were no detectable differences regarding myelination of cerebral and cerebellar white matter in affected and unaffected animals compared to a healthy control (Figures 1A–C). However, hypomyelination was evident in the white

matter of the spinal cord of affected animals compared to unaffected littermates and a healthy control (Figures 1D–F). Affected animals showed a clear reduction in the thickness of the myelin sheaths. In one affected animal few dilated myelin sheaths and vacuoles in the white matter of medulla oblongata and spinal cord were found. Unaffected animals did not show any lesions in medulla oblongata or spinal cord. Two affected piglets and one unaffected animal showed mild, partially perivascular, focal gliosis in brain and spinal cord. In the CNS and the kidneys small foci of extravasation were present in affected and unaffected animals from farm A.

Nuclei of oligodendrocytes were labeled in the white matter of affected and unaffected animals as well as the control animal by immunohistochemistry. Neither affected nor unaffected piglets showed reduced numbers of oligodendrocytes compared to the healthy control. In contrast staining intensity of oligodendrocytes was slightly increased in affected animals compared to the healthy control (Figures 1G–I).

For transmission electron microscopic examination two piglets from farm A (one affected, one clinically unaffected) were used. Tissue samples from the cerebellar white matter, cerebellar peduncles and medulla oblongata of both piglets revealed ultrastructural defects such as alterations of myelin and a variety of membrane-bordered vacuoles or spaces in the cytoplasm of glial cells and within axons. In the cerebellar white matter and medulla oblongata samples of the clinically affected piglet, mild hypomyelination accompanied by myelin breakdown and disruption could be found (Additional files 2A and B). There was also multifocal general separation and severe decompaction of myelin lamellae, formation of myelin balloons and degeneration of axons (Additional files 2A–C). Additionally, intramyelinic vacuoles containing membranous debris, which may represent degenerating dendrites or neuronal cell bodies, were evident. In the cerebellar and medulla oblongata samples of the unaffected littermate only mild ultrastructural alterations, such as vacuole formation, hypomyelination and pathological changes in the myelin sheath could be observed.

Detection of APPV

Using conventional RT-PCR and qRT-PCR targeting the NS5B region we diagnosed the presence of APPV in two retrospective cases (2013) and in six current cases (2015–2016) of CT A-II in Austria. One case occurred 2016 in farm F that had already experienced problems in 2013. More than twenty clinical samples (serum, saliva and CNS material) of healthy pigs from Austrian pig farms, which had never experienced problems with CT, were negatively tested for APPV RNA. APPV was consistently detectable in serum and saliva of CT affected

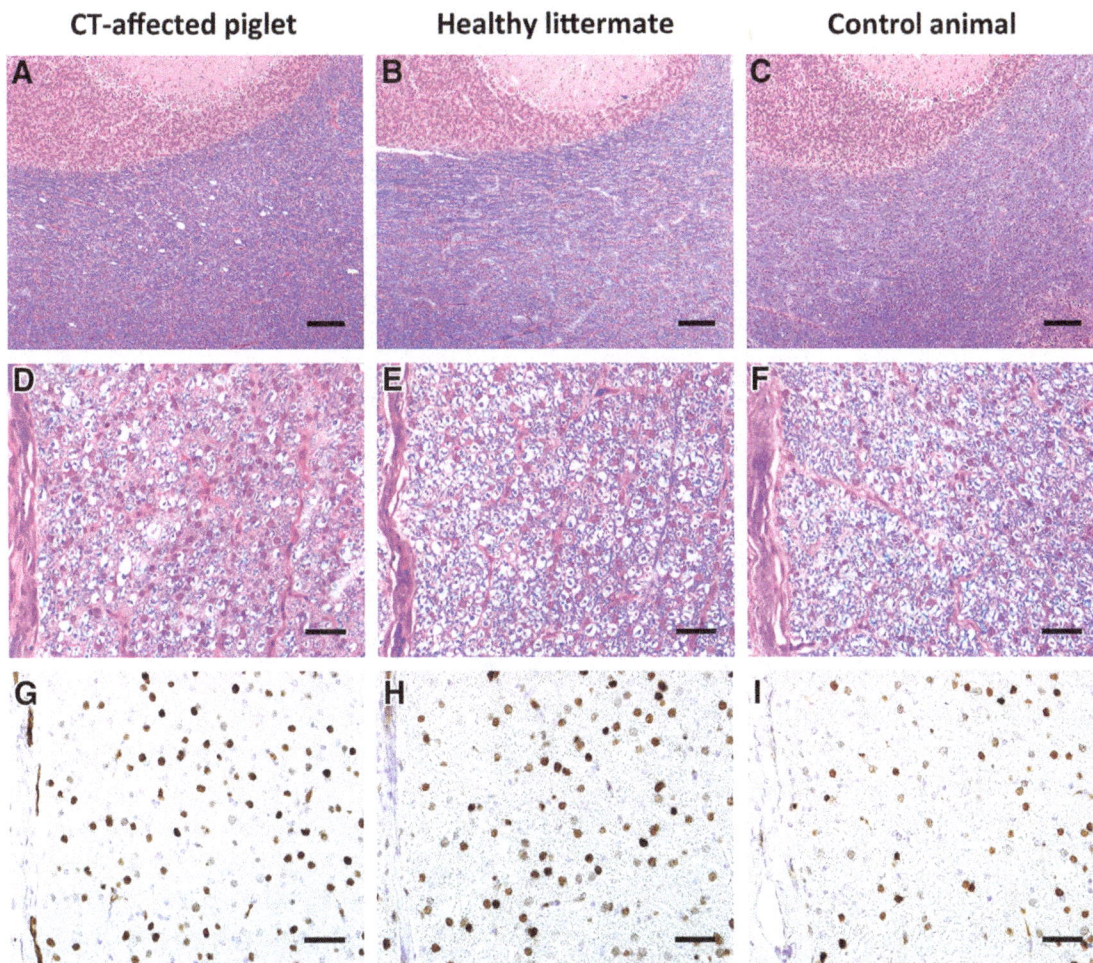

Figure 1 Histological lesions in a CT-affected animal compared to a healthy littermate and a healthy control. Vacuoles in cerebellar white matter in affected animal (**A**), normal white matter in littermate (**B**) and control (**C**), LFB-HE, bar = 150 μm. Hypomyelination in white matter of the thoracic spinal cord in affected animal (**D**), normal myelination in littermate (**E**) and control (**F**), LFB-HE, bar = 40 μm. Detection of oligodendrocytes, increased staining intensity in affected animal (**G**), less intense staining in littermate (**H**) and control (**I**), Olig2-IHC, bar = 40 μm.

piglets. All sampled organs of two three-week old piglets were positive in conventional RT-PCR, except for the spleen. Serum samples of all sows and boars of farm A were tested negative for the presence of APPV nucleic acid by RT-PCR. In a different farm (farm F), we obtained positive RT-PCR results in the saliva of one sow shortly after farrowing of shaking piglets that were APPV positive. These nucleic acids most likely represent viral contaminations of the sow's oral cavity obtained from their infected offspring, as the same animal was negatively tested after weaning.

Characterization of APPV sequences
Initial genetic typing of the field strains was done on the basis of a 770 bp fragment of the NS5B genes. All Austrian strains, except one, were closely related to each other (>99% sequence identity, Figure 2A). Only the APPV strain originating from farm G was more distant, clustering with the corresponding NS5B fragment of an APPV strain from Germany (94% sequence identity, Figure 2A). Interestingly, one farm already clinically affected in 2013 (AUT-2013-Farm F) experienced another outbreak in 2016 (AUT-2016-Farm F) with a very closely related strain (one nt exchange). Significant differences to APPV sequences originating from the US (<91% sequence identity, Figure 2A) were observed. A total of 11.535 nucleotides (nt) were determined for APPV strain AUT 2016 Farm C consisting of 360 nt of the 5′NTR, 268 nt of the 3′NTR and 10908 nt of the coding region (ORF). The 5′-NTR misses 10 nt at the 5′-end compared to the APPV from Iowa ISDVDL2014016573 (KU1942299). The open reading frame contains 3635 codons, as for all other available APPV full-length sequences, and yields an amino acid identity of 97.2% (nucleotide identity 93.3%)

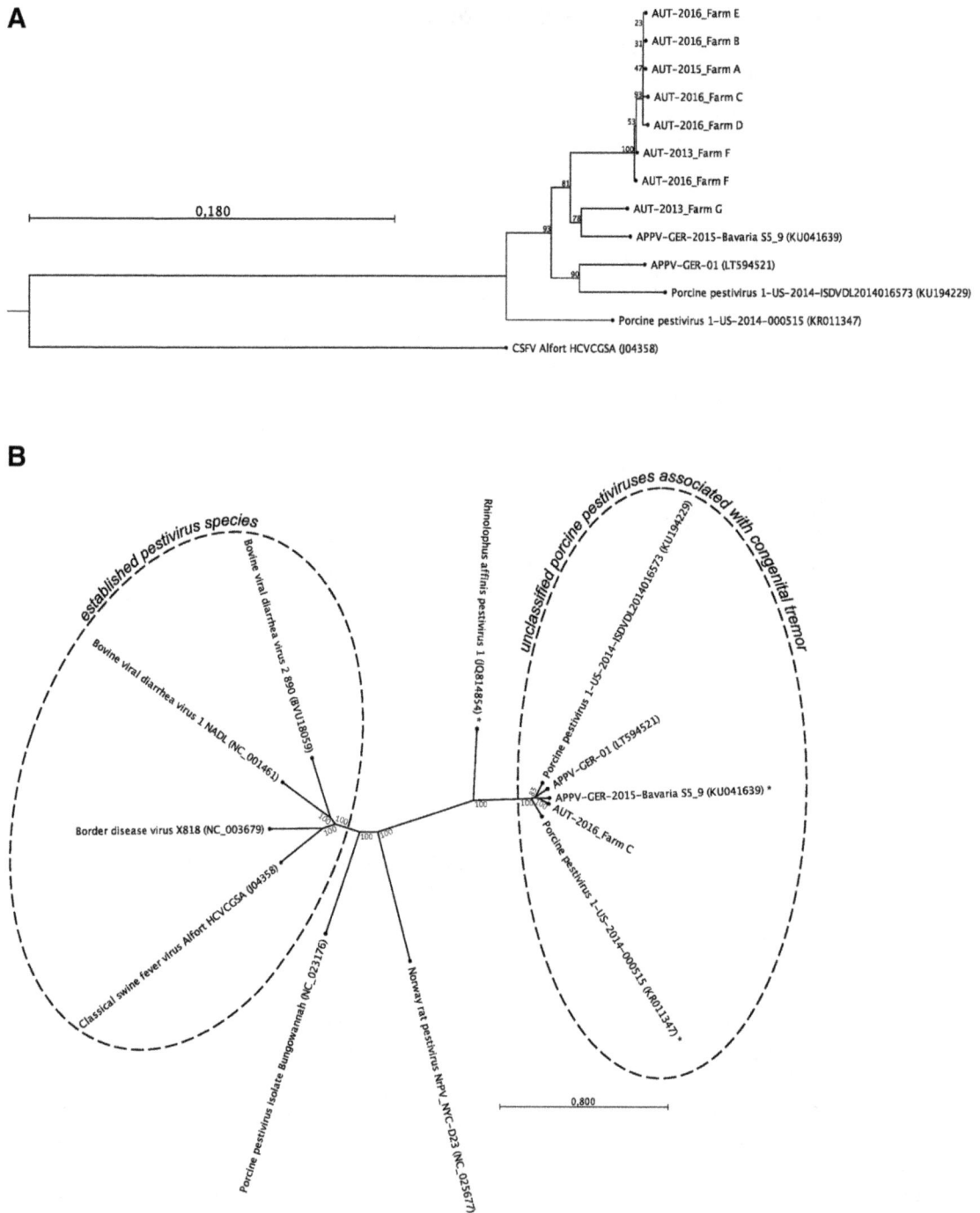

Figure 2 Phylogeny of Austrian APPV strains. Phylogenetic trees were constructed using the neighbor joining method with 1000 replicates. **A** Phylogenetic pairwise comparison of NS5B sequence fragments (770 bps) indicates that APPV strains from Austria are closely related to each other and distinct from recently detected APPV strains from the US and Germany. The tree is rooted to CSFV, which serves as an out-group. **B** Simulation of the phylogenetic relationship of available full-length APPV sequences to the four pestiviral species and ungrouped pestivirus isolates (unrooted tree). Full genomes and truncated genome sequences (indicated by asterisk) branch with bootstrap values of >85% each. The GenBank accession numbers of APPV sequences presented here are: KX778725 (AUT-2015_A), KX778726 (AUT-2016_B), KX778724 (AUT-2016_C), KX778727 (AUT-2016_D), KX778728 (AUT-2016_E), KX778729 (AUT-2013_F), KX778730 (AUT-2016_F), KX778731 (AUT-2013_G).

with the Bavarian strain S5_9 (20), 95.7% (nucleotide identity 89.8%) [5], 94.3% (nucleotide identity 87.2%) with the APPV strain from Kansas, and 95.6% (nucleotide identity 90.0%) with the APPV strain from Iowa. As already reported by others, the distance to the classical pestivirus species (Figure 2B) is considerable with less than 50% nucleotide identity.

Serological reagents and APPV NS3 blocking ELISA

A panel of 120 cross-reactive NS3H specific mAbs, which were established earlier (unpublished data) using recombinant helicase domains of different pestivirus species (CSFV, BVDV-1, BVDV-2, and Bungowannah), was tested for reactivity against the recombinant APPV NS3 helicase (Figure 3A). The NS3H specific antibodies were screened for cross-reactivity using an indirect ELISA. Several antibodies were identified that reacted with the APPV NS3 helicase. The specificity of antibodies WLAP-PV3H1 (1B3) and WLAPPV3H2 (7C10) was confirmed in western blot analysis using crude bacterial lysates. Reactivity with specific protein bands at about 60 kDa after induction of NS3 expression is shown in Figure 3B. Unfortunately, neither of these antibodies was suited for the detection of APPV infection by immunofluorescence. Recombinant APPV GFP-NS3H expressed in BHK cells served as positive control but was not recognized (data not shown). We also tried to use APPV GFP–NS3H expressing cells for the screening of porcine sera for the presence of APPV antibodies. This approach failed due to strong unspecific binding of porcine serum antibodies to BHK cells.

We applied the recombinant APPV NS3H to test different swine sera in an indirect antibody ELISA setup. Sera of RT-PCR negative sows, which had given birth to clinically affected RT-PCR positive piglets, showed strong ELISA signals, while sera of swine originating from unsuspicious farms demonstrated a weak reactivity. Nevertheless, the specificity and sensitivity of the indirect ELISA was insufficient for further use. To set up a more robust assay, the NS3 specific antibodies 7C10 and 1B3 were employed to establish an APPV NS3H blocking ELISA. Only mAb 1B3 gave satisfactory results with regard to sensitivity and specificity when applied in this type of assay. Using the APPV antibody blocking ELISA we analyzed the prevalence of APPV antibodies in farm A (Figure 4). Sows that had given birth to tremor-affected piglets and had a strong reactivity in the indirect ELISA were used as reactive controls. In addition, we included CT affected piglets with high OD values in indirect ELISAs as reactive controls. All of these sows and piglets were highly positive (OD 0.05–0.3) in the NS3H blocking ELISA. Among the 168 sows and two boars of herd A that were tested, 59 sows and one boar displayed

reactivities lower than the threshold (OD 0.5) giving a rate of 35.3% APPV NS3H antibody positive pigs. In addition, we found that sows that had given birth to CT piglets displayed a higher blocking activity than the sows of the affected farm on average. Affinity purified IgGs from blocking ELISA positive animals yielded clear signals in immunofluorescence assays using APPV GFP-NS3H transfected BHK cells as positive control (Additional file 3).

Isolation and propagation of APPV

The availability of APPV specific antibodies as well as qRT-PCR assay allowed us to screen for APPV infection of cultured cells. After initial attempts to isolate APPV had failed and thus confirmed reports of others [6–8], we could show the presence of APPV antigen in SK-6 and PK-15 cells after 5 passages by immunofluorescence (Figure 5) and qRT-PCR. Key to this experiment was the inoculation of cells with an APPV positive serum sample (APPV AUT 646/16) that was obtained from a CT piglet before suckling and hence devoid of colostral antibodies. In contrast to high nucleic acid titers measured in the samples of APPV positive piglets ($>10^6$ GE/mL or swab) and in the cell culture supernatant ($>10^9$ GE/mL), the infectivity of these samples was minute (10^1–10^2 ffu/mL). Virus spread of the APPV isolate in cell culture was very inefficient as indicated by the small size of antigen positive foci (Figure 5).

Long-term monitoring of APPV infected piglets in farm F

Five RT-PCR positive shaking piglets from one affected litter at farm F were chosen for detailed analyses of disease. Three of the piglets were sacrificed at different time points for storage of organ material. For integration in the herd, the health status of one female and one male piglet was assessed over 6 months and consecutive diagnostic tests were conducted to determine the risk of virus shedding and transmission. The piglets showed a mild tremor most obvious at the ear tips and flank as shown in the Additional file 1. CT symptoms improved within several weeks and disappeared completely until 14 weeks of age. The course of viremia, virus shedding via saliva and the APPV NS3H specific antibody titers are presented for both piglets from week 3 to 14 weeks of age (Figure 6). Continuously positive qRT-PCR results in serum and saliva samples demonstrate constant viremia and virus shedding in both animals over the period of 12 weeks. APPV NS3H specific antibodies were present after birth, but vanished in both animals at the age of eight weeks. One of these piglets became a clinically unsuspicious boar that reached sexual maturity. At 6 months of age, high levels of APPV genomes were present in saliva (2.9×10^8 GE/swab) and semen (2.1×10^9 GE/

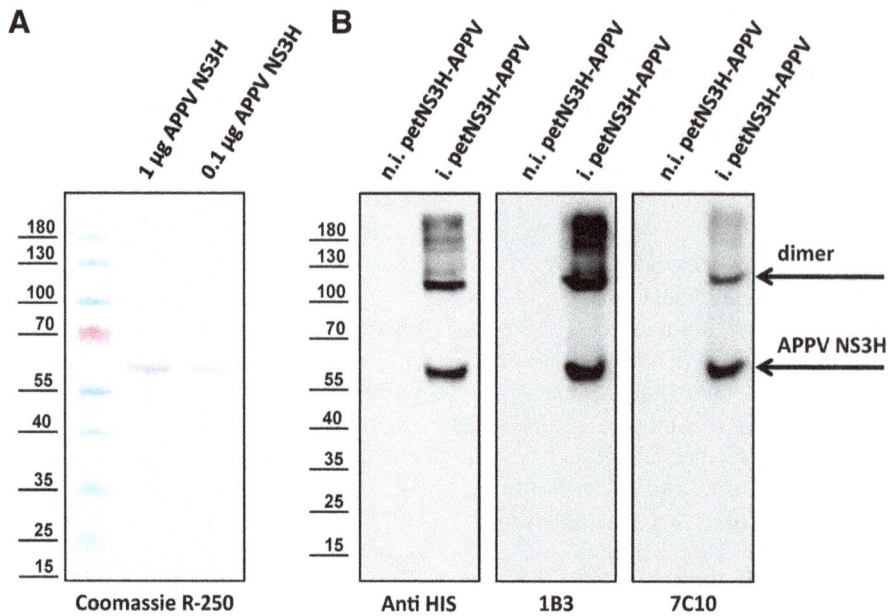

Figure 3 Purification of recombinant APPV NS3H and reactivity of mAbs. A Coomassie blue R-250 stain of the recombinant APPV NS3H protein preparation (calculated molecular mass of NS3H 57.9 kDa). **B** Lysates of non-induced (n.i. petNS3H-APPV) and APPV NS3H expressing bacteria (i. petNS3H-APPV) were probed with different antibodies as indicated.

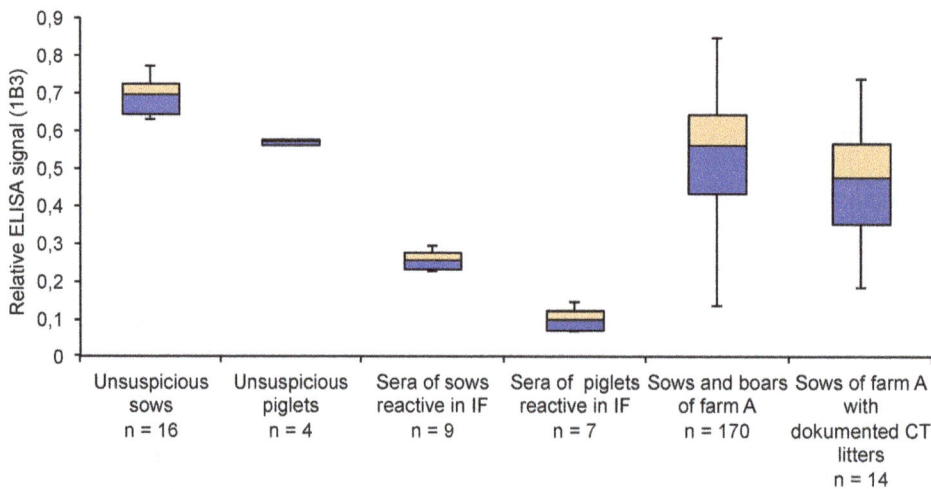

Figure 4 NS3 blocking ELISA results of farm A. The relative signal of the mAb 1B3 is depicted after blocking with porcine sera. Blocking with FCS was used as a reference. Sera of unsuspicious sows and piglets from unaffected farms showed relative intensities >50%. Seroconverted sows that had given birth to APPV infected piglets and their CT-affected piglets have a strong serum blocking activity with signal intensities <30%. The specificity of the ELISA reaction was validated by IF staining of cell expressing APPV-NS3H (Additional file 3). The ELISA intensities of all sows and boars of farm A are shown to demonstrate the mixed reactivity within this affected herd. In addition, the ELISA values of 14 sows, which had a litter with well-documented APPV positive CT cases, are presented separately. The sows with APPV associated CT-litters exhibit a stronger reactivity in the blocking ELISA on average. Using a cut-off value of 50% the seroprevalence in farm A reached 35% (60/170).

mL), while levels in serum remained lower in the boar (2.0×10^7 GE/mL). The serum APPV genome load of the 6-month-old sow was below the detection limit of our qPCR assay (LOD: 3.0×10^6 GE/mL) in two consecutive tests, while high genome loads could still be observed in saliva (1.3×10^9 GE/swab).

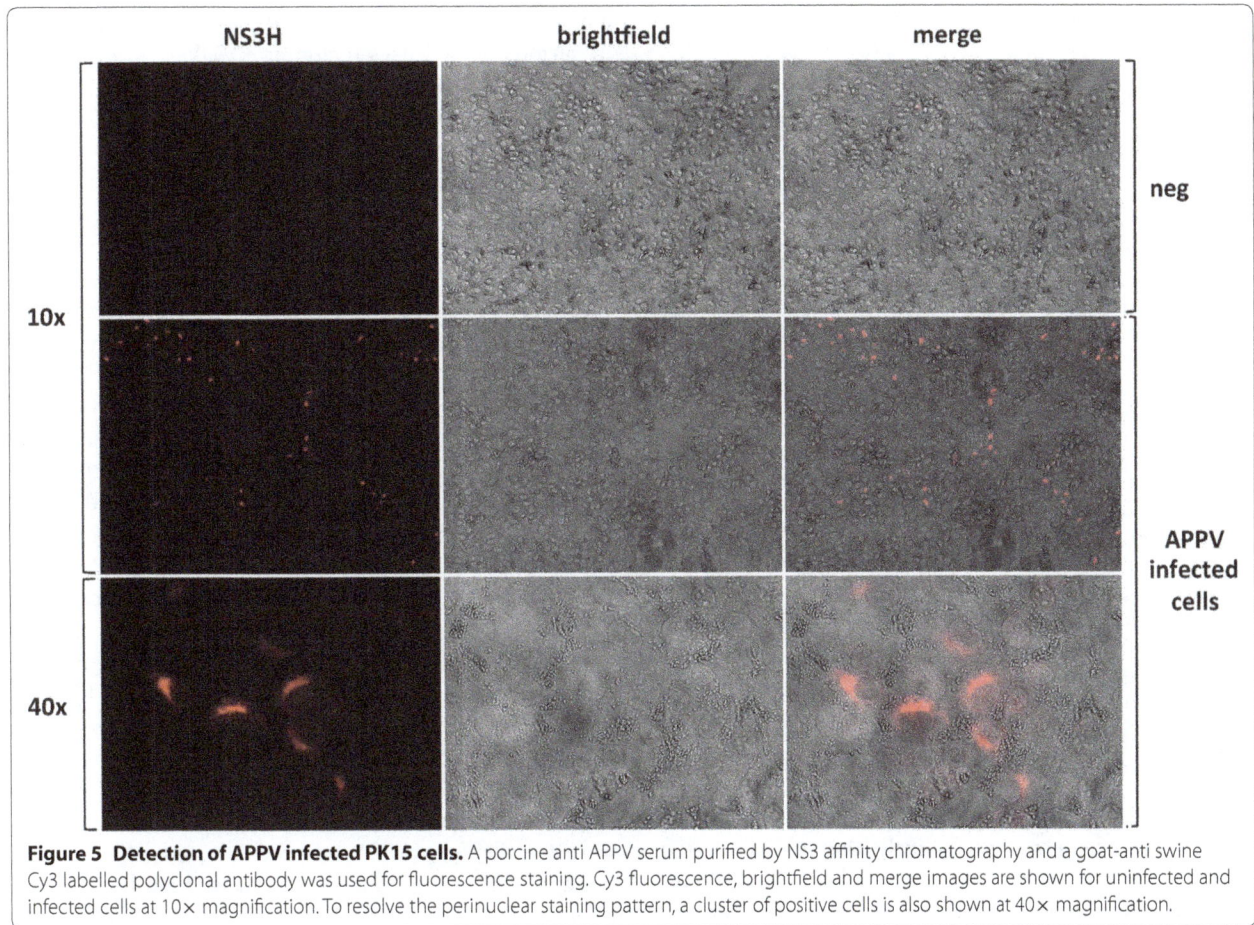

Figure 5 Detection of APPV infected PK15 cells. A porcine anti APPV serum purified by NS3 affinity chromatography and a goat-anti swine Cy3 labelled polyclonal antibody was used for fluorescence staining. Cy3 fluorescence, brightfield and merge images are shown for uninfected and infected cells at 10× magnification. To resolve the perinuclear staining pattern, a cluster of positive cells is also shown at 40× magnification.

Discussion

Outbreaks of CT in several piglet producing farms in Austria between 2013 and 2016 were puzzling as comprehensive analyses of non-infectious noxae (mycotoxins) and known porcine pathogens (Herpes-, Entero-, and Sapoviruses) gave negative or inconclusive results. The discrete histologic lesions present in the spinal cord of infected animals were consistent with hypomyelination. These alterations were quite similar to lesions reported in piglets infected with CSFV [3] and a calf infected with BVDV [24]. The mild vacuolization of the cerebellar white matter of affected animals is in accordance with lesions reported in piglets with CT due to suspected BVDV-related pestivirus infection [25]. Immunohistochemically there was no detectable loss of oligodendrocytes in the spinal cord of affected animals. There was rather an increased expression of Olig 2 present in affected piglets. Furthermore, ultrastructural examination of cerebellar white matter showed not only hypomyelination but myelin disruption and breakdown in affected animals. This is in contrast to ultrastructural lesions reported in piglets with classical swine fever [3] and a calf infected with

BVDV [24]. We therefore conclude that in utero infection with APPV has a deleterious effect on fetal oligodendrocytes, which are present in sufficient numbers. This effect may have an impact on myelin development and function or lead to degeneration of the present myelin. Further research in this regard is crucial to better understand the pathogenesis of the disease.

We analyzed diagnostic samples of CT-affected piglets employing RT-PCRs using primers deduced from the NS5B region of a published novel atypical pestivirus sequence shortly after its availability by the end of 2015 [7]. In all tested cases we amplified APPV specific RT-PCR products that upon sequencing matched well (about 90%) to the published sequence. Apart from one sequence obtained from a CT case from 2013 (farm G), the Austrian isolates show a very high degree of sequence conservation within the analyzed NS5B fragment (>99%) and form a distinct cluster compared to isolates from Germany and the US (Figure 4A). One farm (F) experienced an outbreak in 2013 and 2016. As the analyzed NS5B fragments only contain 1 nt exchange but differ from the isolates of farm A-E in three conserved residues,

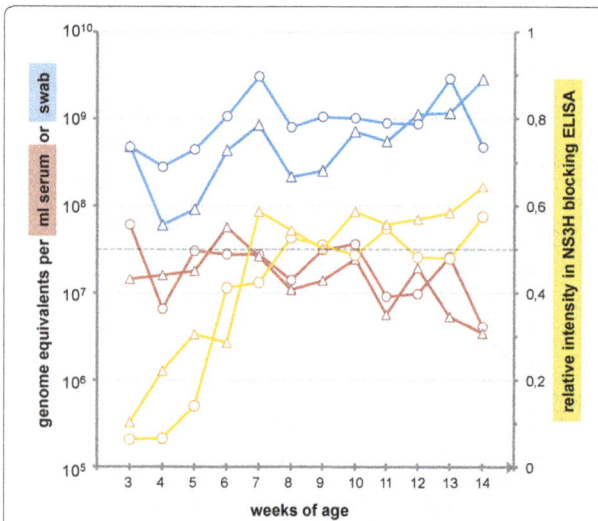

Figure 6 Course of APPV infection in two CT affected piglets.
qRT-PCR values of serum samples (red) and oral swabs (blue) are depicted together with the relative signal intensities of the NS3 blocking ELISA (yellow). The dotted grey line represents the empirical cut-off value of 0.5. Note the constant presence of APPV genomes in both animals in serum and saliva over the period of 12 weeks, whereas APPV specific antibodies could no longer be detected at the age of 8 weeks indicating maternal origin.

viral persistence in this herd is likely. Due to APPV detection on two continents, it seems likely that APPV has a worldwide distribution, especially if one takes into account that the "non-CSFV" clinical picture of CT A-II has been known for decades. APPV most likely has been present in domestic pigs since decades but remained elusive, as diagnostics targeting classical pestiviruses do not cross-react.

While detection of APPV genomes by PCR is straightforward and different RT-PCR protocols have already been developed targeting conserved sites within NS3 or NS5B, there is only one report about the establishment of an E^{rns} based serological assay. Hause et al. determined antibodies against recombinant bacterially expressed APPV E^{rns} in 94% of randomly tested animals, while sera from a specific pathogen free farm yielded no positive reactions [7]. We established a serological assay on the basis of NS3 in analogy to NS3 blocking ELISAs routinely used in CSFV and BVDV serodiagnostic. First indirect ELISA tests with recombinant APPV NS3H coated to plates were sufficient to discern clearly positive (some sows that farrowed CT piglets) from clearly negative sera (non-infected controls from APPV unsuspicious farms) but a more detailed analysis was not possible. NS3 contains at least two indispensable enzymatic functions, protease and helicase and functional protein can easily be produced in *E. coli*. In previous projects we characterized

a panel of 120 cross-specific mAbs against NS3 molecules of various pestiviruses including BVDV-II and Bungowannah virus. We screened these mAbs against the bacterially expressed APPV NS3 helicase domain (60 kDa) using ELISA. One mAb proofed suitable for the application in a highly specific blocking ELISA. In our survey of farm A, which had experienced several farrowings with clinical overt CT in APPV positive piglets, but revealed no APPV RT-PCR positive adults, the reactivity rate was 60/170 (35.3%). These results were quite contrasting the 94% seroprevalence reported earlier in samples initially taken for a PRRSV survey employing an E^{rns} based ELISA. E^{rns} is a highly glycosylated protein with several intramolecular disulfide bonds. Therefore, it is possible that antigen produced in bacteria may not be optimal for diagnostic purposes. Beside the test system, the different APPV strains might vary in their immunological properties explaining differences in seroprevalence between Austria and the US. Future studies will have to compare the reactivities of both ELISA concepts. APPV antigen detection in infected cells or tissues was difficult and required the preparation of NS3 monospecific antibodies extracted from APPV positive pig sera. This procedure was necessary because the NS3 specific mAbs did not react in immunofluorescence or immunohistochemistry applications. The monospecific porcine NS3 antibodies were reactive with APPV infected cultured cells but were not applicable in porcine tissues due to high background caused by the intrinsic presence of porcine IgG. In our hands in situ hybridization also failed to detect APPV genomes in tissues. Likely our method is not sensitive enough and an optimized FISH protocol (as described by Postel et al. [16]) needs to be applied.

As reported earlier [6, 8, 26], clinical signs of CT can be dramatic in piglets, but cease over time. The Austrian cases described in this study were associated with moderately increased piglet mortality. Losses of 2.5 piglets per sow and year in farm A mainly occurred as severe tremor interfered with the piglets' ability to suckle milk. The farmers also reported on some growers with persistent tremor that decreased the productivity. Not surprising for a newly discovered agent, routes of infection, epidemiology of APPV and pathogenesis of CT remain unclear. The evidence for APPV as a causative agent behind CT is robust but Koch's postulates have not been fully fulfilled, yet [8]. Recent infection experiments indicated a trans-placental infection of piglets. Controlled animal experiments are essential to evaluate the clinic signs of intrauterine APPV infection, the impact of APPV on piglet production and the economic importance of this virus. Nevertheless, virus isolation is key to address these questions. As we have shown that APPV can be propagated and persists in porcine cells, animal trials to proof Koch's postulates can now be conducted. Also, cultured isolates are a basic requirement to address questions related to the molecular biology of APPV, such as its low infectivity in vitro or the role of the N-terminal E2 truncation [7].

Up to date we were not able to identify the source of virus introduction into the affected Austrian farms. We could show that persistently infected (PI) animals exist, reach sexual maturity and shed high virus quantities with their saliva and semen in the absence of any clinical signs or antibody response. It is not clear from our study, whether the persistence of APPV is a common phenomenon in CT affected animals. By analogy to other pestiviruses we assume that immunotolerance and virus persistence solely occurs after In utero infection within a defined gestation period yielding a few percent of PI animals. These animals are a reservoir for APPV and a threat for APPV naïve herds. Also, as we showed high viral loads in semen of an adult boar formerly affected by CT, there is a potential for sexual transmission or transmission via artificial insemination. This aspect urgently needs clarification, as it could severely affect the pig industry. Usually a farm experiences CT affected farrowings for a few weeks to a few months, depending on the production scheme, including some sows rearing healthy litters before the clinical signs completely subside. This is indicative of a transient infection process that affects only a few animals clinically in the suitable gestation period, while the others are subclinically infected and mount an antibody response. The serological data of our study at farm A using the NS3H based blocking ELISA show that the farrowing of CT affected piglets is not necessarily inducing detectable antibody levels as indicated by the moderate seroprevalence of 35.3%. We can only speculate on the immunogenicity of our target epitope and it is so far unclear whether the antibody response is stringent. The blocking antibody response could also be transient and vanish within a short period of time. A high prevalence of atypical porcine pestiviruses was found in German pig herds with no obvious link to CT [5]. However, within an immune herd APPV might be present in persistently infected animals without inducing clinical signs. This is in line with the hypothesis that CT in piglets only occurs when naïve sows are infected in a certain gestation period [8].

The discovery of APPV demonstrates that the diversity among the genus pestivirus was underestimated and that it is likely that more "atypical" pestiviruses circulate in domestic and feral populations of pigs and ruminants. Novel pestivirus sequences were also reported for rats (Norway rat pestivirus) in North America and bats (*Rhinolophus affinis* pestivirus) in China [27, 28],

which are distantly related to both classical and atypical porcine pestiviruses. With regard to nomenclature the proposed terms "atypical porcine pestivirus, APPV" [7] or "congenital tremor virus, CTV" [8] are misleading as "atypical" is a more general term already used for other pestiviruses (e.g. BVDV 3). The same is true for CTV, as CT has earlier been linked to certain strains of CSFV or BDV in lambs. As it can be expected that the genus pestivirus will expand in the near future, a more rational terminology would be straightforward. As in herpesviruses (human herpesvirus 1–8) the host species could be combined with a number. According to this strategy CSFV could be termed as Porcine pestivirus 1, Bungowannah virus as Porcine pestivirus 2 and Atypical porcine pestivirus as Porcine pestivirus 3 based on the order of first description. Strict rules for species affiliation regarding sequence identities would further substantiate the concept. Besides terminology, this would also simplify the separation of notifiable and non-notifiable livestock diseases caused by pestiviruses. The biology of APPV, considering its pestivirus-specific traits, such as persistence or in utero infection, as well as its unique properties, such as high genome loads in saliva versus lower to nondetectable levels in serum, points out that there is much more variety than expected within the genus pestivirus.

Additional files

Additional file 1. Movie of CT-affected piglets of farm A. Note the tremor most obvious at the ear tips and flank.

Additional file 2. Electron micrographs of the central nervous system of an affected piglet show severe lesions. (A) Separation and decompaction of myelin sheaths (white asterisk) as well as intraaxonal vacuole formation (x) in the cerebellar white matter, bar = 2.5 μm. (B) Axonal degeneration (black arrow), vacuole formation (x) and myelin balloons (black asterisk) in the medulla oblongata, bar = 2.5 μm. (C) Defects of the myelin lamellae characterized by disruption of lamellae (black arrowhead) and formation of myelin balloons (black asterisk) in the medulla oblongata, bar = 250 nm.

Additional file 3. Validation of NS3H blocking ELISA results. BHK cells expressing GFP-NS3H were incubated with NS3H affinity purified porcine sera and stained by Cy3 conjugated goat anti swine serum. Blocking ELISA positive sows (#1–3) and a negative sow #4 are shown. A brightfield image of the BHK cells (left panel), the GFP (middle panel) and the Cy3 fluorescence (right panel) are presented. A murine anti GFP antibody is applied as a positive control.

Competing interests
The authors declare that they have no competing interests.

Authors' contributions
LS, BW, TV and AL examined the animals at piglet production sites and in the clinic and provided the field samples. BL, CR, LJS, and TR performed the laboratory work and analyzed the data. SH, BRB, ND and HW performed necropsy, histological, immunohistochemical and ultrastructural examinations on CT animals and wrote parts of the manuscript. BL, TR, CR, LJS, LS interpreted the results and designed the figures. BL wrote the manuscript. All authors read and approved the final manuscript.

Acknowledgements

The authors thank involved Austrian farmers for cooperation and the respective practitioners for their participation in the study. The authors want to thank the Animal Health Service of Upper Austria (Tiergesundheitsdienst Oberösterreich – TGD OÖ), for partially funding this study.

Author details

[1] Department for Farm Animals and Veterinary Public Health, University Clinic for Swine, University of Veterinary Medicine Vienna, Veterinaerplatz 1, 1210 Vienna, Austria. [2] Department of Pathobiology, Institute of Virology, University of Veterinary Medicine Vienna, Veterinaerplatz 1, 1210 Vienna, Austria. [3] Department of Pathobiology, Institute of Pathology and Forensic Veterinary Medicine, University of Veterinary Medicine Vienna, Veterinaerplatz 1, 1210 Vienna, Austria. [4] Traunkreis Vet Clinic, Großendorf 3, 4551 Ried im Traunkreis, Austria.

References

1. Blakemore WF, Harding JD, Done JT (1974) Ultrastructural observations on the spinal cord of a Landrace pig with congenital tremor type AIII. Res Vet Sci 17:174–178
2. Blakemore WF, Harding JD (1974) Ultrastructural observations on the spinal cords of piglets affected with congenital tremor type AIV. Res Vet Sci 17:248–255
3. Bradley R, Done JT, Hebert CN, Overby E, Askaa J, Basse A, Bloch B (1983) Congenital tremor type AI: light and electron microscopical observations on the spinal cords of affected piglets. J Comp Pathol 93:43–59
4. Done JT, Woolley J, Upcott DH, Hebert CN (1986) Porcine congenital tremor type AII: spinal cord morphometry. Br Vet J 142:145–150
5. Beer M, Wernike K, Drager C, Hoper D, Pohlmann A, Bergermann C, Schroder C, Klinkhammer S, Blome S, Hoffmann B (2016) High prevalence of highly variable atypical porcine pestiviruses found in Germany. Transboun Emerg Dis. doi:10.1111/tbed.12532
6. Postel A, Hansmann F, Baechlein C, Fischer N, Alawi M, Grundhoff A, Derking S, Tenhundfeld J, Pfankuche VM, Herder V, Baumgartner W, Wendt M, Becher P (2016) Presence of atypical porcine pestivirus (APPV) genomes in newborn piglets correlates with congenital tremor. Sci Rep 6:27735
7. Hause BM, Collin EA, Peddireddi L, Yuan F, Chen Z, Hesse RA, Gauger PC, Clement T, Fang Y, Anderson G (2015) Discovery of a novel putative atypical porcine pestivirus in pigs in the USA. J Gen Virol 96:2994–2998
8. Arruda BL, Arruda PH, Magstadt DR, Schwartz KJ, Dohlman T, Schleining JA, Patterson AR, Visek CA, Victoria JG (2016) Identification of a divergent lineage porcine pestivirus in nursing piglets with congenital tremors and reproduction of disease following experimental inoculation. PLoS One 11:e0150104
9. Bielefeldt Ohmann H (1988) BVD virus antigens in tissues of persistently viraemic, clinically normal cattle: implications for the pathogenesis of clinically fatal disease. Acta Vet Scand 29:77–84
10. Barlow RM (1980) Morphogenesis of hydranencephaly and other intracranial malformations in progeny of pregnant ewes infected with pestiviruses. J Comp Pathol 90:87–98
11. Anderson CA, Higgins RJ, Smith ME, Osburn BI (1987) Border disease. Virus-induced decrease in thyroid hormone levels with associated hypomyelination. Lab Invest 57:168–175
12. Clarke GL, Osburn BI (1978) Transmissible congenital demyelinating encephalopathy of lambs. Vet Pathol 15:68–82
13. Anderson CA, Higgins RJ, Waldvogel AS, Osburn BI (1982) Tropism of border disease virus for oligodendrocytes in ovine fetal brain cultures. In: Barlow RM, Patterson DS (eds) Border disease of sheep; a virus-induced teratogenic disorder. Parey, Berlin, pp 81–87
14. Anderson CA, Sawyer M, Higgins RJ, East N, Osburn BI (1987) Experimentally induced ovine border disease: extensive hypomyelination with minimal viral antigen in neonatal spinal cord. Am J Vet Res 48:499–503
15. Tao J, Liao J, Wang Y, Zhang X, Wang J, Zhu G (2013) Bovine viral diarrhea virus (BVDV) infections in pigs. Vet Microbiol 165:185–189
16. Kirkland PD, Frost MJ, Finlaison DS, King KR, Ridpath JF, Gu X (2007) Identification of a novel virus in pigs–Bungowannah virus: a possible new species of pestivirus. Virus Res 129:26–34
17. Kirkland PD, Read AJ, Frost MJ, Finlaison DS (2015) Bungowannah virus–a probable new species of pestivirus–what have we found in the last 10 years? Anim Health Res Rev 16:60–63
18. Lamp B, Riedel C, Roman-Sosa G, Heimann M, Jacobi S, Becher P, Thiel HJ, Rumenapf T (2011) Biosynthesis of classical swine fever virus nonstructural proteins. J Virol 85:3607–3620
19. Isken O, Langerwisch U, Schonherr R, Lamp B, Schroder K, Duden R, Rumenapf TH, Tautz N (2014) Functional characterization of bovine viral diarrhea virus nonstructural protein 5A by reverse genetic analysis and live cell imaging. J Virol 88:82–98
20. Riedel C, Lamp B, Heimann M, Konig M, Blome S, Moennig V, Schuttler C, Thiel HJ, Rumenapf T (2012) The core protein of classical swine fever virus is dispensable for virus propagation in vitro. PLoS Pathog 8:e1002598
21. Gilmartin AA, Lamp B, Rumenapf T, Persson MA, Rey FA, Krey T (2012) High-level secretion of recombinant monomeric murine and human single-chain Fv antibodies from Drosophila S2 cells. Protein Eng Des Sel 25:59–66
22. Callens N, Brugger B, Bonnafous P, Drobecq H, Gerl MJ, Krey T, Roman-Sosa G, Rumenapf T, Lambert O, Dubuisson J, Rouille Y (2016) Morphology and molecular composition of purified bovine viral diarrhea virus envelope. PLoS Pathog 12:e1005476
23. Lamp B, Riedel C, Wentz E, Tortorici MA, Rumenapf T (2013) Autocatalytic cleavage within classical swine fever virus NS3 leads to a functional separation of protease and helicase. J Virol 87:11872–11883
24. Porter BF, Ridpath JF, Calise DV, Payne HR, Janke JJ, Baxter DG, Edwards JF (2010) Hypomyelination associated with bovine viral diarrhea virus type 2 infection in a longhorn calf. Vet Pathol 47:658–663
25. Segalés J, Granberg F, Liu L, Cabezón O, Rosell R, Belák S (2012) Is congenital tremor type AII of pigs associated to bovine viral diarrhoea virus (BVDV) and/or a BVDV-related pestivirus? IPVS Congress VO- 036:106
26. Vandekerckhove P, Maenhout D, Curvers P, Hoorens J, Ducatelle R (1989) Type A2 congenital tremor in piglets. Zentralbl Veterinarmed A 36:763–771
27. Wu Z, Ren X, Yang L, Hu Y, Yang J, He G, Zhang J, Dong J, Sun L, Du J, Liu L, Xue Y, Wang J, Yang F, Zhang S, Jin Q (2012) Virome analysis for identification of novel mammalian viruses in bat species from Chinese provinces. J Virol 86:10999–11012
28. Firth C, Bhat M, Firth MA, Williams SH, Frye MJ, Simmonds P, Conte JM, Ng J, Garcia J, Bhuva NP, Lee B, Che X, Quan PL, Lipkin WI (2014) Detection of zoonotic pathogens and characterization of novel viruses carried by commensal Rattus norvegicus in New York City. MBio 5:e01933–01914

2

Enhancing the toolbox to study IL-17A in cattle and sheep

Sean R. Wattegedera[1*], Yolanda Corripio-Miyar[1,2], Yvonne Pang[1], David Frew[1], Tom N. McNeilly[1], Javier Palarea-Albaladejo[3], Colin J. McInnes[1], Jayne C. Hope[2], Elizabeth J. Glass[2] and Gary Entrican[1,2]

Abstract

The development of methods to detect cytokine expression by T cell subsets in ruminants is fundamental to strategic development of new livestock vaccines for prevention of infectious diseases. It has been possible to detect T cell expression of IFN-γ, IL-4 and IL-10 in ruminants for many years but methods to detect expression of IL-17A are relatively limited. To address this gap in capability we have cloned bovine and ovine IL-17A cDNAs and expressed biologically-active recombinant proteins in Chinese Hamster Ovary (CHO) cells. We used the transfected CHO cells to screen commercially-available antibodies for their ability to detect IL-17A expression intracellularly and in culture supernates. We demonstrate that an ELISA for bovine IL-17A detects native ovine IL-17A. Moreover, the constituent polyclonal antibodies (pabs) in the ELISA were used to enumerate peripheral blood mononuclear cells (PBMC) expressing IL-17A from cattle and sheep by ELISpot. We identified two monoclonal antibodies (mabs) that detect recombinant intracellular IL-17A in CHO cells by flow cytometry. One of these mabs was used to detect native intracellular IL-17A expression in PBMC in conjunction with cell surface phenotyping mabs [CD4+ve, CD8+ve and Workshop Cluster 1 (WC-1)+ve gamma-delta (γδ)] we show that distinct T cell subsets in cattle (defined as CD4+ve, CD8+ve or WC-1+ve) and sheep (defined as CD4+ve or WC-1+ve) can express IL-17A following activation. These novel techniques provide a solid basis to investigate IL-17A expression and define specific CD4+ve T cell subset activation in ruminants.

Introduction

Interleukin(IL)-17 was first described in 1993 as a novel transcript in a T cell hybridoma clone and named cytotoxic T lymphocyte associated antigen 8 (CTLA-8) [1]. It was subsequently renamed IL-17A and it is one of the IL-17 family of six related homodimeric cytokines [IL-17A, -B, -C, -D, -E (also known as IL-25) and -F] that are involved in acute and chronic inflammatory responses in humans and murine models as reviewed by Gu et al. [2]. IL-17A is the "signature cytokine" secreted by the Th-17 CD4+ve T cell subset [3]. Activation of Th-17-type responses are important not only for host immune control of extracellular bacterial and fungal infections but are also associated with chronic inflammation and autoimmunity. Detailed knowledge of IL-17A biology in humans has led to the targeted development of immunotherapeutic monoclonal antibodies (mabs) to block IL-17A and the IL-17RA receptor for the treatment and control of psoriasis, multiple sclerosis and rheumatoid arthritis [4].

However, as for many immunological parameters, our knowledge of IL-17A production and its function in veterinary species is very limited compared to humans and biomedical rodent models [5] despite cloning of bovine IL-17A in 2006 [6]. In farmed ruminant species, there are published studies that measure mRNA encoding bovine IL-17 family members. These include IL-17A expression in purified protein derivative-stimulated peripheral blood mononuclear cells (PBMC) from cattle with macroscopic lung lesion pathology following experimental *Mycobacterium bovis* infection [7]; IL-17A and IL-17F in afferent lymph cells in response to liposomal vaccine preparations [8]; and IL-17A, IL-17C, IL-17E and IL-17F in the udder of lactating cows infected with *Escherichia coli* [9]. Measurement of IL-17 family members at the protein level in ruminant species has been limited by the

*Correspondence: Sean.Wattegedera@moredun.ac.uk
[1] Moredun Research Institute, International Research Centre, Pentlands Science Park, Bush Loan, Penicuik, Scotland EH26 0PZ, UK
Full list of author information is available at the end of the article

paucity of species-specific reagents with the exception of one commercially-available ELISA kit to detect bovine IL-17A (Kingfisher Biotech). Using this ELISA, Flynn et al. [10] have shown the capacity of *Neospora caninum*-infected bovine macrophages to stimulate IL-17A production in naive CD4+ve T cells while Tassi et al. [11] have shown the presence of IL-17A in milk from lactating cattle infected by *Streptococcus uberis*.

The detection and biological function of other IL-17 family members in ruminants is less well characterised. Bougarn et al. [12] and Roussel et al. [9] reported the up-regulation of mRNA encoding the chemokines CCL2 and CCL20 in primary bovine mammary epithelial cells by recombinant bovine IL-17A and IL-17F, consistent with activities of the human and rodent orthologues. In 2011, Gossner et al. [13] sequenced two variant IL-17E (IL-25) sequences from ovine gastric lymph nodes. Most of the cattle, sheep and goat IL-17 family sequences have been published (Additional file 1) but only recombinant IL-17A is commercially available at present for all three species, with IL-17F also available for cattle. To improve our capability to study IL-17A biology in sheep and cattle we have screened a panel of commercial antibodies for ability to recognise recombinant bovine and ovine IL-17A expressed in mammalian cells and further evaluated their performance in a range of techniques for detection of the native cytokine in T cell subsets.

Materials and methods
Animals
Four Texel-cross ewes of approximately 3 years of age, six Greyface ewes 2–4 years of age and three male Holstein–Friesian cattle 8–12 months of age were maintained off pasture by the Bioservices Division at Moredun Research Institute (MRI) in helminth-free conditions. In addition, four female Holstein–Friesian cattle of approximately 2 years of age were maintained off pasture at Dryden Farm, The Roslin Institute (RI) at The University of Edinburgh. All animal procedures were approved by the Ethics Committees at MRI and RI and performed to Home Office Guidelines under Project Licences PPL 60/4394, PPL 60/3854, PPL 60/4380 and PPL 60/4391. Venous blood was collected into heparinised vacutainers (Becton–Dickinson, Oxford, UK) or into syringes containing sodium heparin (final concentration 20 U/mL, Sigma-Aldrich, Dorset, UK). PBMC were isolated from heparinised sheep and cattle blood by density centrifugation using established protocols [14] and used for molecular cloning, mitogen re-stimulation assays and ELISpot assays. For analysis of cytokine expression by specific T cell subsets, an additional red blood cell lysis step was applied to the PBMC following density centrifugation using a lysis buffer containing 10 mM $KHCO_3$, 150 mM

NH_4Cl, 0.1 mM EDTA pH 8.0 for 5 min at room temperature (RT).

Cloning, sequencing and bioinformatic analyses of IL-17A
We have observed that Concanavalin A (ConA) stimulates ruminant PBMC and found it very effective at upregulating mRNA expression of inflammatory (IFN-γ) and regulatory (IL-10) cytokines from 6 to 96 h [15] and considered this time-frame ideal for acquiring template cDNA for bovine and ovine IL-17A. PBMC from one male calf (male Holstein–Friesian) and one ewe (Texel-cross) were seeded into six-well flat bottom plates (Corning Costar, Scientific Laboratory Supplies Ltd, Coatbridge, UK) at a concentration of 1×10^6 cells/mL in RPMI-1640 (Gibco, Life Technologies, Paisley, UK) supplemented with 0.1% 2-mercaptoethanol (Sigma-Aldrich), 1% L-glutamine and 10% heat-inactivated fetal bovine serum (FBS, Gibco) and stimulated with the T cell mitogen ConA (Sigma-Aldrich) at 5 µg/mL for 72 h in a humidified incubator 37 °C/5% CO_2. Cells were lysed by the addition of 1 mL of cell lysis buffer containing 0.1% v/v beta-mercaptoethanol. Total RNA was isolated using the RNeasy Mini Kit (Qiagen Inc., Manchester, UK) following the manufacturer's instructions and cDNA was prepared by reverse transcription using SuperScript® III Reverse Transcriptase (Invitrogen, Life Technologies, Paisley, UK) to serve as a template for the cloning of the *IL-17A* genes. The gene encoding bovine (bov) IL-17A was amplified using specific primers encoding the full length sequences (for cattle bovIL17apEExsF2: CAA TAA GCT TCC ATG GCT TCT ATG AGA ACT TC and bovIL17apEExsR3: TCT GCC CGG GTC TTA AGC CAA ATG GCG) flanked by restriction enzymes sites *Hind*III and *Sma*I to facilitate sub-cloning into pEE14 expression vector (Lonza, Slough, UK). At the start of the study no ovine IL-17A sequence was available so primers based on the bovine and caprine IL-17A sequences were used to clone the ovine gene (cahIL17apEExsF2: CAA TAA GCT TCC ATG GCG TCT ATG AGA ACT GC and ovIL17xsR2: TCT GCC CGG GTC TTA AGC CAC ATG GCG GAC) along with the restriction enzymes sites *Hind*III and *Sma*I to facilitate sub-cloning. BovIL-17A cDNA sequence derived from ConA-stimulated PBMC was identical to the previously reported sequence (NM_001008412.2). The sequence of ovIL-*17A* derived in this study (LN835312, European Nucleotide Archive record) has a 100% identity with the *ovIL-17A* (XP_004018936.1) predicted from genomic DNA.

Conventional PCR protocols were undertaken to amplify the full length genes in a reaction containing: 1 µL of cDNA, 2.5 µL of 10× PCR buffer, 1.5 µL of $MgCl_2$, 0.5 µL 10 mM dNTP, 0.1 µL of a mix of 10:1 Taq DNA polymerase (5 U/mL) (Bioline, UK) and Pfu DNA polymerase (5 U/

mL) (Promega, Madison, USA) and PCR water (Sigma-Aldrich) to a volume of 25 μL. The PCR conditions for the amplification of both bovIL-17A and ovIL-17A consisted of an initial denaturation of 5 min at 95 °C, followed by 40 cycles of 94 °C for 30 s, 60 °C for 30 s and 72 °C for 1 min. The PCR products were visualised on a 1% w/v agarose gel containing SYBR® Safe DNA gel stain (Invitrogen, Life Technologies) using a UV light box and purified using a QIAquick Gel Extraction Kit (Qiagen Inc.) before ligation into pGEM-T Easy Cloning Vector (Promega).

After the transformation into XL1-Blue Competent Cells (Stratagene, Agilent Technologies Division, USA), the cells were grown on Luria–Bertani (LB) agar (Sigma-Aldrich) supplemented with X-Gal and 10 mM IPTG overnight at 37 °C. White colonies were selected and grown overnight in 5 mL of LB medium with ampicillin (100 μg/mL, Sigma-Aldrich), in a shaking incubator at 37 °C. Plasmid DNA from four independent colonies of bovIL-17A and ovIL-17A cDNAs was purified using a QIAprep Plasmid DNA Miniprep kit (Qiagen Inc.) following the manufacturer's instructions and then sequenced to confirm the full length sequences using the T7 and SP6 sequencing primers (Eurofins Genomics, Ebersberg, Germany).

Bovine IL-17A and ovIL-17A cDNAs were compared for similarity using the Basic Local Alignment Search Tool (BLAST 2.5.1, [16, 17]). The predicted amino acid sequences were then analysed for the presence of a signal peptide using Signal 4.1 [18, 19]. The mature protein sequences were aligned with the corresponding sequences from a variety of vertebrates including representative mammal, reptile and avian species using Clustal Omega [20, 21]). A matrix of pair-wise identity at the amino acid level was generated using Clustal 2.1. Evolutionary sequence comparisons were undertaken using 13 selected mammalian and other sequences with the multiple alignment generated using Clustal Omega. Prior to running the phylogenetic analysis the most appropriate amino acid substitution model was obtained by running the model selection module of TOPALi v2.5 [22]. The evolutionary relationships between the sequences were inferred using Mr. Bayes launched from TOPALI v2.5 using the Jones–Taylor–Thornton plus gamma (JTT + G) model with two runs each of 1 250 000 generations with a burn in period of 20% and sampling frequency of 1000.

Expression vector construct production

The pEE14 vector was linearized and the confirmed bovIL-17A/ovIL-17A excised from pGEM-T Easy clones by double digestion using HindIII and SmaI at 37 °C for 3 h in 30 μL reactions. The digests were run in a 1% w/v agarose gel and bands excised and purified with a QIAquick Gel Extraction kit (Qiagen Inc.). The cDNA and linearized expression vector were then ligated in 1:3 ratio of insert/vector using T4 DNA ligase (Promega) at 4 °C overnight. Ligated products were transformed into competent JM109 cells (Promega), and seeded into LB plates with ampicillin (100 μg/mL). Positive colonies were grown overnight in 5 mL of LB medium with ampicillin in a shaking incubator at 37 °C. Plasmid DNA was purified as above and quantified using the Nanodrop spectrophotometer (NanoDrop Technologies, Thermo Fisher Scientific, MA, USA). Plasmid constructs were sequenced (Eurofins) to verify the integrity of the bovIL-17A and ovIL-17A sequences.

Expression and quantification of recombinant bovine IL-17A and ovine IL-17A

Chinese Hamster Ovary (CHO) cells were used as the expression system for the cloned cytokine cDNAs. The CHO cells were maintained in Glasgow's modified Dulbecco's Medium (GMEM, Sigma-Aldrich) supplemented with minimum essential medium non-specific amino acids (Gibco), 1 mM sodium pyruvate (Gibco), 410 μM glutamic acid (Sigma-Aldrich) with 450 μM L-asparagine (Sigma-Aldrich), 1.3 mM adenosine (Sigma-Aldrich), nucleosides (1.2 mM guanosine, 1.4 mM cytidine, 1.4 mM uridine and 495 μM thymidine, all Sigma-Aldrich), 10% heat-inactivated FBS (PAA Gold, Little Chalfont, UK) and 2 mM L-glutamine (Sigma-Aldrich), designated parent CHO medium [23]. CHO cells were subcultured twice weekly in 75 cm^2 vent-capped tissue culture flasks (Corning Costar, Scientific Laboratory Supplies Ltd) using 0.05% trypsin in versene/EDTA (Gibco and Sigma-Aldrich) for detachment. For transfection, cells were seeded at 3×10^5 cells/well in a six well plate (Nunc, Roskilde, Denmark) and incubated overnight at 37 °C/5% CO$_2$. Cells were then transfected with 3 μg of the plasmid vector pEE14 containing cDNA encoding either bovIL-17A or ovIL-17A cDNA using Lipofectamine 2000 (Invitrogen, Life Technologies Ltd) according to the manufacturer's instructions. Transfected CHO cells were initially established in transfectant CHO medium comprising GMEM containing 7.5% dialysed (d) glutamine-free heat-inactivated FBS (Invitrogen) and 25 μM methionine sulfoximine (MSX; Sigma-Aldrich).

Cells that survived the selective MSX inhibitor were subsequently amplified with increasing concentrations of MSX prior to cloning by limiting dilution to establish stable, cloned transfectant cell lines as previously described [24]. The supernatants from the IL-17A-transfected CHO cells were tested for the presence of rIL-17A using a commercial bovine IL-17A ELISA with quantifiable reference standards (Kingfisher Biotech, Minneapolis, USA).

Validation of transfected CHO cells expressing recombinant bovine IFN-γ and ovine IFN-γ

Existing transfected CHO cell lines expressing rbovIFN-γ and rovIFN-γ were used as positive controls for detection of intracellular IFN-γ. The CHO-expressed rbovIFN-γ and rovIFN-γ were evaluated by an in-house ELISA using the anti-bovine IFN-γ mab clones CC330 and CC302 (Bio-Rad Laboratories, Oxford, UK) and commercial rbovIFN-γ (Pierce Endogen, Rockford, USA) as a quantifiable reference standard. The biological activities of the rbovIFN-γ and rovIFN-γ were confirmed using a viral inhibition bioassay as described by Entrican et al. [25].

Bulk recombinant cytokine production and functional determination of recombinant bovine and ovine IL-17A

For bulk recombinant cytokine production and matched negative-control supernatant, transfected and parent CHO cell lines were maintained routinely in 225 cm^2 flasks and sub-cultured twice weekly at a 1:10 ratio as previously described. Multiple flasks with sub-confluent cell monolayers from each cell line were grown prior to the preparation of serum-free conditioned medium as previously described [24], clarified by centrifugation at 1000 g at 4 °C for 10 min and stored at −80 °C until required. The CHO-expressed rbov and rovIL-17A were tested for their capacity to stimulate CXCL8 production in vitro using an Embryonic Bovine Lung cell line (EBL, kindly provided by Dr. Amin Tahoun and Professor David Gally, RI) and the ovine ST-6 cell line [26]. The EBL cells were subcultured in Dulbecco's Modified Eagle Medium (DMEM, Invitrogen) containing 10% heat-inactivated FBS (PAA) defined as culture medium, using 75 cm^2 vent-capped tissue culture flasks (Corning Costar, Scientific Laboratory Supplies Ltd). The ST-6 cells were similarly subcultured in Iscove's Modified Eagle Medium (IMDM, Gibco, Life Technologies) containing 10% heat-inactivated FBS (PAA). Cells were adjusted to 1×10^5/mL in culture medium and seeded in triplicate, at 500 μL/well in 48 well plates (Corning Costar, Scientific Laboratory Supplies Ltd) then cultured in a humidified incubator at 37 °C/5% CO_2 overnight. The culture medium was then replaced with either serum-free conditioned CHO medium containing rbov or rovIL-17A adjusted to 100 ng/mL or serum-free conditioned medium from untransfected CHO cells at an equivalent dilution. The resultant supernatants from the treated EBL and ST-6 cells were harvested 24 h later and stored at −20 °C until analysis for the presence of CXCL8 by ELISA. This ELISA protocol has been described elsewhere in detail [27] and is based on a murine anti-ovine CXCL8 mab 8M6 as a capture and rabbit anti-sheep CXCL8 polyclonal antibody for detection (Bio-Rad Laboratories). This ELISA has also been shown to detect native bovine CXCL8 [28, 29].

Generation of native ovine IL-17A

PBMC from six ewes (2–4 year old Greyface breed) were cultured at 2×10^6 cell/mL in 100 μL of IMDM supplemented with 10% heat-inactivated FBS, 50 μg/mL gentamicin and 50 μM 2-mercaptoethanol in the presence or absence of 100 μL per well ConA (5 μg/mL) in a 96 well U-bottom plate (Nunc) in a humidified incubator at 37 °C/5% CO_2. Quadruplicate wells were set up for each treatment for the six animals. The culture supernatants from the technical replicates were harvested and pooled together after 96 h and stored at −20 °C prior to analysis by the commercial anti-bovine IL-17A ELISA (Kingfisher Biotech).

IL-17A ELISpot

MultiScreen-IP Filter Plates (Merck Millipore, Hertfordshire, UK) were activated by addition of 70% ethanol (Fisher Scientific, Loughborough, UK) for a maximum of 2 min. Plates were washed five times with sterile ddH$_2$O and then incubated with 50 μL/well of 5 μg/mL rabbit polyclonal anti-bovine IL-17A antibody (product code PB0274B-100, Kingfisher Biotech) for 18 h at 4 °C. Simultaneously, PBMC from three cattle (8–12 month old Holstein–Friesian) and three ewes (3 year old Texel-cross) were re-suspended in RPMI 1640 medium containing 10% heat-inactivated FBS, 2 mM L-glutamine, 100 U/mL penicillin, 100 μg/mL streptomycin and 50 μM 2-mercaptoethanol (RPMI culture medium) at a concentration of 2×10^6 cells/mL and stimulated with either 5 μg/mL ConA or culture medium alone for 18 h or for the last treatment culture medium for 12 h replaced with 50 ng/mL phorbol 12-myristate 13-acetate (PMA, Sigma-Aldrich) and 1 μg/mL ionomycin (ionomycin calcium salt from *Streptomyces conglobatus*, Sigma-Aldrich) for the final 6 h in a humidified incubator at 37 °C/5% CO_2. The plates were set up for three technical replicates for each treatment for each animal.

Following incubation with the coating antibody, the ELISpot filter plate was washed five times with sterile PBS and subsequently incubated with 100 μL/well RPMI culture medium for 30 min at RT. Medium was removed and 2×10^5 stimulated or unstimulated cells were added to each well, with each treatment in triplicate wells for each animal. The plate was incubated overnight at 37 °C/5% CO_2. The cells were removed from the ELISpot plate wells and discarded. The plate was washed five times with PBS and 0.5 μg/mL biotinylated rabbit polyclonal anti-bovine IL-17A antibody (product code number PB0277B-50, Kingfisher Biotech) in PBS with 0.5% FBS was added to the wells and incubated for 2 h at RT. After a further five washes with PBS, wells were incubated with a 1:1000 dilution of streptavidin conjugated to horse radish peroxidase (Sigma-Aldrich) in PBS with

0.5% FBS for 1 h at RT. After a final five washes with PBS, wells were incubated with SureBlue™ TMB Microwell Peroxidase Substrate (KPL, Maryland, USA) for 10 min at RT. Reactions were stopped by washing wells five times with ddH$_2$O and the plate was left to dry overnight prior to analysis using an AID EliSpot Reader HR (AID Auto-immun Diagnostika GmbH, Straßberg, Germany) using AID EliSpot software version 4.0.

Evaluation of commercial antibodies for intracellular detection of IL-17A

The cloned, transfected CHO cells served as source of constitutive IL-17A expression for evaluation of antibod-ies and the CHO parent cells served as negative control cells. CHO cells were cultured as described above. For flow cytometry, cells were pelleted by centrifugation at 626 g at 4 °C for 2 min and washed three times in cold PBS before being fixed in 0.5 mL of 1% paraformaldehyde (PFA, Sigma-Aldrich) at RT for 10 min. Cells were washed once more in cold PBS and adjusted to 1 × 10^7 cells/mL in PBS/0.05% (w/v) sodium azide (Sigma-Aldrich) and stored at 4 °C. The transfected CHO cells were prepared in advance and have been shown to be stable (without significant changes to detection of recombinant proteins by ICS or cell autofluorescence) when stored at +4 °C for several weeks (data not shown). Transfectant CHO cells stored in this way have been used to evaluate commercial antibodies for their capacity to bind recombinant ovine TNF-α [30] and recombinant ovine FoxP3 [31]. Prior to staining the cells underwent an overnight permeabilisa-tion and block step. Cells were pelleted by centrifugation at 626 g for 2 min at 4 °C then resuspended to 10^7 cells/ mL in PBS containing 5% heat-inactivated FBS (PAA Gold), 0.05% (w/v) NaN$_3$ (Sigma-Aldrich), 0.2% (w/v) saponin (Sigma-Aldrich) (permeabilisation buffer) plus 20% normal goat serum (Merck Millipore) (combined permeabilisation and blocking buffer) and maintained overnight at 4 °C consistent with our established protocol using transfectant CHO cells [30, 31].

The permeabilised and blocked CHO cells were then transferred to 96 well U-bottom plate (BD Falcon, Mas-sachusetts, USA), 50 μL of cell suspension per well per labelling antibody. The cells were pelleted by centrifuga-tion at 626 g for 2 min at 4 °C, aspirated in permeabilisa-tion buffer and then 100 μL primary antibody or isotype/ equivalent matched control antibody or permeabilisation buffer alone was added for 30 min at 4 °C. A full detailed list of the commercial anti-IL-17A antibodies used in this study is provided in Table 1 and these were used accord-ing to the manufacturer's recommendations. A list of isotype-matched or equivalent polyclonal antibodies used as appropriate negative controls is shown in detail in Table 2. Cells were then washed by centrifugation at

626 g for 2 min at 4 °C three times in permeabilisation buffer. The secondary antibody consisting of 100 μL per well goat anti-mouse-IgG-phycoerythrin (PE) conjugated (Invitrogen, USA) at 1 μg/mL in permeabilisation buffer for cells labelled with the primary mabs or 100 μL per well goat anti-rabbit IgG alexafluor 488 at 1 μg/mL for cells labelled with the primary pabs. Cells labelled using the RPE-conjugated anti-IL-17A mab were incubated in 100 μL per well in permeabilisation buffer alone for 30 min at 4 °C. Cells were washed twice in permeabilisa-tion buffer then finally washed in PBS prior to fixation in 200 μL of 1% PFA and stored at 4 °C in the dark prior to acquisition.

Cells were acquired for flow cytometric analyses using the MacsQuant flow cytometer (Miltenyi Biotech, Ger-many) and analysed using the MacsQuantify Software v2.7. 20 000–50 000 events were collected and the sub-sequent gating strategy shown in Additional file 2 fol-lowed. Briefly, after removing artefacts with gating P1 (Additional file 2A), P1/P2 was applied to the main popu-lation to exclude debris (Additional file 2B) followed by P1/P2/P3 for doublet discrimination (Additional file 2C). The positive threshold setting in the phycoerythrin or alexafluor 488 channels P1/P2/P3/P4 were set using the isotype or equivalent control for each CHO cell line (Additional file 2D). Overlaying histogram plots of P1/ P2/P3 were used to compare anti-IL-17A antibodies with appropriate isotype or equivalent controls (Addi-tional file 2E). Gated percentage numbers (P1/P2/P3/P4) and median fluorescence region values (P1/P2/P3) were measured for each antibody. Delta median fluorescence intensity (deltaMFI) was calculated by deducting the median mab isotype or pab control median fluorescence region value from the anti-IL-17A antibody median flu-orescence region value. The summarised data are pre-sented in Additional file 3.

IL-17A and IFN-γ expression by bovine and ovine T cell subsets

PBMC were prepared from whole blood from four cat-tle (2 year old female Holstein–Friesian) and four sheep (3 year old Texel-cross), resuspended in RPMI-1640 cul-ture medium, counted using Trypan Blue (ThermoFisher Scientific, Utah, USA) and adjusted to 1 × 10^7 cells/mL. 2 × 10^7 cells were stimulated with PMA (50 ng/mL), ionomycin (1 μg/mL), brefeldin A (10 μg/mL) diluted in RPMI culture medium for 4 h in sterile centrifuge tubes in a humidified incubator at 37 °C/5% CO$_2$.

Cells were pelleted by centrifugation at 258 g for 5 min at 4 °C and washed in PBS and samples reserved as con-trols for the live/dead stain for flow cytometric analyses. 1 × 10^7 cells were stained using the violet live/dead Fix-able Dead Cell Stain Kit (Life Technologies) according to

Table 1 Commercial anti-IL-17A antibodies evaluated by intracellular staining for capacity to bind recombinant bovine and ovine IL-17A

Primary antibody used in the intracellular staining (CHO cells)	Clone	Commercial supplier and product code in brackets	Antibody isotype	Immunogen	Specificity	Antibody conjugation if present
A.1	N/A rabbit derived polyclonal antibody. Lot number BO1431JK	Kingfisher Biotech (PB0274B-100)	IgG1	Recombinant bovine IL-17A	Bovine	None
B.1	eBio64Dec17	eBiosciences (12-7179-41)	IgG1	Recombinant human IL-17A	Human	PE
C.1	MT44.6	Mabtech (3520-3-250)	IgG1	Recombinant human IL-17A	Human, rhesus and cynomolgus macaques and common marmoset monkeys	None
C.2	MT241	Mabtech (3520M-3-250)	IgG1	Recombinant human IL-17A	Human, rhesus and cyn-omolgus macaques	None
C.3	MT2770	Mabtech (3521-14-250)	IgG1	Recombinant mouse IL-17A	Mouse	None
C.4	MT504	Mabtech (3520-6-250)	IgG1	Recombinant human IL-17A	Human, rhesus and cynomolgus macaques and common marmoset monkeys	Biotin
D.1	41809	R & D Systems IC317P	IgG2b	Recombinant human IL-17A amino acids 20-155	Human	PE
D.2	41802	R & D Systems (IC3171P)	IgG1	Recombinant human IL-17A amino acids 20-155	Human	PE

All details of antibody clone, product code, immunogen, host specificity and antibody conjugate have been taken from supplier datasheets. Each antibody has been assigned a code where the capital letter denotes the commercial supplier and the integer an individual pab or a mab clone. The commercial antibodies were used in conjunction with an appropriate control antibody (see Table 2, denoted by the equivalent letter but in lowercase) for the intracellular staining protocol described in "Evaluation of commercial antibodies section".

Table 2 Isotype control mabs and control pab used in the evaluation of the commercial anti-IL-17A antibodies

Control antibody used in the intracellular staining (CHO cells)	Clone	Source	Immunogen/host raised in	Isotype	Antibody conjugation, if present
a	N/A	Professor Waithaka Mwangi, A & M University, Texas, USA	Bovine CD34 construct/rabbit	Rabbit IgG	None
b, c and d	VPM 21	Moredun	Border disease virus/mouse	Mouse IgG1	None
d	VPM22	Moredun	Border disease virus/mouse	Mouse IgG2b	None

The two mabs VPM21 and VPM22 (both MRI, Edinburgh, UK) and control pab (raised against bovine CD34; A & M University, Texas, USA) were derived from non-commercial sources. The hybridoma cell lines were grown in-house to generate mabs that were then adjusted for concentration to match that of the anti-IL-17A mabs listed in Table 1. The antibodies were assigned a code letter in lower case that corresponds with the commercial antibodies listed in Table 1 (denoted by the equivalent uppercase letter) for the intracellular staining protocol followed in "Evaluation of commercial antibodies section".

the manufacturer's protocol. Cells were fixed in 1% PFA for 10 min at RT. PBMC were permeabilised overnight as described above for the CHO cells (which also served as positive controls for the PBMC intracellular cytokine staining). 1×10^6 permeabilised PBMC were transferred into each well of a 96 well U-bottom plate (BD Falcon, Massachusetts, USA) then pelleted by centrifugation. A combined cell surface phenotyping and intracellular cytokine staining step was undertaken with directly-conjugated mabs and the appropriate isotype-matched and FMO controls in a volume of 100 μL per well for 30 min at RT (Table 3). Cells were pelleted, washed once in permeabilisation buffer and then once in PBS before final resuspension in 150 μL PBS. A minimum of 50 000 events were acquired using an LSRFortessa™ cell analyzer (Becton–Dickinson) and analysed using FlowJo vX for Windows 7

using the gating strategies shown in Additional file 4 (cattle cells) and Additional file 5 (sheep cells).

Statistical analyses

The various datasets were analysed separately for statistical interpretation and the methods used will be outlined sequentially. The IL-17A bioassay datasets for the differential CXCL8 expression in technical replicates stimulated with rbovIL-17A, rovIL-17A and CHO UTF control supernatant was statistically assessed using Kruskal–Wallis tests for both bovine (EBL) and ovine (ST-6) cell lines. The native IL-17A expression of ovine PBMC from six animals in re-recall assays with ConA was analysed using the two-tailed Mann–Whitney test.

The ELISpot data were modelled by fitting a Poisson generalised linear mixed model (GLMM) by maximum

Table 3 Commercial antibodies used in the detection of native intracellular IL-17A and IFN-γ by bovine and ovine T cell subsets

Antibody clone	Commercial supplier and product code in brackets	Antibody isotype	Target antigen	Host specificity	Antibody conjugation	Antibody dilution
CC8	Bio-Rad Laboratories (MCA1653PE)	IgG2a	CD4	Bovine	Phycoerythrin	1:20
44.38	Bio-Rad Laboratories (MCA2213PE)	IgG2a	CD4	Ovine	Phycoerythrin	1:20
CC58	Bio-Rad Laboratories (MCA1654PE)	IgG1	CD8β	Bovine	Phycoerythrin	1:20
CC15	Bio-Rad Laboratories (MCA838PE)	IgG2a	WC-1	Bovine	Phycoerythrin	1:200
CC302	Bio-Rad Laboratories (MCA1783A647)	IgG1	IFN-γ	Bovine	Alexafluor-647	1:200
eBio64DEC17	eBiosciences (17-7179)	IgG1	IL-17A	Human	APC	1:20
F8-11-13	Bio-Rad Laboratories (MCA1209PE)	IgG1	Recognised rat cell surface marker	Rat	Phycoerythrin	1:20
MRC OX-34	Bio-Rad Laboratories (MCA929PE)	IgG2a	Rat cell surface marker	Rat	Phycoerythrin	1:20

All details of antibody clones, product code, immunogen, host specificity and antibody conjugate are taken from datasheets provided by the commercial suppliers. The antibodies were used at the described dilutions for the cell phenotyping and intracellular cytokine staining described in "Expression of intracellular IL-17A and IFN-γ by bovine and ovine T cell subsets section".

likelihood to the IL-17A SFU/10^6 production, using log-arithmic link function and Laplace approximations to calculate log-likelihoods. The model included treatment (ConA, medium and PMA/ionomycin), species (bovine, ovine) and their interaction as fixed effects and animal identification as a random effect in order to account for both within- and between-animal variability. An observation-level random effect term was specified to account for data over-dispersion. The statistical significance of the fixed effect terms was assessed using p values derived from type II Wald Chi square tests. Linear hypothesis tests were defined from the GLMM in order to conduct pair-wise comparisons of means between treatments and species. The associated p values were adjusted for false discovery rate (FDR) following Benjamini–Hochberg's procedure [32].

A principal component analysis (PCA) was conducted to investigate the overall relationships between commercial antibodies and specific binding capacity to rbov and rovIL-17A on the basis of the six metrics considered simultaneously. This statistical technique projects the information in multi-variable/-parameter datasets onto low dimensions, typically two dimensions, which is useful here to facilitate meaningful comparisons and clustering of the commercial antibodies by means of optimal linear combinations (principal components, PCs) of the original metrics, that are represented visually in a biplot [33, 34]. For example, Hemmink et al. [35] have used PCA to analyse immunological datasets following an influenza pathogenesis study in pigs showing the correlation of cytokine production, with viral titre over time. Our antibody screening results were displayed using a biplot based on the two first PCs (those accounting for the highest percentage of the total observed data variability) to facilitate discussion and ranking of the commercial antibodies. Finally, in the bovine and ovine T cell subset phenotyping and combined intracellular staining datasets, the total percentage IL-17A and IFN-γ expression for cattle and sheep PBMC were used to statistically assess the significance of differences in expression between species using two-tailed Mann–Whitney tests allowing for ties.

Statistical test significance was assessed at the 5% significance level. The statistical analyses were conducted on the R system for statistical computing v3.2.

Results
Genetic relationships of mammalian IL-17A sequences
BovIL-17A and ovIL-17A cDNA coding sequences were 462 nucleotides in length and shared 97% identity. The predicted amino acid sequences including the signal peptide corresponded to 153 amino acids. According to SignalP 4.1, both bovIL-17A and ovIL-17A signal peptides account for the first 23 amino acids and the mature

peptides are 130 amino acids in length. The pair-wise identity matrix of the bovIL-17A and ovIL-17A with other published mature peptide sequences revealed identities of between 48.4 and 89.5% to the chicken and wild Bactrian camel respectively (Additional file 6). Further analysis revealed over 99% identity between the bovine, ovine and caprine IL-17A amino acid sequences and a high degree of identity to human IL-17A (bovine and ovine 76.2%; caprine 75.8%). Evolutionary sequence comparisons using 13 selected mammalian and other sequences were inferred using Mr. Bayes launched from TOPALI v 2.5 using the Jones–Taylor–Thornton plus gamma (JTT + G) model, as shown in Figure 1. The sequences cluster to three groups with the caprine, bovine, ovine and swine sequences in one cluster. Given the pair-wise identities and the evolutionary relationships between the human and bovine and ovine sequences, we speculated that there would be a strong likelihood of mabs produced against human IL-17A binding to the bovine and ovine orthologues and that this could be definitively determined using the mammalian CHO expression system.

Expression, detection and biological function of recombinant ruminant IL-17A
The Kingfisher Biotech bovine IL-17A VetSet is a pab-based ELISA for detection of bovine IL-17A and based on the homology between the bovine and ovine orthologues, we predicted that it would detect both of the expressed recombinant proteins. Figure 2A shows titration curves for supernatant from transfected CHO cells expressing rbovIL-17A and rovIL-17A demonstrating the dynamic range that the rbov and rovIL-17A can be detected at using this commercial ELISA test. No signal was detected in supernatant from untransfected CHO cells (data not shown). The supernatant from the CHO line expressing rovIL-17A titrated over a wider range of concentrations than the rbovIL-17A-expressing CHO line. Quantification of the supernatants using the Vetset kit recombinant bovine IL-17A standard revealed that rovIL-17A and rbovIL-17A supernatants had concentrations of 8809 and 1660 ng/mL respectively.

We next established that the expressed recombinant proteins were functionally active. The supernatants were adjusted to 100 ng/mL for direct comparison of their ability to stimulate CXCL8 expression in a bovine (EBL) and ovine (ST-6) cell line (Figures 2B and C respectively). The magnitude of CXCL8 production by the two cell lines was notably different, with higher levels observed in the ovine ST-6 cell line compared to the bovine EBL cell line, irrespective of whether they were stimulated with rbovIL-17A or rovIL-17A. One effect of rIL-17A is shown by the mean up-regulation of CXCL8 over the background

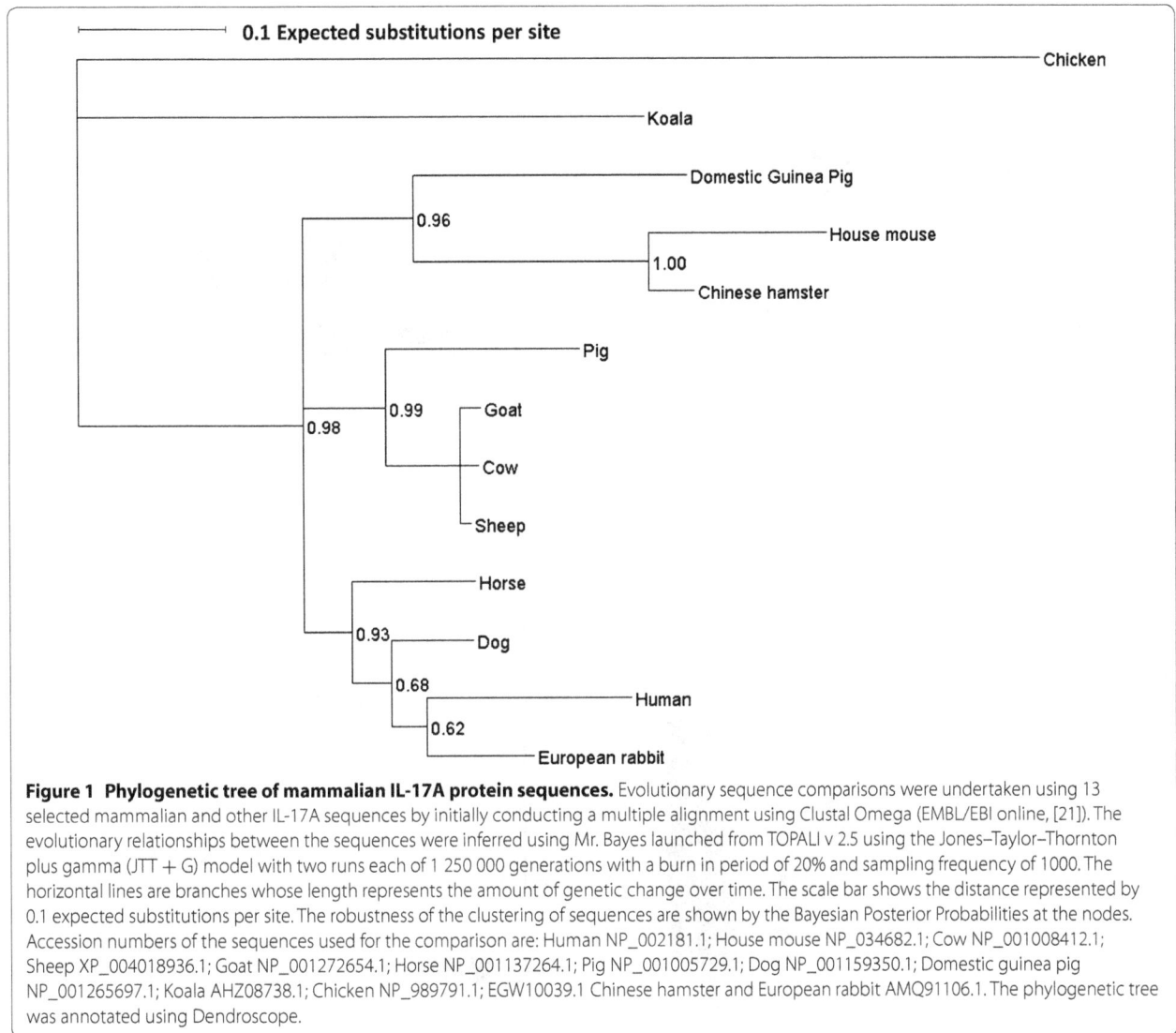

Figure 1 Phylogenetic tree of mammalian IL-17A protein sequences. Evolutionary sequence comparisons were undertaken using 13 selected mammalian and other IL-17A sequences by initially conducting a multiple alignment using Clustal Omega (EMBL/EBI online, [21]). The evolutionary relationships between the sequences were inferred using Mr. Bayes launched from TOPALI v 2.5 using the Jones–Taylor–Thornton plus gamma (JTT + G) model with two runs each of 1 250 000 generations with a burn in period of 20% and sampling frequency of 1000. The horizontal lines are branches whose length represents the amount of genetic change over time. The scale bar shows the distance represented by 0.1 expected substitutions per site. The robustness of the clustering of sequences are shown by the Bayesian Posterior Probabilities at the nodes. Accession numbers of the sequences used for the comparison are: Human NP_002181.1; House mouse NP_034682.1; Cow NP_001008412.1; Sheep XP_004018936.1; Goat NP_001272654.1; Horse NP_001137264.1; Pig NP_001005729.1; Dog NP_001159350.1; Domestic guinea pig NP_001265697.1; Koala AHZ08738.1; Chicken NP_989791.1; EGW10039.1 Chinese hamster and European rabbit AMQ91106.1. The phylogenetic tree was annotated using Dendroscope.

levels produced by EBL cells ($p = 0.027$) or ST-6 cells ($p = 0.027$) exposed to supernatant from untransfected CHO cells. The rovIL-17A stimulated more CXCL8 production than rbovIL-17A in both cell types. Having shown that the bovine IL-17A Vetset ELISA detects rovIL-17A, consistent with publically-available cross-species reactivity information, it was important to confirm that it could also detect and quantify native ovine IL-17A. Culture supernatants from ovine PBMC incubated for 96 h in the presence or absence of ConA were assessed for the presence of IL-17A by the Vetset ELISA. A low level of endogenous IL-17A was found in unstimulated cells, which was statistically significantly upregulated in response to ConA stimulation ($p = 0.002$, Figure 2D).

Enumeration of ruminant cells expressing IL-17A by ELISpot

Quantification of cytokines in cell culture supernatants is one method for characterising the polarisation of cellular immune responses and another is the enumeration of cells expressing individual cytokines. Given the ELISA results above, we decided to use the pabs from the Vetset ELISA to develop an IL-17A ELISpot to determine the frequency of IL-17A-producing cells in activated PBMC from cattle and sheep. Figures 3A and B show three technical replicates of PBMC from one cow and one sheep stimulated by ConA or PMA/ionomycin. Consistency of the technical replicates was clearly visible, as was the almost complete absence of IL-17A-secreting cells in the unstimulated controls. Note that these cells were

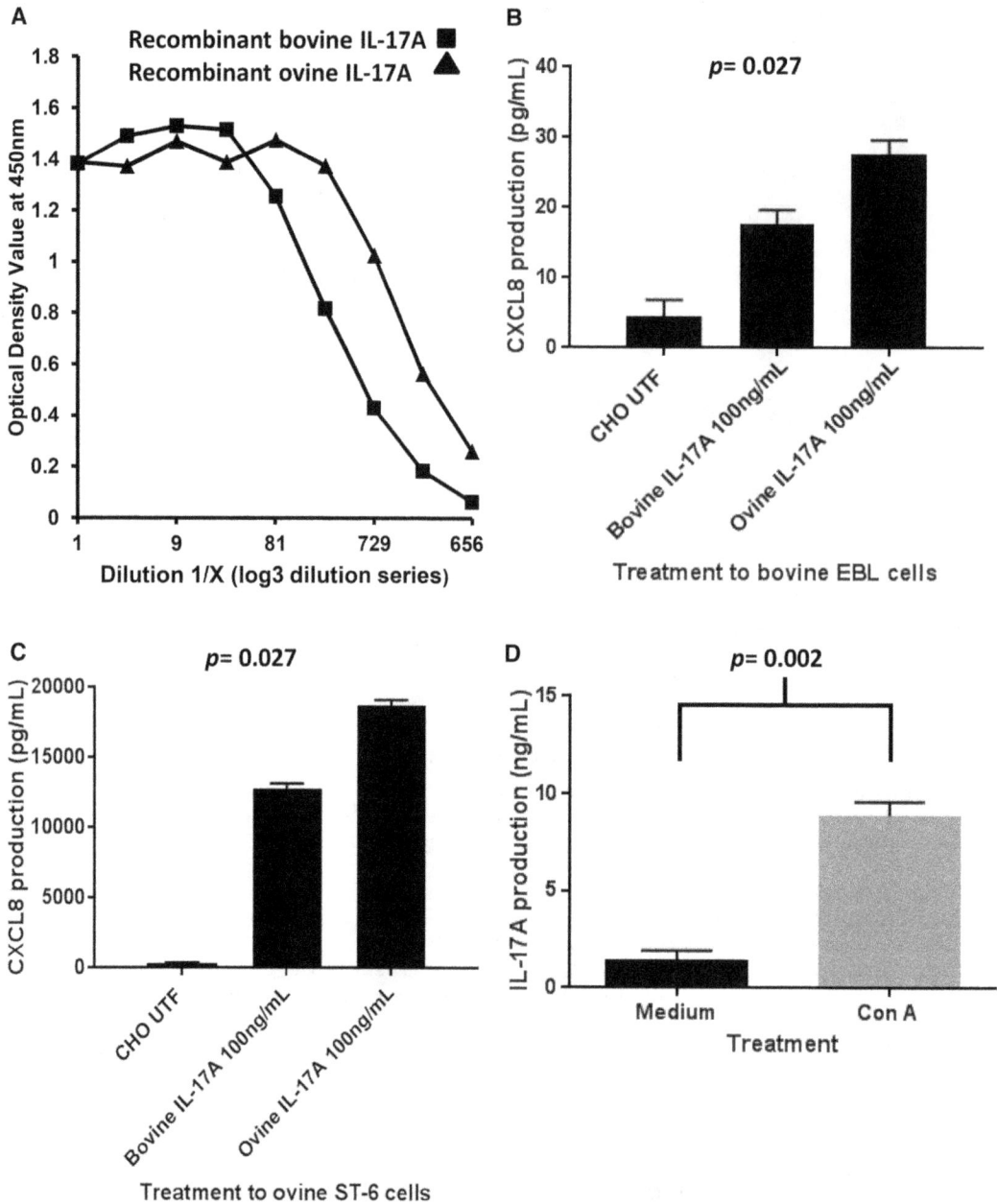

Figure 2 Measurement and biological function of recombinant bovine and ovine IL-17A and detection of native ovine IL-17A by ELISA. A Detection of rbov and rovIL-17A by ELISA. The supernatants from transfected CHO cells expressing rbovIL-17A or rovIL-17A, or control parent untransfected line (UTF) were serially diluted (Log$_3$ dilutions) and evaluated using the commercial bovIL-17A ELISA. Data presented are optical density (OD) values from the Spectrophotometer at 450 nm. The X-axis displays Dilution 1/X and the Y-axis gives the OD value. Readings from UTF supernatant were below the limit of detection. **B** Functional activity of rbov and rovIL-17A on bovine embryonic lung cells. Bovine embryonic lung (EBL) cells were stimulated with 100 ng/mL CHO-expressed rbovIL-17A or rovIL-17A or UTF CHO negative control supernatant. Following 24 h incubation, culture supernatants were collected from triplicate cultures then tested for CXCL8 by ELISA. The X-axis displays the bioassay treatments and the Y-axis shows CXCL8 production in pg/mL. Data are the arithmetic mean of three technical replicates with error bars representing the standard error from one of three experiments. CXCL8 expression between treatments was statistically assessed using Kruskal–Wallis test. **C** Functional activity of rbov and rovIL-17A on ovine ST-6 cells. Ovine ST-6 cells were stimulated with 100 ng/mL CHO-expressed rbovIL-17A or rovIL-17A or UTF CHO supernatant. Following 24 h incubation and culture supernatants collected, tested and analysed as described in Figure 2B. CXCL8 expression between treatments was statistically assessed using Kruskal–Wallis test. **D** Detection of native ovIL-17A by ELISA. Ovine PBMC were cultured at 2×10^6 cells/mL with or without 5 μg/mL ConA. Culture supernatants were analysed for IL-17A using the bovIL-17A ELISA. Data represent the arithmetic mean of PBMC from six ewes and error bars represent standard error. Data were analysed statistically for significance using the two-tailed Mann–Whitney test.

only cultured for 18 h as opposed to 96 h for the ELISA analyses where a positive signal was detected in supernatants of unstimulated cells. Figure 3C shows the average number of spots from activated PBMC from three cattle and three sheep. The average number of spots in cattle and sheep PBMC was similar when activated by PMA/ionomycin [1789.74 Spot Forming Units (SFU) $\pm$ 314.42 vs 1731.72 SFU $\pm$ 304.29, $p = 0.895$], whereas the mean frequency of IL-17A-producing cells was statistically significantly lower in cattle PBMC compared to sheep PBMC when activated with ConA (546.95 SFU $\pm$ 96.32 vs 1130.53 SFU $\pm$ 198.76, $p = 0.004$).

Identification of antibodies that detect recombinant intracellular bovine and ovine IL-17A by flow cytometry

While the ELISpot provides the capability to enumerate the frequency of IL-17A-producing cells and estimates cell-level production determined by spot-size, flow cytometry can provide additional information on the relative levels of IL-17A produced per cell and also identify the phenotype of the producing cell. We used the transfected CHO cells as stable expressers of IL-17A to screen a panel of available mabs and pabs (Table 1) for their ability to detect intracellular bovine and ovine IL-17A. Although the rbovIL-17A and rovIL-17A transfectant CHO cells are derived from the same parent untransfected CHO cells, all three cell lines have different size and granularity properties. To define specific cross-reactive staining of the antibody panel, it was necessary to draw multiple parameter comparisons by overlaying histograms of isotype-matched or appropriate pab controls and calculating the percentages of cells in the gated positive regions from P1/P2/P3/P4 and the deltaMFIs of the entire cell population using the median fluorescence region values within the P1/P2/P3 region relative to appropriate control antibodies (Additional file 2). A

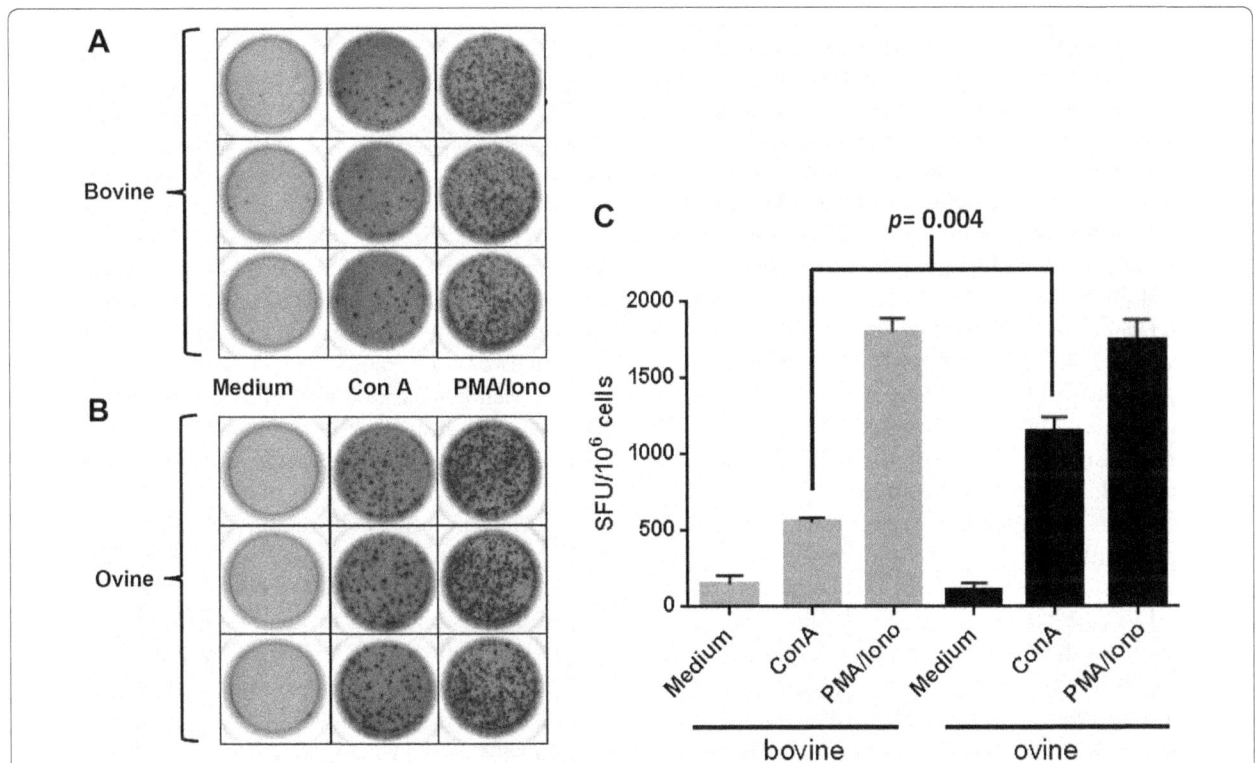

Figure 3 Detection of single-cell expression of ruminant IL-17A by ELISpot. Plates and PBMC were prepared and cultured as described in "IL-17A ELISpot section". ELISpot images shown are representative of PBMC from one of three cattle (**A**) and one of three sheep (**B**) activated with ConA and PMA/ionomycin. The average number of spot-forming units (SFU) with standard errors are shown for 10^6 PBMC from all three cattle (grey bars) and sheep (black bars), stimulated under the different conditions (**C**). Data were modelled by fitting a Poisson generalised linear mixed model (GLMM) by maximum likelihood to the IL-17A SFU/10^6 values, using logarithmic link function and Laplace approximations to calculate log-likelihoods. The model included treatment (medium control, ConA and PMA/ionomycin), species (bovine, ovine) and their interaction as fixed effects and animal identification as a random effect in order to account for both within- and between-animal variability. An observation-level random effect term was specified to account for data over-dispersion. The statistical significance of the fixed effect terms was assessed using p values derived from type II Wald Chi square tests. Linear hypothesis tests were defined from the GLMM in order to conduct pair-wise comparisons of means between treatments and species. The associated p values were adjusted for false discovery rate (FDR) following Benjamini–Hochberg's procedure.

summary of the numerical percentage positivity and deltaMFIs for all of the commercial IL-17A antibodies screened against the UTF CHO, rbov IL-17A CHO and rov IL-17A CHO cells can be found in Additional file 3 which provides six measures to evaluate specific capacity to bind the IL-17A cytokine through intracellular staining.

As we had previously confirmed that the Vetset pabs detected both recombinant and native bovine and ovine IL-17A by ELISA and ELISpot, we first evaluated the unconjugated pab for intracellular staining of the CHO cells using an anti-rabbit second-stage conjugate. Although positive staining was observed in the transfected CHO cells, there was also a considerable background signal with the untransfected CHO cells, possibly reflective of the use of a pab control antibody (Figure 4A). We then screened the panel of seven mabs (listed in Table 1) against the CHO transfectants. Only two (eBio64DEC17 and MT504) of the seven mabs tested were found to specifically cross-react with rbovIL-17A and rovIL-17A in the CHO cells (Figures 4B and C). Both of these mabs were raised against recombinant human IL-17A. Clone eBio64DEC17 clone gave a higher percentage binding in the positive region and deltaMFI values (38.7%+ve/deltaMFI of 1.03 to the bovIL-17A CHO cells and 92.9%+ve/deltaMFI of 6.07 to the ovIL-17A CHO cells respectively) relative to the isotype-matched mab control (displayed in Figure 4B and metrics shown Additional file 3). The respective values for MT504 were 61.7%+ve/deltaMFI 1.27 and 96.0%+ve/deltaMFI 6.72 (displayed in Figure 4C and metrics shown in Additional file 3). Note the absence of non-specific staining with these mabs on the untransfected control (UTF) CHO cells (displayed in Figures 4B and C). Mab 41809 has a negligible proportion of cells in the positive region whereas mab 41802 gave a high degree of non-specific staining using the UTF CHO cells (deltaMFI of 2.45 and 94.1% of cells in the positive region) compared to the combined isotype controls (Figure 4D). Both mabs have high percentage positivity for bovIL-17A and ovIL-17A based on the region boundary (displayed in Figure 4D and metrics shown Additional file 3), but the very low deltaMFIs (41809: 0.14 (rbov) and 1.12 (rov) and 41802: 0.11 (rbov) and 0.2 (rov) respectively) indicating poor specificity with bovIL-17A and ovIL-17A.

The six metrics used to assess antibody binding to rbov and rovIL-17A (numerical percentage in positive upper region and deltaMFIs for the three CHO cell lines) were represented along with the antibodies in a PCA biplot providing an additional objective way to rank them displayed in Additional file 7. Data for the unconjugated pab were excluded as it was the only non-mab and appeared to be distorting the overall representation of the other antibodies when included in the PCA analyses. The biplot planar representation based on the two first PCs (on the horizontal, PC1, and vertical axes, PC2, respectively) explained 87.37% of the variability of the original data set. The distances between the antibodies (represented by symbol points) spatially reflect their similarity in regards to the original six metrics (represented by axes, with arrows indicating directions of higher values). The mabs eBio64DEC17 and MT504 associate together linking to the highest values of the rbovIL-17A and rovIL-17A deltaMFI variables. The mabs MT44.6, MT241 and MT2270 overlap linking to the lowest values in the rbovIL-17A and rovIL-17A MFI variables. Mab 41809 has a negligible proportion of cells in the positive region whereas Mab 41802 gave a high degree of non-specific staining using the UTF CHO cells (deltaMFI of 2.45 and 94.1% of cells in the positive region) compared to the combined isotype controls (Figure 4D). The angles between axes are representative of the types of correlation between the corresponding metrics. Hence, the small angles observed between the axes for bovIL-17A %, CHO UTF deltaMFI, CHO UTF % and ovIL-17A % on the one hand, and those for ovIL-17A deltaMFI and bovIL-17A deltaMFI on the other hand, are indicative of high correlations within each of these two sets of metrics. The angle of approximately 90° between these two sets of metrics reflects negligible correlation between them. Together our dataset suggests that bovIL-17A and ovIL-17A deltaMFI metrics provide a more reliable measure of specific IL-17A binding than %# bovIL-17A and %# ovIL-17A respectively.

Of all of the antibodies listed in Table 1, only the MT504 mab clone is available in a form that is compatible with use in tissue culture and not stored in a buffer containing sodium azide. As this mab gave positive staining on the transfected CHO cells by flow cytometry, we assessed its potential to neutralise the bioactivity of rbovIL-17A and rovIL-17A. 1 µg/mL of mab MT504 was mixed with 50 ng/mL of rbovIL-17A and rovIL-17A for 2 h at 37 °C then tested for induction of CXCL8 expression in ovine ST-6 cells as described previously in "Bulk recombinant cytokine production and functional determination of recombinant bovine and ovine IL-17A section" and shown in Figure 2C. The pre-mixing of the mab with recombinant IL-17A resulted in 65.3 and 62.8% decreases in CXCL8 release for rbovIL-17A and rovIL-17A respectively indicating the ability of mab MT504 to neutralise the biological activity of ruminant IL-17A (Additional file 8).

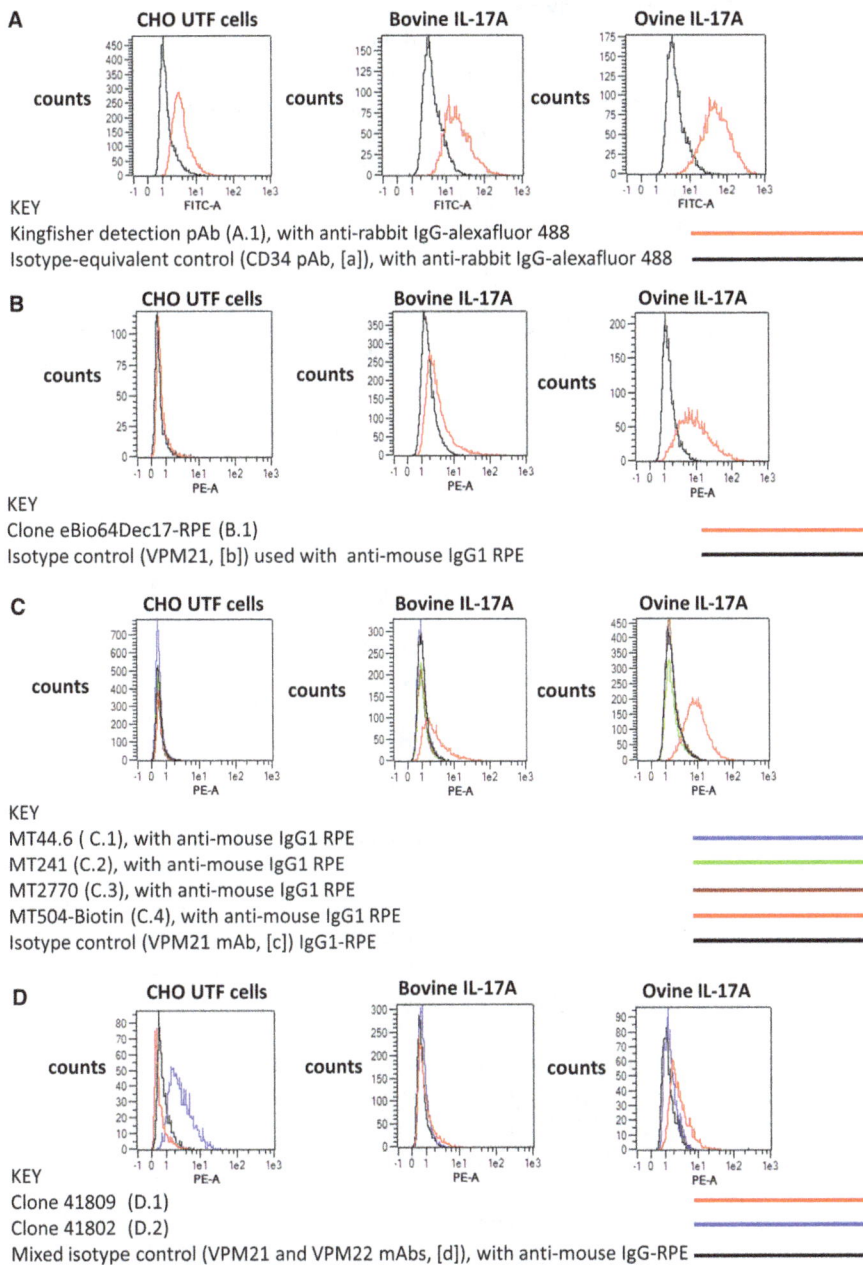

Figure 4 Evaluation of commercial antibodies for the intracellular detection of recombinant bovine and ovine IL-17A. The eight commercial antibodies listed in Table 1 were tested against fixed, permeabilised untransfected (UTF) CHO cells and CHO cells transfected with cDNA encoding bovIL-17A or ovIL-17A for their capacity to detect intracellular recombinant IL-17A by flow cytometry. Results are shown for one polyclonal antibody (pab) produced against bovIL-17A (**A**) and seven monoclonal antibodies (mabs) produced against human or mouse IL-17A (**B–D**). Profiles of the relevant control antibodies listed in Table 2 are included in the overlapping histograms. Events were acquired on the Macs-Quant according to the gating strategy described previously (in brief) and shown in Additional file 2. Line colours representing different antibody treatments are given in parentheses: **A** Primary rabbit anti-bovine IL-17A pab PB0274B-100 at 1 μg/mL (A.1, red) or negative control primary anti-bovine CD34 pab (in-house) at an estimated 1 μg/mL equivalent (a, black) then detected with a secondary goat anti-rabbit alexafluor 488 at 1 μg/mL; **B** Directly conjugated mouse anti-human IL-17A eBio64DEC17-phycoerythrin (PE) mab (IgG1) at 2.5 μg/mL (B.1, red) and control IgG1 VPM21 mab (in-house) at an estimated 2.5 μg/mL equivalent (b, black) and detected with goat anti-mouse PE at 1 μg/mL; **C** Primary mouse anti-IL-17A mabs MT44.6 (C.1, blue), MT241 (C.2, green), MT2770 (C.3, brown) and MT504 (C.4, red) [all IgG1] at 0.5 μg/mL and control IgG1 VPM21 mab (in-house) at an estimated 0.5 μg/mL equivalent (black), all detected with goat anti-mouse PE at 1 μg/mL; **D** Primary mouse anti-human IL-17A mabs #41809 (D.1, red) (IgG2b) and #41802 (D.2, blue) (IgG1) at 2.5 μg/mL and a mixture of control mabs VPM21 (IgG1) and VPM22 (IgG2b) at an estimated 2.5 μg/mL equivalent (d, black), all detected with goat anti-mouse PE at 1 μg/mL.

Expression of intracellular IL-17A and IFN-γ by bovine and ovine T cell subsets

PBMC from cattle and sheep were activated with PMA/ionomycin and the expression of intracellular cytokines by different T cells subsets was measured by double staining. Representative plots of the double staining of activated PBMC (one of four biological replicates) showed that CD4+ve, CD8β+ve (dim) and WC-1+ve cells from cattle whereas CD4+ve and WC-1+ve cells from sheep are capable of expressing intracellular IL-17A (Figures 5 and 6). Compared to the activated bovine PBMC, there are insufficient events to confirm the presence of CD8+ve(dim) cells expressing IL-17A in activated ovine PBMC. The proportions of cells expressing IL-17A are lower than those expressing IFN-γ in both cattle (Figure 5) and sheep (Figure 6), with the exception of the WC-1+ve cells in cattle which were proportionally greater for IL-17A. The bovine PBMC occupying the WC-1+ve IFN-γ+ve region in Figure 5F are mostly artefactual and non-specific (rectangular population crossing the region boundary for WC-1+ve region). However, under these stimulatory conditions, cattle PBMC proportionately expressed more IL-17A compared to sheep PBMC (Figure 7A; $p = 0.020$) whereas for IFN-γ the converse was true (Figure 7B; $p = 0.021$).

Discussion

Since the discovery of two types of murine T cell clones with distinct cytokine expression [36], our knowledge of the cytokine profiles and function of the extended family of Th subsets has greatly expanded. In the process of gaining a deeper understanding of how the different CD4+ve Th subsets are induced to protect against different infections, it has become clear that they are no longer considered to be mutually-exclusive or irreversibly committed, but demonstrate a degree of plasticity and cross-regulation (reviewed by Zhu et al. [3]). Single-cell technologies are providing further insights into T cell biology and regulation of immune responses [37] which underpins novel strategic approaches to disease control and vaccine design.

Of the CD4+ve Th subsets described in mice, there appears to be a particular plasticity between Th-17 and Th-1 cells. In a model of diabetes purified Th-17 cells adoptively transferred into recipient mice have been shown to convert to Th-1-type cells secreting IFN-γ [38]. This close relationship of Th-1-type and Th-17-type responses and the cytokines that contribute to their differentiation, namely IL-12 and IL-23, that share the common p40 subunit, underlines the importance of being able to identify T cell cytokine profiles in target species. While the capability to study IFN-γ-related responses in farmed ruminants is advanced, there are relatively few reports describing the cellular expression and function of the IL-17 cytokine family.

Bougarn et al. [12] described the cloning of bovine IL-17A and IL-17F and the expression of biologically-active recombinant proteins in insect cells that could induce expression of a range of cytokines and chemokines (including CXCL8) in primary bovine mammary epithelial cells. We have taken the approach of comparing cattle and sheep by cloning and stably expressing bovine and ovine IL-17A in CHO cells. The rbovIL-17A and rovIL-17A were shown to be functionally active as they stimulated CXCL8 expression in fibroblasts and epithelial cells. The sequence identity of the mature bovine IL-17A protein with the ovine orthologue IL-17A is 100% which is reflected by their reciprocal species cross-reactivity (Figures 2B and C).

There have been several publications reporting the expression of mRNA encoding bovine IL-17A (and other IL-17 family members) as measured by RT-PCR [9, 39, 40]. There have also been publications reporting the quantification of IL-17A protein in cattle using the anti-bovIL-17A ELISA Vetset marketed by Kingfisher Biotech [10, 11, 39, 41, 42]. A principal objective of our study was to use the transfected CHO cells and their expressed recombinant proteins as defined standards to identify cross-reactive antibodies and to further refine methods to detect bovIL-17A and ovIL-17A. We have demonstrated for the first time the ability of the Kingfisher bovIL-17A Vetset to detect and quantify native ovIL-17A in the culture supernatants of mitogen-activated sheep PBMC (Figure 2D). The bovIL-17A Vetset ELISA antibodies have been used in an ELISpot to identify IL-17A-secreting CD4+ve and gamma-delta (γδ)T cells in cattle [43]. We have added to that capability by using these antibodies in an ELISpot to quantify the frequency of both bovIL-17A- and ovIL-17A-secreting cells in populations of activated PBMC (Figure 3). Our results show that PMA/ionomycin is a more potent stimulator of IL-17A in PBMC than ConA which is consistent with observations in human PBMC [44]. ConA induced a higher mean frequency of IL-17A-secreting cells from sheep PBMC than cattle, the reasons for which are unclear (Figure 3) but may include variability associated with age, breed and environment.

As described above, the ability to identify and quantify cytokine expression at the single-cell level by flow cytometry is invaluable for characterising cellular immune responses and informs on vaccine delivery strategies. The transfected CHO cells revealed that the bovIL-17A Vetset antibodies that were utilised successfully in ELISA and ELISpot were not optimal for intracellular IL-17A flow cytometric staining due to non-specific binding to untransfected cells (Figure 4A). We therefore focussed

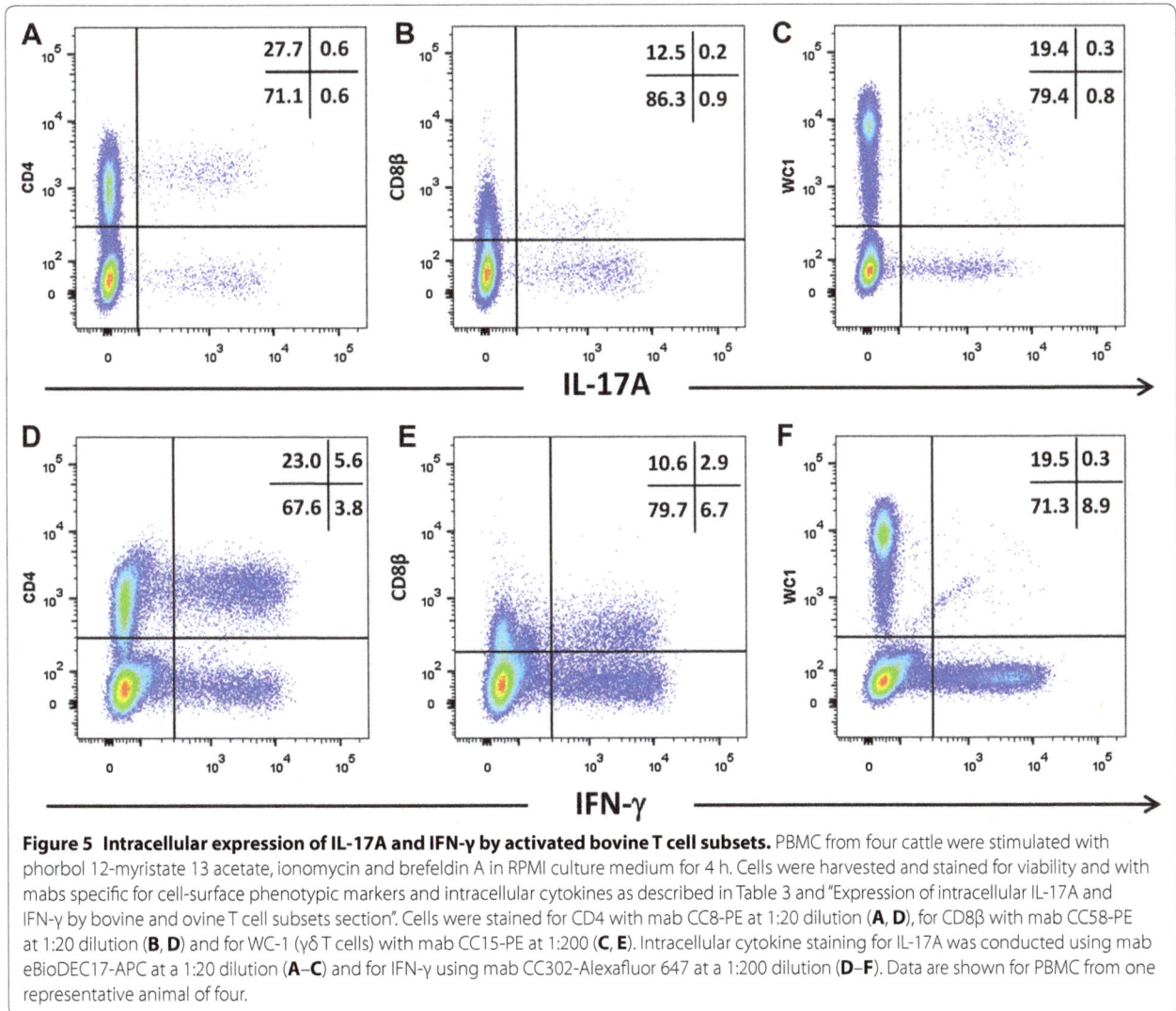

Figure 5 Intracellular expression of IL-17A and IFN-γ by activated bovine T cell subsets. PBMC from four cattle were stimulated with phorbol 12-myristate 13 acetate, ionomycin and brefeldin A in RPMI culture medium for 4 h. Cells were harvested and stained for viability and with mabs specific for cell-surface phenotypic markers and intracellular cytokines as described in Table 3 and "Expression of intracellular IL-17A and IFN-γ by bovine and ovine T cell subsets section". Cells were stained for CD4 with mab CC8-PE at 1:20 dilution (**A**, **D**), for CD8β with mab CC58-PE at 1:20 dilution (**B**, **D**) and for WC-1 (γδ T cells) with mab CC15-PE at 1:200 (**C**, **E**). Intracellular cytokine staining for IL-17A was conducted using mab eBioDEC17-APC at a 1:20 dilution (**A–C**) and for IFN-γ using mab CC302-Alexafluor 647 at a 1:200 dilution (**D–F**). Data are shown for PBMC from one representative animal of four.

on screening a panel of seven anti-human or anti-mouse IL-17A mabs for ability to detect cattle and sheep IL-17A intracellularly. One of these mabs (eBio64DEC17) has been reported to detect intracellular IL-17A in sheep lymphocytes [45] and cattle, sheep and goat PBMC [46]. In these previous studies the cross-reactivity is implied as there was no validation against a specific control where IL-17A was known to be expressed. We have shown in a number of studies that stably transfected CHO cells constitutively express high levels of recombinant cytokines [30] and the transcription factor FoxP3 [31]. We have previously shown that brefeldin A increases intracellular accumulation of cytokine in the transfectants but does alter not the percentage positivity of the cells [47]. The intracellular cytokine staining of activated lymphocytes tends to be lower than the transfectants. Consequently, amplifying the signal even further in the CHO cells would

not help select antibodies for native staining or give a better indication of their working dilutions for activated lymphocytes. In the present study, we found that eBio-64DEC17 and another anti-human IL-17A mab (MT504) gave high deltaMFI values for bovIL-17A and ovIL-17A (Figures 4B and C), findings that were objectively confirmed using the PCA biplot analysis (Additional file 7). We demonstrate that deltaMFIs and to a lesser extent percentage of cells (in relation to appropriate control antibodies) can be used to objectively rank antibodies for their capacity to bind. MT504 clone is available in a tissue culture compatible format and was capable of neutralising rbovIL-17A and rovIL-17A function in vitro (Additional file 8). This mab adds to the panel of antibodies available to neutralise ruminant cytokine function which includes mabs 3C2 for ovine GMCSF [24], CC320 for bovine IL-10 [48] and CC326 for bovine IL-12 [49].

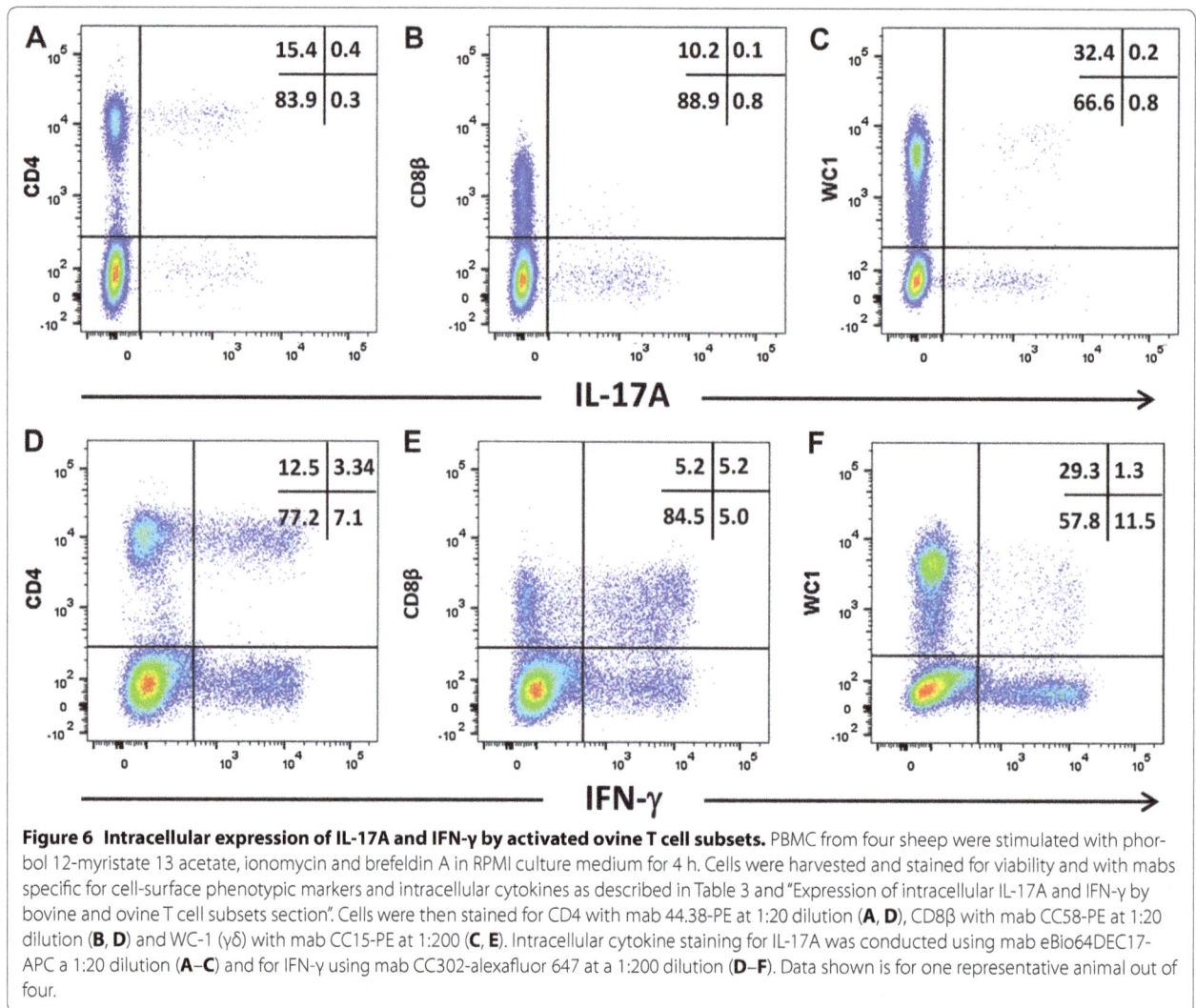

Figure 6 Intracellular expression of IL-17A and IFN-γ by activated ovine T cell subsets. PBMC from four sheep were stimulated with phorbol 12-myristate 13 acetate, ionomycin and brefeldin A in RPMI culture medium for 4 h. Cells were harvested and stained for viability and with mabs specific for cell-surface phenotypic markers and intracellular cytokines as described in Table 3 and "Expression of intracellular IL-17A and IFN-γ by bovine and ovine T cell subsets section". Cells were then stained for CD4 with mab 44.38-PE at 1:20 dilution (**A, D**), CD8β with mab CC58-PE at 1:20 dilution (**B, D**) and WC-1 (γδ) with mab CC15-PE at 1:200 (**C, E**). Intracellular cytokine staining for IL-17A was conducted using mab eBio64DEC17-APC a 1:20 dilution (**A–C**) and for IFN-γ using mab CC302-alexafluor 647 at a 1:200 dilution (**D–F**). Data shown is for one representative animal out of four.

We compared intracellular staining for IL-17A using mab eBio64DEC17 with intracellular staining for IFN-γ in combination with cell-surface phenotyping to compare cytokine expression in activated cattle and sheep PBMC. Since the cytokines and the receptors involved in the production of IL-17A and IFN-γ share common components, it is important to know if distinctive T cell subsets expressing these cytokines exist in ruminants as they appear to in other mammalian species. We found that the major T cell subsets (CD4+ve and WC-1+ve) can express IL-17A (Figures 5 and 6), consistent with reports in humans [50] and mice [51, 52]. We found CD8+ve IL-17A for cattle PBMC but had insufficient cells to confirm their presence in PMA/ionomycin-stimulated ovine PBMC. Further evidence ideally in an antigen-driven setting is required to determine the existence of this cell population in sheep. There was a higher mean proportion of activated cattle PBMC expressing IL-17A than sheep

PBMC, the converse being true for IFN-γ (Figure 7). The reason for this difference is unclear. The expression of bovine and ovine IL-17A by CD4+ve and WC-1+ve/γδT cell subsets is consistent with other studies using a combination of flow cytometry and ELISpot [43, 45]. Only 0.2% of total WC-1+ve/γδT cells from activated ovine PBMC expressed IL-17A in our study, whereas around 6% of total WC-1+ve/γδT cells were constitutively IL-17A+ve from skin-draining lymph. This difference is possibly reflective of the altered capacity for surveillance and mobilisation at the skin to cutaneous infection [45]. Our data show that activated bovine CD8+ve(dim) T cells also have the capacity to produce intracellular IL-17A, the first report of this phenomenon in ruminants, but consistent with reports of human CD8+ve T cells (reviewed by Srenathan et al. [51]).

IL-17A has an important role particularly at mucosal barriers such as the skin, lung and intestinal tract where

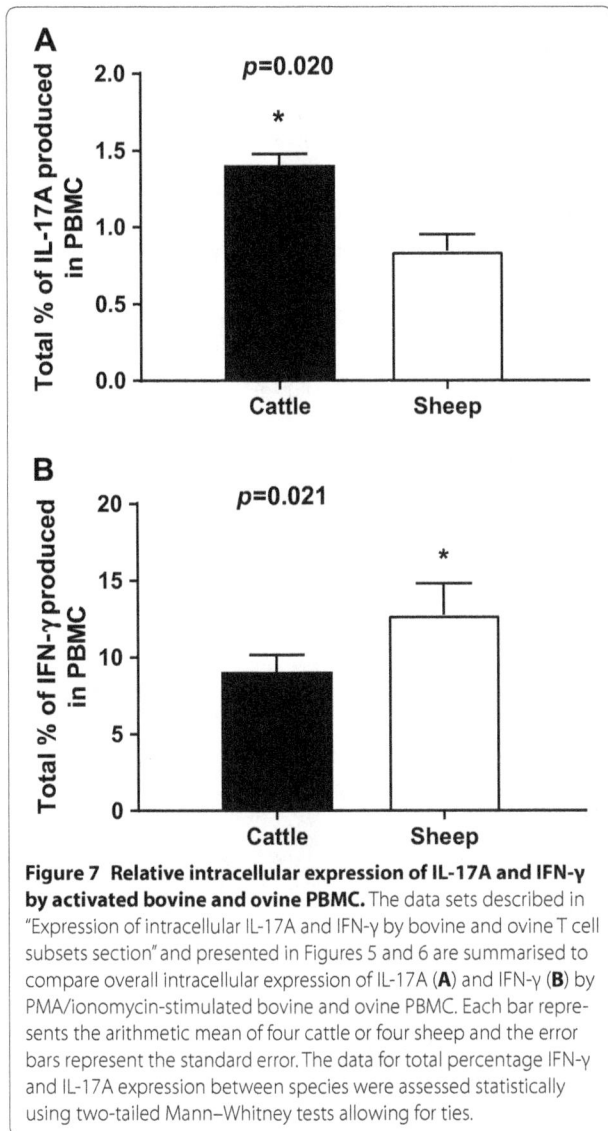

Figure 7 Relative intracellular expression of IL-17A and IFN-γ by activated bovine and ovine PBMC. The data sets described in "Expression of intracellular IL-17A and IFN-γ by bovine and ovine T cell subsets section" and presented in Figures 5 and 6 are summarised to compare overall intracellular expression of IL-17A (**A**) and IFN-γ (**B**) by PMA/ionomycin-stimulated bovine and ovine PBMC. Each bar represents the arithmetic mean of four cattle or four sheep and the error bars represent the standard error. The data for total percentage IFN-γ and IL-17A expression between species were assessed statistically using two-tailed Mann–Whitney tests allowing for ties.

its production can be crucial to the control or exacerbation of inflammation in humans or mice [53]. The new tools and assays developed in this study will enable greater investigation of mucosal compartments in ruminants to improve understanding of host response to infection in situ. The capability to measure both IL-17A and IFN-γ by intracellular staining will help determine if the Th-cell plasticity observed in Th-17 cells converting to a Th-1 IFN-γ-secreting phenotype in mice [38] can occur in ruminant species.

The validation and quality assurance of antibodies is currently a topic of great interest with several opinion articles discussing their impact on scientific advancement including inability to reproduce published data, the duplication of effort for testing reagents in specific assays

and time lost due to use of unreliable reagents [54–56]. This is especially important in veterinary immunology as investment in immunological reagent development is relatively low [57].

In this study we have developed the capacity to measure native ovine IL-17A in liquid phase by ELISA and identify positive secreting cells by ELISpot using existing pabs from the commercial bovine ELISA. We have used molecular cloning techniques to generate stable mammalian CHO cells expressing recombinant IL-17A (constitutive positive and UTF negative controls) for screening a panel of commercial anti-IL-17A antibodies. Using PCA on six parameters we have represented the species cross-reactivity data identifying two suitable mabs for intracellular staining for sheep and cattle cells. We are able to identify CD4, CD8β and WC-1+ γδ T cells from activated bovine and ovine PBMC and block IL-17A activity. We took the approach of screening existing antibodies for detection of bovine and ovine IL-17A rather than embark on the production of new pabs or mabs against our recombinant proteins. This approach has the ethical advantage of avoiding immunisation schedules and therefore animal usage. There is always the possibility that higher affinity antibodies could be made against the homologous cytokine for each species by immunisation, but in balance we have shown that mabs produced against human cytokines can cross-react with ruminant cytokines. Confidence in the specific labelling is provided with the use of sufficiently robust controls. In summary, the tools we describe here for IL-17A will improve our ability to characterise inflammatory immune responses in ruminants and our understanding of host-pathogen interactions to inform on rational vaccine development.

Additional files

Additional file 1. Bovine, ovine and caprine IL-17 family sequences in publically accessible databases. A list of the known IL-17 family orthologue sequences is shown where all sequences are full unless otherwise stated. The source of the sequence is stated either from mRNA/cDNA or predicted from genome annotation and the National Center for Biotechnology Information (NCBI, accessed 04/03/2017) accession numbers are as stated below: Cow (*Bos taurus*): IL-17-A EU682381.1; IL-17B NM_001192045.1; IL-17C XM_010826654.2; IL-17D transcript variant X1 XM_015465706.1; IL-17E/IL-25 XM_015464998.1 and IL-17F NM_001192082.1. Sheep (*Ovis aries*): IL-17A XM_004018887.3; IL-17B transcript variant X1 XM_012178770.2; IL-17C transcript variant X1 XM_012189660.2; IL-17D no accession record; IL-17E/IL-25 NM_001195219.1 and IL-17F XM_004018888.3. Goat (*Capra hircus*): IL-17A GU269912.1; IL-17B XM_005683151.3; IL-17C XM_005683151.3; IL-17D transcript variant X1 XM_018056543.1; IL-17E/IL-25 XM_018054603.1 and IL-17F XM_005696412.2.

Additional file 2. Gating strategy used for the evaluation of commercial antibodies to bind intracellular recombinant bovine and ovine IL-17A in fixed cells. Cells were acquired for flow cytometric analyses using the MacsQuant flow cytometer and analysed using the MacsQuantify Software. 20 000–50 000 events were collected and the following gating strategy was followed. Cells in the plot of Forward Scatter-Area (FSC-A) against the high dynamic range over time (HDR-T) are gated in P1 to exclude any non-specific artefacts (**A**). The P1/P2 gate represents Side Scatter-Area (SSC-A) plotted against FSC-A set to identify the main cell population and exclude debris (**B**). Single cells were gated (P1/P2/P3) using FSC-Height (H) vs FSC-A for doublet discrimination (**C**). Finally, the cells of interest were identified in the phycoerythrin or alexafluor 488 channel vs SSC-A (P1/P2/P3/P4) where regions were set using the isotype or equivalent control for each CHO cell line to establish threshold gates (**D**). Overlaying histogram plots of phycoerythrin or alexafluor 488 using (P1/P2/P3) gating strategy selecting for all cells in the region (equivalent to cells above and below region boundary in plot **D**) (**E**) were used to compare anti-IL-17A antibodies with appropriate isotype or equivalent controls presented in Figure 4. Gated percentage numbers above the region boundary (P1/P2/P3/P4) and median fluorescence region values (P1/P2/P3) were measured for each antibody in the relevant fluorochrome channel phycoerythrin or alexafluor 488. Delta median fluorescence intensity (deltaMFI) was calculated by deducting the median fluorescence region value for mab isotype control or pab control from the anti-IL-17A antibody value for the appropriate fluorochrome channel. The summarised data are presented in Additional file 3.

Additional file 3. Summary of commercial IL-17A antibody evaluation for capacity to bind intracellular recombinant bovine and ovine IL-17A in fixed Chinese Hamster Ovary cells. Control antibodies are listed in lower case, the anti-IL-17A antibodies are listed in upper case. Using the gating strategy described in brief in evaluation of commercial antibodies subsection (displayed in Additional file 2) the following data are shown: P1/P2/P3/P4 percentage of cells above the region boundary line of phycoerythrin or alexafluor 488 channels vs Side Scatter-Area (denoted #%); P1/P2/P3 median fluorescence region value (phycoerythrin or alexafluor 488 channels); and delta median fluorescence intensity (deltaMFI) calculated by taking the median fluorescence region values (phycoerythrin or alexafluor 488 channels) for the commercial IL-17A antibody and deducting the median fluorescence region value of the appropriate isotype or equivalent control antibody in the same fluorochrome channel) for the CHO UTF, bovIL-17A and ovIL-17A transfected, fixed CHO cells.

Additional file 4. Gating strategy for the identification of activated bovine T cell subsets expressing intracellular IL-17A and IFN-γ. Activated bovine PBMC were stained for viability, cell surface markers and intracellular cytokines according to the protocol outlined in "Expression of intracellular IL-17A and IFN-γ by bovine and ovine T cell subsets section" using antibodies listed in Table 3 and acquired using an LSRFortessa™ cell analyzer (Becton–Dickinson). Cells were gated to eliminate dead cells using the Vioblue Live/Dead® Fixable Dead Cell Stain Kit, Side Scatter Height (SSC-H) vs Vioblue channel (A) and to include only single cells Forward Scatter Height (FSC-H) vs FSC-Area (FSC-A) (B). Gated single cells used for subsequent two-colour cell phenotyping and intracellular cytokine staining (C). Quadrant region boundaries were set based on isotype-matched directly conjugated antibody controls (FITC vs APC/ Alexafluor 647 channels, D) and (Phycoerythrin vs APC/Alexafluor 647 channels, E) and fluorescence minus one (FMO) controls for each cell marker (WC-1, F; CD4, G; CD8β, H) and for each cytokine IL-17A, I-J and IFN-γ, K-L). Data are shown for one representative animal of four.

Additional file 5. Gating strategy for the identification of activated ovine T cell subsets expressing intracellular IL-17A and IFN-γ. Activated ovine PBMC were stained for viability, cell surface markers and intracellular cytokines according to the protocol outlined in "Expression of intracellular IL-17A and IFN-γ by bovine and ovine T cell subsets section" using antibodies listed in Table 3 and acquired using an LSRFortessa™ cell analyzer (Becton Dickenson). Cells were gated to eliminate dead cells using the Vioblue Live/Dead Stain® Fixable Dead Cell Stain Kit, Side Scatter Height (SSC-H) vs Vioblue channel (A) and to include only single cells Forward Scatter Height (FSC-H) vs FSC-Area (FSC-A) (B). Gated single cells used for subsequent two-colour cell phenotyping and intracellular cytokine staining (C). Quadrant region boundaries were set based on isotype-matched directly conjugated antibody controls (FITC vs APC/ Alexafluor 647 channels, D) and (Phycoerythrin vs APC/Alexafluor 647

channels, E) and fluorescence minus one (FMO) controls for each cell marker (WC-1, F; CD4, G; CD8β, H) and for each cytokine IL-17A, I-J and IFN-γ, K-L). Data are shown for one representative animal of four.

Additional file 6. IL-17A sequence pair-wise identity matrix. BovIL-17-A and ovIL-17A cDNAs encoding the mature proteins were aligned with the corresponding sequences from a variety of vertebrates including representative mammal, reptile and avian species and the protein pair-wise identity matrix was derived using Clustal 2.1.

Additional file 7. Principal components analysis biplot of binding of commercial antibodies to transfected Chinese Hamster Ovary cells stably-expressing recombinant bovine or ovine IL-17A. A principal component analysis (PCA) was conducted to investigate the structure of relationships between commercial monoclonal antibody clones to IL-17A and the six metrics used to assess antibody staining. These metrics were the binding to transfected CHO cells stably expressing rbovIL-17A, rovIL-17A or the untransfected CHO negative control (UTF) cells [numerical percentage of (%) cells] in the upper positive region (% CHO UTF, % bovIL-17A and % ovIL-17A) and delta median fluorescence intensity (deltaMFI) values for the same three CHO cell lines. Data used in the PCA is taken from Additional File 6. PCA reduced the dimension of the data set by means of optimal linear combinations (principal components, PCs) of the six metrics aimed to retain as much of the original data variability as possible. The results were displayed using a correlation biplot based on the two first PCs (those accounting for the highest percentage of the total variability) to facilitate discussion and ranking of the commercial antibodies.

Additional file 8. Neutralisation of recombinant bovine and ovine IL-17A activity on ovine cells by commercial mab. Ovine ST-6 cells were set up as described in "Bulk recombinant cytokine production and functional determination of recombinant bovine and ovine IL-17A section" but using 96 well flat bottom plates. The following treatments were pre-incubated at 37 °C for 2 h in a water bath: IMDM culture medium only (unstimulated cells), rovIL-17A (50 ng/mL), rovIL-17A (50 ng/mL) + MT504 monoclonal antibody (mab, 1 μg/mL), rbovIL-17A (50 ng/mL) and rbovIL-17A (50 ng/mL) + MT504 mab (1 μg/mL). The treatments were then added to the ovine cells for 24 h and harvested and assayed as previously described. The X-axis displays the neutralisation bioassay treatments and the Y-axis shows levels of CXCL8 in pg/mL. Data are the arithmetic mean of three technical replicate samples from one representative experiment of two. The percentage neutralisation values displayed on the graph have been calculated by firstly deducting the unstimulated (IMDM culture medium control) value from all other treatment values. The value for rbovIL-17A neutralisation with MT504 mab was calculated by: 100 minus [(rbovIL-17A/MT504 mab minus background value) divided by (rbovIL-17A minus background value) multiplied by 100]. Percentage neutralisation for rovIL-17A was calculated by substituting rbovIL-17A for rovIL-17A values into equation above.

Competing interests

Bio-Rad Laboratories distributes and markets ruminant immunological reagents produced by The Moredun Research Institute and by The Roslin Institute at the University of Edinburgh. Both organizations receive royalties from Bio-Rad Laboratories from the sale of these ruminant immunological reagents.

Authors' contributions

SW, YC-M, EG, JH, CM and GE conceived the study and participated in its design. YC-M and YP undertook the cloning and expression work. SW and YP undertook the screening of the IL-17A antibodies. SW performed the IL-17A bioassay and neutralisation experiments. DF, TMN and SW designed and performed the ELISpot assays, SW and YC-M performed the combined intracellular staining and cell surface phenotyping. JP-A devised and conducted the statistical analyses. All authors contributed to the writing and reviewing of the manuscript. All authors read and approved the final manuscript.

Acknowledgements

This work was conducted jointly at the Moredun Research Institute and The Roslin Institute at the University of Edinburgh as part of the Biotechnology and Biological Sciences Research Council (BBSRC) Industrial Partnership Award "The route to identification of immunological correlates of protection in ruminants" Industrial Partnership Award with Bio-Rad Laboratories (grant numbers BB/I019863/1; BB/I020519/1). SW, DF, TMN, CMI, GE and JPA were also funded by the Scottish Government Rural and Environment Science and Analytical Services (RESAS). JH and EJG were also supported by the BBSRC Institute Strategic Programme Grant ISP3 "Innate Immunity & Endemic Disease" [BB/J004227/1]. The authors acknowledge that this scientific manuscript has been prepared following the principles laid out in the Animal Research: Reporting of In Vivo Experiments (ARRIVE) guidelines [58].

Author details
[1] Moredun Research Institute, International Research Centre, Pentlands Science Park, Bush Loan, Penicuik, Scotland EH26 0PZ, UK. [2] The Roslin Institute and Royal (Dick) School of Veterinary Studies, The University of Edinburgh, Easter Bush, Midlothian, Scotland EH25 9RG, UK. [3] Biomathematics and Statistics Scotland, JCMB, The King's Buildings, Peter Guthrie Tait Road, Edinburgh, Scotland EH9 3FD, UK.

References

1. Rouvier E, Luciani MF, Mattei MG, Denizot F, Golstein P (1993) CTLA-8, cloned from an activated T cell, bearing AU-rich messenger RNA instability sequences, and homologous to a herpesvirus saimiri gene. J Immunol 150:5445–5456
2. Gu C, Wu L, Li X (2013) IL-17 family: cytokines, receptors and signaling. Cytokine 64:477–485
3. Zhu J, Yamane H, Paul WE (2010) Differentiation of effector CD4 T cell populations (*). Annu Rev Immunol 28:445–489
4. van den Berg WB, McInnes IB (2013) Th17 cells and IL-17A -focus on immunopathogenesis and immunotherapeutics. Semin Arthritis Rheum 43:158–170
5. Mensikova M, Stepanova H, Faldyna M (2013) Interleukin-17 in veterinary animal species and its role in various diseases: a review. Cytokine 64:11–17
6. Riollet C, Mutuel D, Duonor-Cerutti M, Rainard P (2006) Determination and characterization of bovine interleukin-17 cDNA. J Interferon Cytokine Res 26:141–149
7. Blanco FC, Bianco MV, Meikle V, Garbaccio S, Vagnoni L, Forrellad M, Klepp LI, Cataldi AA, Bigi F (2011) Increased IL-17 expression is associated with pathology in a bovine model of tuberculosis. Tuberculosis 91:57–63
8. Burke ML, Veer M, Pleasance J, Neeland M, Elhay M, Harrison P, Meeusen E (2014) Innate immune pathways in afferent lymph following vaccination with poly(I:C)-containing liposomes. Innate Immun 20:501–510
9. Roussel P, Cunha P, Porcherie A, Petzl W, Gilbert FB, Riollet C, Zerbe H, Rainard P, Germon P (2015) Investigating the contribution of IL-17A and IL-17F to the host response during Escherichia coli mastitis. Vet Res 46:56
10. Flynn RJ, Marshall ES (2011) Parasite limiting macrophages promote IL-17 secretion in naive bovine CD4(+) T-cells during Neospora caninum infection. Vet Immunol Immunopathol 144:423–429
11. Tassi R, McNeilly TN, Fitzpatrick JL, Fontaine MC, Reddick D, Ramage C, Lutton M, Schukken YH, Zadoks RN (2013) Strain-specific pathogenicity of putative host-adapted and nonadapted strains of Streptococcus uberis in dairy cattle. J Dairy Sci 96:5129–5145
12. Bougarn S, Cunha P, Gilbert FB, Harmache A, Foucras G, Rainard P (2011) Staphylococcal-associated molecular patterns enhance expression of immune defense genes induced by IL-17 in mammary epithelial cells. Cytokine 56:749–759
13. Gossner A, Peers A, Venturina V, Hopkins J (2011) Expressed gene sequences of two variants of sheep interleukin-25. Vet Immunol Immunopathol 139:319–323
14. Wattegedera S, Sills K, Howard CJ, Hope JC, McInnes CJ, Entrican G (2004) Variability in cytokine production and cell proliferation by mitogen-activated ovine peripheral blood mononuclear cells: modulation by interleukin (IL)-10 and IL-12. Vet Immunol Immunopathol 102:67–76
15. Wattegedera SR, Watson DM, Hope JC, Kaiser P, Sales J, McInnes CJ, Entrican G (2010) Relative quantitative kinetics of interferon-gamma and interleukin-10 mRNA and protein production by activated ovine peripheral blood mononuclear cells. Vet Immunol Immunopathol 136:34–42
16. Basic Local Alignment Search Tool (BLAST 2.5.1). https://blast.ncbi.nlm.nih.gov/Blast.cgi?PROGRAM=blastn&PAGE_TYPE=BlastSearch&LINK_LOC=blasthome. Accessed 21 Dec 2016
17. Altschul SF, Gish W, Miller W, Myers EW, Lipman DJ (1990) Basic local alignment search tool. J Mol Biol 215:403–410
18. Petersen TN, Brunak S, von Heijne G, Nielsen H (2011) SignalP 4.0: discriminating signal peptides from transmembrane regions. Nat Methods 8:785–786
19. Signal 4.1 Server. http://www.cbs.dtu.dk/services/SignalP/. Accessed 21 Dec 2016
20. Sievers F, Higgins DG (2014) Clustal omega. Curr Protoc Bioinform 48:3.13.1–3.13.16
21. Clustal Omega. http://www.ebi.ac.uk/Tools/msa/clustalo/. Accessed 21 Dec 2016
22. Milne I, Lindner D, Bayer M, Husmeier D, McGuire G, Marshall DF, Wright F (2009) TOPALi v2: a rich graphical interface for evolutionary analyses of multiple alignments on HPC clusters and multi-core desktops. Bioinformatics 25:126–127
23. Bebbington CR (1995) Use of vectors based on gene amplification for the expression of cloned genes in mammalian cells, 2nd edn. In: DNA cloning 4, mammalian systems. Oxford University Press, Oxford, pp 85–112
24. Entrican G, Deane D, MacLean M, Inglis L, Thomson J, McInnes C, Haig DM (1996) Development of a sandwich ELISA for ovine granulocyte/macrophage colony-stimulating factor. Vet Immunol Immunopathol 50:105–115
25. Entrican G, McInnes CJ, Rothel JS, Haig DM (1992) Kinetics of ovine interferon-gamma production: detection of mRNA and characterisation of biological activity. Vet Immunol Immunopathol 33:171–178
26. Norval M, Head KW, Else RW, Hart H, Neill WA (1981) Growth in culture of adenocarcinoma cells from the small intestine of sheep. Br J Exp Pathol 62:270–282
27. Rothel JS, Corner LA, Lightowlers MW, Seow HF, McWaters P, Entrican G, Wood PR (1998) Antibody and cytokine responses in efferent lymph following vaccination with different adjuvants. Vet Immunol Immunopathol 63:167–183
28. Caswell JL, Middleton DM, Sorden SD, Gordon JR (1998) Expression of the neutrophil chemoattractant interleukin-8 in the lesions of bovine pneumonic pasteurellosis. Vet Pathol 35:124–131
29. Doull L, Wattegedera SR, Longbottom D, Mwangi D, Nath M, Glass EJ, Entrican G (2015) Late production of CXCL8 in ruminant oro-nasal turbinate cells in response to Chlamydia abortus infection. Vet Immunol Immunopathol 168:97–102
30. Kwong LS, Thom M, Sopp P, Rocchi M, Wattegedera S, Entrican G, Hope JC (2010) Production and characterization of two monoclonal antibodies to bovine tumour necrosis factor alpha (TNF-α) and their cross-reactivity with ovine TNF-alpha. Vet Immunol Immunopathol 135:320–324
31. Rocchi MS, Wattegedera SR, Frew D, Entrican G, Huntley JF, McNeilly TN (2011) Identification of CD4+ CD25 high Foxp3+ T cells in ovine peripheral blood. Vet Immunol Immunopathol 144:172–177
32. Benjamini Y, Hochberg Y (1995) Controlling the false discovery rate: a practical and powerful approach to multiple testing. J R Stat Soc Series B Stat Methodol 57:289–300
33. Ringnér M (2008) What is principal component analysis? Nat Biotechnol 26:303–304
34. Meng C, Zeleznik OA, Thallinger GG, Kuster B, Gholami AM, Culhane AC (2016) Dimension reduction techniques for the integrative analysis of multi-omics data. Brief Bioinform 17:628–641
35. Hemmink JD, Morgan SB, Aramouni M, Everett H, Salguero FJ, Canini L, Porter E, Chase-Topping M, Beck K, Loughlin RM, Carr BV, Brown IH, Bailey M, Woolhouse M, Brookes SM, Charleston B, Tchilian E (2016) Distinct immune responses and virus shedding in pigs following aerosol, intra-nasal and contact infection with pandemic swine influenza A virus, A(H1N1)09. Vet Res 47:103
36. Mosmann TR, Cherwinski H, Bond MW, Giedlin MA, Coffman RL (1986) Two types of murine helper T cell clone. I. Definition according to profiles of lymphokine activities and secreted proteins. J Immunol 136:2348–2357
37. Proserpio V, Mahata B (2016) Single-cell technologies to study the immune system. Immunology 147:133–140
38. Bending D, De la Pena H, Veldhoen M, Phillips JM, Uyttenhove C, Stockinger B, Cooke A (2009) Highly purified Th17 cells from BDC2.5NOD mice convert into Th1-like cells in NOD/SCID recipient mice. J Clin Investig 119:565–572

39. Rainard P, Cunha P, Ledresseur M, Staub C, Touze JL, Kempf F, Gilbert FB, Foucras G (2015) Antigen-specific mammary inflammation depends on the production of IL-17A and IFN-γ by bovine CD4+ T lymphocytes. PLoS One 10:e0137755

40. Waters WR, Maggioli MF, Palmer MV, Thacker TC, McGill JL, Vordermeier HM, Berney-Meyer L, Jacobs WR Jr, Larsen MH (2015) Interleukin-17A as a biomarker for bovine tuberculosis. Clin Vaccine Immunol 23:168–180

41. Peckham RK, Brill R, Foster DS, Bowen AL, Leigh JA, Coffey TJ, Flynn RJ (2014) Two distinct populations of bovine IL-17(+) T-cells can be induced and WC1(+)IL-17(+)gammadelta T-cells are effective killers of protozoan parasites. Sci Rep 4:5431

42. Baquero MM, Plattner BL (2016) Bovine WC1(+) gammadelta T lymphocytes modify monocyte-derived macrophage responses during early *Mycobacterium avium* subspecies paratuberculosis infection. Vet Immunol Immunopathol 170:65–72

43. McGill JL, Sacco RE, Baldwin CL, Telfer JC, Palmer MV, Waters WR (2014) Specific recognition of mycobacterial protein and peptide antigens by gammadelta T cell subsets following infection with virulent *Mycobacterium bovis*. J Immunol 192:2756–2769

44. Lenarczyk A, Helsloot J, Farmer K, Peters L, Sturgess A, Kirkham B (2000) Antigen-induced IL-17 response in the peripheral blood mononuclear cells (PBMC) of healthy controls. Clin Exp Immunol 122:41–48

45. Geherin SA, Lee MH, Wilson RP, Debes GF (2013) Ovine skin-recirculating gammadelta T cells express IFN-gamma and IL-17 and exit tissue independently of CCR7. Vet Immunol Immunopathol 155:87–97

46. Dorneles EM, Araujo MS, Teixeira-Carvalho A, Martins-Filho OA, Lage AP (2015) Cross-reactivity of anti-human cytokine monoclonal antibodies used as a tool to identify novel immunological biomarkers in domestic ruminants. Genet Mol Res 14:940–951

47. Entrican G (2002) New technologies for studying immune regulation in ruminants. Vet Immunol Immunopathol 87:485–490

48. Kwong LS, Hope JC, Thom ML, Sopp P, Duggan S, Bembridge GP, Howard CJ (2002) Development of an ELISA for bovine IL-10. Vet Immunol Immunopathol 85:213–223

49. Hope JC, Kwong LS, Entrican G, Wattegedera S, Vordermeier HM, Sopp P, Howard CJ (2002) Development of detection methods for ruminant interleukin (IL)-12. J Immunol Methods 266:117–126

50. Tsai H-C, Wu R (2013) Cholera toxin directly enhances IL-17A production from human CD4(+) T cells. J Immunol 191:4095–4192

51. Srenathan U, Steel K, Taams LS (2016) IL-17+ CD8+ T cells: differentiation, phenotype and role in inflammatory disease. Immunol Lett 178:20–26

52. Ono T, Okamoto K, Nakashima T, Nitta T, Hori S, Iwakura Y, Takayanagi H (2016) IL-17-producing gammadelta T cells enhance bone regeneration. Nat Commun 7:10928

53. Song X, He X, Li X, Qian Y (2016) The roles and functional mechanisms of interleukin-17 family cytokines in mucosal immunity. Cell Mol Immunol 13:418–431

54. Bradbury A, Pluckthun A (2015) Reproducibility: standardize antibodies used in research. Nature 518:27–29

55. Polakiewicz RD (2015) Antibodies: the solution is validation. Nature 518:483

56. Freedman LP (2015) Antibodies: validate recombinants too. Nature 518:483

57. Entrican G, Lunney JK, Rutten VP, Baldwin CL (2009) A current perspective on availability of tools, resources and networks for veterinary immunology. Vet Immunol Immunopathol 128:24–29

58. Kilkenny C, Browne WJ, Cuthill IC, Emerson M, Altman DG (2010) Improving bioscience research reporting: the ARRIVE guidelines for reporting animal research. PLoS Biol 8:e1000412

3

Permissiveness of bovine epithelial cells from lung, intestine, placenta and udder for infection with *Coxiella burnetii*

Katharina Sobotta[1], Katharina Bonkowski[1], Elisabeth Liebler-Tenorio[1], Pierre Germon[2], Pascal Rainard[2], Nina Hambruch[3], Christiane Pfarrer[3], Ilse D. Jacobsen[4] and Christian Menge[1*]

Abstract

Ruminants are the main source of human infections with the obligate intracellular bacterium *Coxiella* (*C.*) *burnetii*. Infected animals shed high numbers of *C. burnetii* by milk, feces, and birth products. In goats, shedding by the latter route coincides with *C. burnetii* replication in epithelial (trophoblast) cells of the placenta, which led us to hypothesize that epithelial cells are generally implicated in replication and shedding of *C. burnetii*. We therefore aimed at analyzing the interactions of *C. burnetii* with epithelial cells of the bovine host (1) at the entry site (lung epithelium) which govern host immune responses and (2) in epithelial cells of gut, udder and placenta decisive for the quantity of pathogen excretion. Epithelial cell lines [PS (udder), FKD-R 971 (small intestine), BCEC (maternal placenta), F3 (fetal placenta), BEL-26 (lung)] were inoculated with *C. burnetii* strains Nine Mile I (NMI) and NMII at different cultivation conditions. The cell lines exhibited different permissiveness for *C. burnetii*. While maintaining cell viability, udder cells allowed the highest replication rates with formation of large cell-filling Coxiella containing vacuoles. Intestinal cells showed an enhanced susceptibility to invasion but supported *C. burnetii* replication only at intermediate levels. Lung and placental cells also internalized the bacteria but in strikingly smaller numbers. In any of the epithelial cells, both Coxiella strains failed to trigger a substantial IL-1β, IL-6 and TNF-α response. Epithelial cells, with mammary epithelial cells in particular, may therefore serve as a niche for *C. burnetii* replication in vivo without alerting the host's immune response.

Introduction

Coxiella (*C.*) *burnetii* is a Gram-negative, obligate intracellular pathogen and causative agent of Q fever, a widely distributed zooanthroponosis [1]. The disease appears as an acute, flu-like and self-limiting illness, or manifests as a chronically progressing infection (e.g., endocarditis, premature delivery in pregnant women). *C. burnetii* has a broad host spectrum, which includes birds, reptiles, arthropods and domestic and wild mammals. Sources of human infections often are infected sheep, goats or cattle [2]. In livestock, *C. burnetii* infection is inapparent in most cases [1]. If disease manifests, referred to as

Coxiellosis, reproductive disorders such as abortions, stillbirth in goats and sheep or delivery of weak newborns in cattle were observed [3]. The main route of *C. burnetii* transmission is via inhalation of infected aerosols or dust, especially when contaminated with *C. burnetii* birth products (placental membranes and fluids) of goat and sheep, but also by feces and milk [4, 5]. An unprecedented large Q-fever outbreak occurred from 2007 to 2011 in the Netherlands, where more than 4000 human cases were notified and approximately 52 000 ruminants were culled as part of the countermeasures taken to control the epidemic [6].

Main shedding of *C. burnetii* with about 10^9 bacteria per gram placenta is observed during parturition in sheep and goat [1]. Coxiella organisms are primarily detected in trophoblast cells in the placentomes [2, 7, 8]. Shedding of bacteria by milk of asymptomatic cattle was observed

*Correspondence: christian.menge@fli.de
[1] Institute of Molecular Pathogenesis, Friedrich-Loeffler-Institut (FLI), Naumburger Strasse 96a, 07743 Jena, Germany
Full list of author information is available at the end of the article

to persist for several months [9]. Dairy cows seem to be more chronically infected with *C. burnetii* than small ruminants. Guatteo et al. [10] could also show that Coxiella shedding was scarce and sporadic in feces of cattle, whereas permanent and sporadic shedding was observed by milk. PCR analysis of bovine bulk tank milk samples detected more than 10^2 *C. burnetii* DNA equivalents per milliliter [11]. Muskens et al. [12] believe that the localization of the pathogen in the bovine udder is the critical factor for a secretion of bacteria into the milk but it is currently unknown which cell types facilitate persistence and replication of *C. burnetii* in the mammary gland.

The chain of events implicated in *C. burnetii* transmission between animals of the reservoir species have poorly been studied at the cellular level. Mononuclear phagocytes, e.g., macrophages and monocytes, are considered the major host cells during natural infection [1]. We recently showed that Coxiella organisms invade primary bovine monocyte-derived and alveolar macrophages in vitro and slowly replicate in these cells without significantly activating them [13]. Even though alveolar macrophages probably represent the first target cell for *C. burnetii* when entering the body, it is highly likely that alveolar epithelial cells also become exposed to and infected by these bacteria in the early stages of the infection as described in rodent models [14, 15]. At the site of entry, the lung epithelium therefore may determine the character of the subsequent immune response in concert with alveolar macrophages. It is also perceivable that epithelial cells at the exit sites are determinative for persistence in and bacterial transmission of *C. burnetii* from the reservoir host [1, 4].

In general, *C. burnetii* is able to grow in a number of cell types, like Vero cells or fibroblast cells [1]. All these cell types poorly mirror the natural cell environment to investigate infection processes in domestic animals. Therefore the present study aimed at developing an in vitro cell system deploying bovine epithelial cell lines from lung, placenta, gut and udder tissues. We studied the permissiveness and host cell response of different epithelial cells with two Coxiella strains: a virulent strain (Nine Mile I), expressing full-length lipopolysaccharide ("smooth LPS"), and an avirulent strain (NM phase II). NMII lacks the full O-polysaccharide I chain and sugars located in the LPS I outer core (called "rough LPS") [16].

Materials and methods
Epithelial cell culture

Source, origin and characteristics of bovine epithelial cells used in this study are provided in Table 1. The epithelial origin of all cell lines deployed was confirmed by detection of cytokeratin and zonula occludens protein (ZO-2) via fluorescence microscopy and western blot analysis (data not shown). Cell culture media were obtained from Life Technologies (Darmstadt, Germany). The basis culture medium of the bovine udder epithelial cells (PS) was supplemented with Insulin-like growth factor 1 (10 ng/mL; Peprotech, Hamburg, Germany), Fibroblast growth factor (5 ng/mL Peprotech), Epidermal growth factor (5 ng/mL; Sigma, Taufkirchen, Germany), Hydrocortisone (1 µg/mL; Sigma), 20 mM HEPES buffer (Fisher Scientific, Schwerte, Germany) and 2 mM L-Glutamine (Life Technologies) [17]. Maintenance media were supplemented with 10% fetal bovine serum [FBS, Fisher Scientific; heat-inactivated (56 °C for 30 min)]. Test media used in experiments for invasion analysis, cell vitality test and cytokine analysis contained 1% FBS. Epithelial cells were grown and maintained in an atmosphere of 5% CO_2 at 37 °C. Detachment of the cells was done with Trypsin/EDTA solution [NaCl 0.8% (w/v), KCl

Table 1 Cell lines used in this study

Code	Clone	Origin		Culture medium	Source	Reference
		Organ	Donor			
L	BEL-26	Lung	Fetal	Dulbecco's Modified Eagle Medium (DMEM, 1.0 g/mL glucose)	CCLV[a]	(−)
G	FKD-R 971	Jejunum	Fetal	Iscove's Modified Dulbecco's Medium (IMDM)/Ham's F12 nutrient mix [1:1]	CCLV[a]	(−)
Pm	BCEC	Maternal placenta	Mature/pregnant	DMEM (4.5 g/mL glucose)/Ham's F12 nutrient mix [1:1]	TiHo[b]	[35]
Pf	F3	Fetal placenta	Mature/pregnant	DMEM (4.5 g/mL glucose)/Ham's F12 nutrient mix [1:1]	TiHo[b]	[36]
U	PS	Udder	Mature	Advanced DMEM/Ham's F12 nutrient mix [1:1] + additional components[d]	INRA[c]	[17]

[a] Collection of Cell Lines in Veterinary Medicine (CCLV) at Friedrich-Loeffler-Institut (Isle of Riems), Germany; cell line FKD-R 971 was generated by Roland Riebe (RIE 971).

[b] Christiane Pfarrer, Department of Anatomy, University of Veterinary Medicine, Hannover, Germany.

[c] Pascal Rainard, ISP, INRA, Université Tours, Nouzilly, France.

[d] See "Materials and methods".

0.08% (v/v), Dextrose 0.1% (w/v), Na_2HCO_3 0.058% (w/v), Trypsin 0.05% (w/v), EDTA 0.02% (w/v)] for 5 min at 5% CO_2 at 37 °C. Cells were seeded into 96-, 24- or 6-well plates with 1×10^4, $4–10 \times 10^4$ and $2–3 \times 10^5$ cells, respectively, and cultured for 2–3 days to reach a confluent cell monolayer.

Coxiella (C.) burnetii infection and sampling

Cells were infected with *C. burnetii* strain "Nine Mile phase I RSA 493" (NMI) and "Nine Mile phase II clone 4" (NMII) (phase I-LPS and phase II-LPS expressing variants, respectively) in multi-well cell culture plates at 37 °C and 5% CO_2. Both *C. burnetii* strains were supplied, propagated and purified as previously described [13].

Once cells had formed a monolayer, cell numbers from a reference well were determined by detaching with Trypsin/EDTA solution and subsequent microscopic cell counting with a Neubauer chamber. Cells were infected with a multiplicity of infection (MOI) of 100 or mock infected with NaCl solution. *C. burnetii* inocula were left in the cultures for 7 days (infection strategy A; Figure 1). Alternatively, non-internalized bacteria were removed 24 h after inoculation by washing two to three times with pre-warmed (37 °C) 1× PBS and fresh culture test medium (1% FBS) was added (infection strategy B). During each set of experiments, supernatants (extracellular fraction) and cells (cell-associated fraction) were sampled directly after inoculation at time point "0 h" ("regained inoculum"; experimental settings A_1, B_1), after 24 h ("1 day"; experimental settings A_2, B_2) or after 7 days ("7 days"; (experimental settings A_3 and B_3) from separate wells. To this end, wells were washed two to three times with warm 1× PBS and cells were detached by incubation with Trypsin/EDTA solution. To inactivate *C. burnetii*, samples were treated with three freeze (−80 °C)/thaw cycles and subsequently incubated for 30 min at 95 °C. For detection of host cell immune response, cells were inoculated following infection strategy B_2 or B_3, or stimulated with LPS of *E. coli* O111:B4 (5 μg/mL) as a control. Cells were harvested for RNA isolation 1 and 7 days post-infection (pi). Total RNA was extracted with RNeasy Mini Kit (Qiagen, Hilden, Germany) according to the instructions of the manufacturer. To avoid DNA contamination RNA was purified with the RNase-free DNase set (Qiagen). For immunofluorescence microscopy studies, infected cells were inoculated following strategy B_3.

Immunofluorescence microscopy

Cells were cultured in 24-well plates (Corning® Costar®, Sigma) until at least 80% confluence was reached and infected with NMI and NMII with a MOI of 100 as described above. Cell vitality was monitored by MTT and LDH assay (according to manufacturer's instructions). After 7 days of infection (see above), cells were fixed

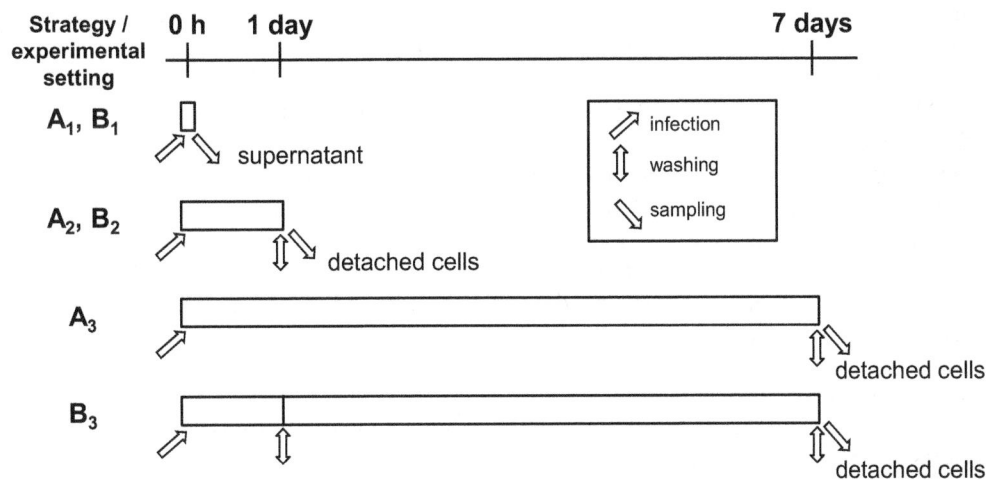

Figure 1 Study design. Invasion and replication of *C. burnetii* in bovine epithelial cell lines were quantified applying two different infection strategies differing in the time the inocula were left with the cells. Strategy B included a washing step after 1 day; in strategy A, inocula were not removed for the duration of the experiment. "Invasion B" refers to the quantitation of cell-associated *C. burnetii* genome equivalents (GE) 24 h after inoculation (values obtained in experimental setting B_2), "invasion A" to the quantitation of cell-associated GE after 7 days (values obtained in experimental setting A_3), each normalized to the GE numbers detected in the supernatant regained immediately after inoculation (time point "0 h"; values obtained in experimental settings A_1 and B_1). Thus the invasion was calculated as follows: (A) x = (A_3 × 100%)/A_1 and (B) x = (B_2 × 100%)/B_1. Replication efficiency was calculated as the fold-increase in the number of cell-associated GE from day 1 (values obtained in experimental setting A_2 and B_2) to values at day 7 (obtained in experimental setting A_3 and B_3). Thus the replication efficiency was calculated as follows: (A) = A_3/A_2 and (B) = B_3/B_2. Arrow depict sampling event, i.e. taking off the supernatant, washing the cell monolayer and detachment of the cells.

with 4% formaldehyde for 24 h and stored at 4 °C. Cells were washed with $1\times$ PBS and permeabilized with 100% ice cold methanol for 1 min followed by incubation with 50 nM NH$_4$Cl for 15 min and PBS/FBS solution (1% FBS) for 30–45 min in the dark at room temperature to block unspecific binding sites. Cells were stained for 30 min at room temperature using an Anti-Coxiella antibody [1:5000 in PBS/FCS] (kindly provided by Anja Lührmann, Friedrich-Alexander-Universität Erlangen-Nürnberg, Germany) followed by incubation (30 min–1 h) with a fluorochrome-conjugated secondary antibody [1:500 in PBS/FCS] [Anti-rabbit IgG (H + L), F(ab') 2 Fragment (Alexa Fluor$^®$ 594 Conjugate), New England Biolabs, Frankfurt, Germany], counterstained with 4',6-diamidino-2-phenylindole (DAPI) for 5 min at room temperature followed by washing with $1\times$ PBS. To characterize the replication compartment of *C. burnetii*, infected cells were labeled with the acidic marker LysoTracker Red DND-99 (Invitrogen, Darmstadt, Germany). After infection, cells were incubated with LysoTracker (1:5000 in test media) for 2 h at 37 °C following fixation as described above. The cells were mounted in DABCO (1,4-diazabicyclo[2.2.2]-octane, 2% in Glycerol). Samples were viewed under a fluorescence microscope [Olympus CK40; camera: Leica DFC420C, software: Leica Application Suite (LAS) Version 3.7.0 (Build: 681)]. Cultures incubated in PBS without primary antibodies served as negative controls.

Transmission electron microscopy (TEM)

Cells were cultured in 6-well plates (Corning$^®$ Costar$^®$, Sigma) and infected with infection strategy B$_3$ as described above. The culture supernatant was removed and cells were fixed with 2.5% glutaraldehyde in cacodylate buffer (0.1 M, pH 7.2) for 2 h at 4 °C, detached with a cell scraper from the culture plate, collected in a reaction tube and centrifuged to obtain a cell pellet [18]. The cell pellet was embedded in 2% agarose and sectioned to 1 mm^3 cubes. Cubes were post fixed in 2% osmium tetroxide and embedded in araldite Cy212. Ultrathin sections (85 nm) were stained with uranyl acetate and lead citrate. They were examined at an accelerating voltage of 80 kV by transmission electron microscopy (Tecnai12, FEI, Eindhoven, Netherlands).

Quantitative real-time PCR for determination of intracellular *C. burnetii* genome equivalents (GE)

To estimate the number of cell associated bacteria, DNA from the cell containing fraction of the cultures of infection strategy A and B was purified with the Invisorb$^®$ DNA Cleanup-Kit (Stratec, Birkenfeld, Germany) according to manufacturer's instructions. The number of genome equivalents (GE) was monitored by quantitation of the isocitrate dehydrogenase (*icd*) gene by quantitative

real-time PCR (qPCR) [19]. The *icd* gene is highly conserved within the species *C. burnetii* and occurs as single copy in the Coxiella genome. Ct values of technical duplicates varied by less than 0.51 and were used to calculate GE considering values obtained with an entrained *icd* harbouring plasmid standard. Invasion rate and replication efficiency were calculated from four biological replicates (independent cell cultures, tested in two technical replicates each) as described in the legend to Figure 1.

Flow cytometry analysis

Cells (4×10^5 cells/well, 24 well plates) were detached by Trypsin/EDTA solution and transferred to microtiter plates (V-shape; Greiner Bio-One GmbH, Frickenhausen, Germany) and pelletized by centrifugation ($400 \times g$, 4 min and 4 °C). For detection of CR3 [CD11b, MM12A, diluted 1:250 (VMRD, Pullman, WA, USA)] and $\alpha_V\beta_3$ [CD61, diluted 1:100 (AbD Serotec, Düsseldorf, Germany)], cells were incubated with 50 µL diluted primary antibody for 20 min. After washing (washing buffer: $1\times$ PBS, 0.5% FCS), cells were incubated with secondary antibody antimouse IgG1-APC (Southern Biotech, Birmingham, USA) diluted 1:1000 in $1\times$ PBS for 20 min. Finally cells were washed again and analyzed with BD FACSCanto$^{™}$II (Becton–Dickinson, Heidelberg, Germany). Data was analyzed with BD FACSDIVA$^{™}$ software (version 6).

Reverse transcription and cytokine-specific real time PCR

Equal amounts of RNA from each sample were reversely transcribed into cDNA as described previously [13]. Levels of relative gene expression of different cytokines in comparison to GAPDH as housekeeping gene were determined by quantitative real-time SYBR Green-based (Applied Biosystems, Waltham, USA) PCR (qPCR) using ABI Prism$^®$7500 (Applied Biosystems). All primers (Table 2) were run at an annealing temperature of 60 °C. The reaction profile applied was: denaturation (10 min, 95 °C), annealing (1 min, 60 °C; 39 cycles) and melting step (15, 60 °C). Ct values for GAPDH-specific mRNA were not subject to variation along the incubation period and values from infected cells did not differ from non-infected control cells (data not shown). Relative gene

Table 2 Sequences of primers used in this study

Primer	Sequence 5'–3'
GAPDH	F: GCG ATA CTC ACT CTT CTA CCT TCG A R: TCG TAC CAG GAA ATG AGC TTG AC
IL-1β	F: ACC TGA ACC CAT CAA CGA AAT G R: TAG GGT CAT CAG CCT CAA ATA ACA
IL-6	F: CTG AAG CAA AAG ATC GCA GAT CTA R: CTC GTT TGA AGA CTG CAT CTT CTC
TNF-α	F: TCT TCT CAA GCC TCA AGT AAC AAG T R: CCA TGA GGG CAT TGG CAT AC

expression levels were calculated by using relative expression software REST [20].

Statistical analysis
Unless otherwise indicated, Mann–Whitney U test was used to compare two different samples. A p value of ≤ 0.05 ("a" or "*") show a statistically significant difference at the 95% confidence level, a p value of ≤ 0.01 ("b" or "**") at the 99% confidence level.

Results
Bovine udder epithelial cells exhibited highest permissiveness for *C. burnetii* propagation
Bovine epithelial cells from different tissues varied in their susceptibility to *C. burnetii* invasion and support of replication (Figure 2). In the experimental setting in which the inocula were left with the cells for 7 days (strategy A), higher numbers of genome equivalents (GE) of *C. burnetii* NMI and NMII were found cell-associated relative to the number in the regained inoculum (upper left graphs in Figures 2A and B; "invasion A") only in the udder (U) epithelial cell line. The intestinal epithelial cell line (G) allowed moderate invasion of both NM strains. Regardless of the strain, very few bacteria were detected inside lung (L) and placental cells with fetal placental cells (Pf) containing more bacteria than maternal placental cells (Pm) which exhibited the lowest permissiveness for *C. burnetii* propagation throughout. Invasion rates in epithelial cell lines were not significantly different for NMI and NMII.

NMI and NMII, both showed a very low invasiveness within the first 24 h after inoculation (lower left graphs in Figures 2A and B; "invasion B") under the experimental conditions applied. The udder epithelial cell line was only slightly more susceptible to incorporate *C. burnetii* than the lung and placental cell lines but differences did not reach statistical significance. Interestingly, although numbers markedly varied between biological replicates, intestinal epithelial cells exhibited the highest susceptibility for *C. burnetii* invasion within the first 24 h after inoculation.

Increases in *C. burnetii*-specific GE numbers during 7 days of culture following strategy A (upper right graphs in Figures 2A and B), reflect efficacy of *C. burnetii* replication but may also be influenced by invasion events having occurred later than 24 h. In order to dissect these two phenomena, excess, i.e., not yet cell-bound *C. burnetii* particles were removed 24 h after inoculation ("strategy B"; lower right graphs in Figures 2A and B). GE numbers were then quantified at day 7 and calculated relative to the numbers found cell-associated after 24 h of culture. It became apparent that udder epithelial cells were most effective in supporting replication of NMI and

NMII ("replication B"): while numbers of NMI increased by approx. 16 000-fold from day 1 to day 7, numbers of NMII increased by approx. 330-fold ($p = 0.032$). Replication efficiency of NMI and NMII in intestinal epithelial cells was not significantly different from lung and maternal placental cells but fetal placental cells exhibited an intermediate support of *C. burnetii* replication.

Large Coxiella containing vacuoles (CCV) were formed in gut and udder epithelial cells without affecting viability of the cell cultures
Immunofluorescence microscopy was applied to investigate the number and distribution of Coxiella organisms within epithelial cells 7 days after inoculation of monolayers (Figure 3). In corroboration of *icd* qPCR results, single cells, uniformly distributed within the monolayers of lung and placental epithelial cells harbored *C. burnetii* and bacterial accumulations were very small. Inoculation of cultures with NMI and NMII yielded comparable results. Monolayers of gut cells showed more infected cells but Coxiella clusters within cells also were small. The highest amount of bacterial accumulations was observed in udder cells, they were more closely spaced and filled up the whole cell. As reported for other *C. burnetii*-susceptible cell types, CCVs in udder epithelial cells induced by either of the *C. burnetii* strains presented as acidic compartments (Figure 4). In addition, small acidified vesicles were observed inside the infected cells next to the CCV (data not shown). A strong fluorescent signal of the LysoTracker Red dye inside the formed vacuoles indicated that phagosomal–lysosomal fusion had occurred.

By transmission electron microscopy numerous CCV were detected in udder and very few in intestinal cells at day 7 pi (Figures 5 and 6). Findings were comparable after infection with strains NMI and NMII. CCV were filled at a variable degree with large cell variants (LCV) representing the metabolically active form and small cell variants (SCV) representing the dormant form of *C. burnetii*. LCV had diameters of up to 400 nm and finely granular cytoplasma; SCV were about 150 nm in diameter, more electron dense and often had a highly electron dense central core. LCV and SCV were surrounded by a Gram-negative cell envelope formed by an inner membrane, a delicate cell wall, a periplasmic space and an outer membrane. The presence of both SCV as well as LCV indicates that *C. burnetii* undergoes a complete life cycle in udder and intestinal cells. CCV in udder cells were large and displaced most of the cytoplasm (Figure 5). Very large CCV which were often ruptured and contained few *C. burnetii* predominated. Since the cellular cytoplasm surrounding these CCV was very thin, their rupture may be artificial due to mechanical forces during processing.

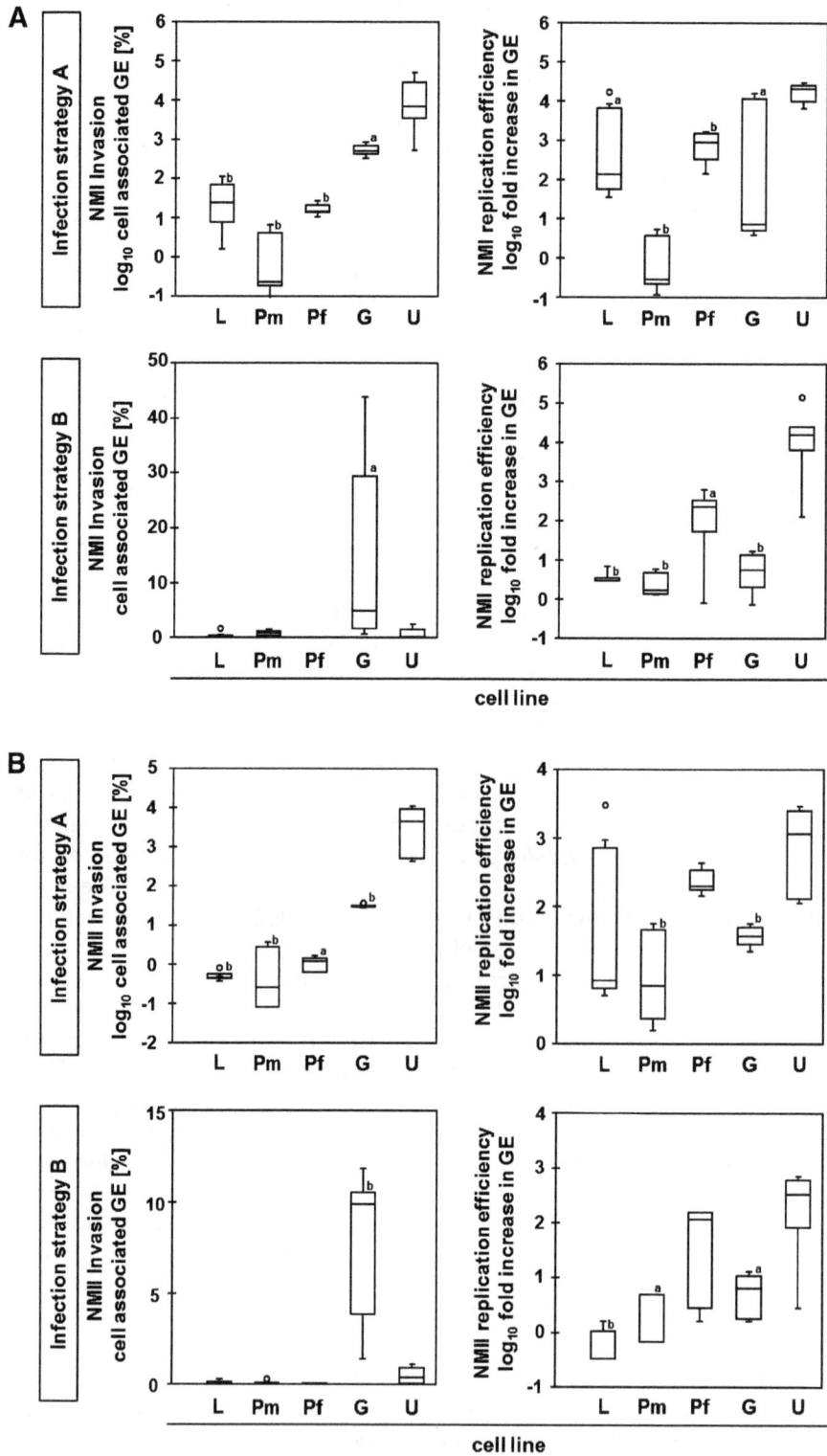

Figure 2 Invasion and replication efficiency of *C. burnetii* in different bovine epithelial cell lines. Efficiencies were determined following the study design described in Figure 1. The relative numbers of cell-associated genome equivalents of *C. burnetii* (GE) of NMI (**A**) and of NMII (**B**) were determined by *icd* qPCR. Significant differences between udder cells and other epithelial cell lines were determined by Mann–Whitney U test (a: $p \leq 0.05$; b: $p \leq 0.01$); L—Bel-26 (lung), Pm—BCEC (maternal placenta), Pf—F3 (fetal placenta), G—FKD-R 971 (jejunum), U—PS (udder).

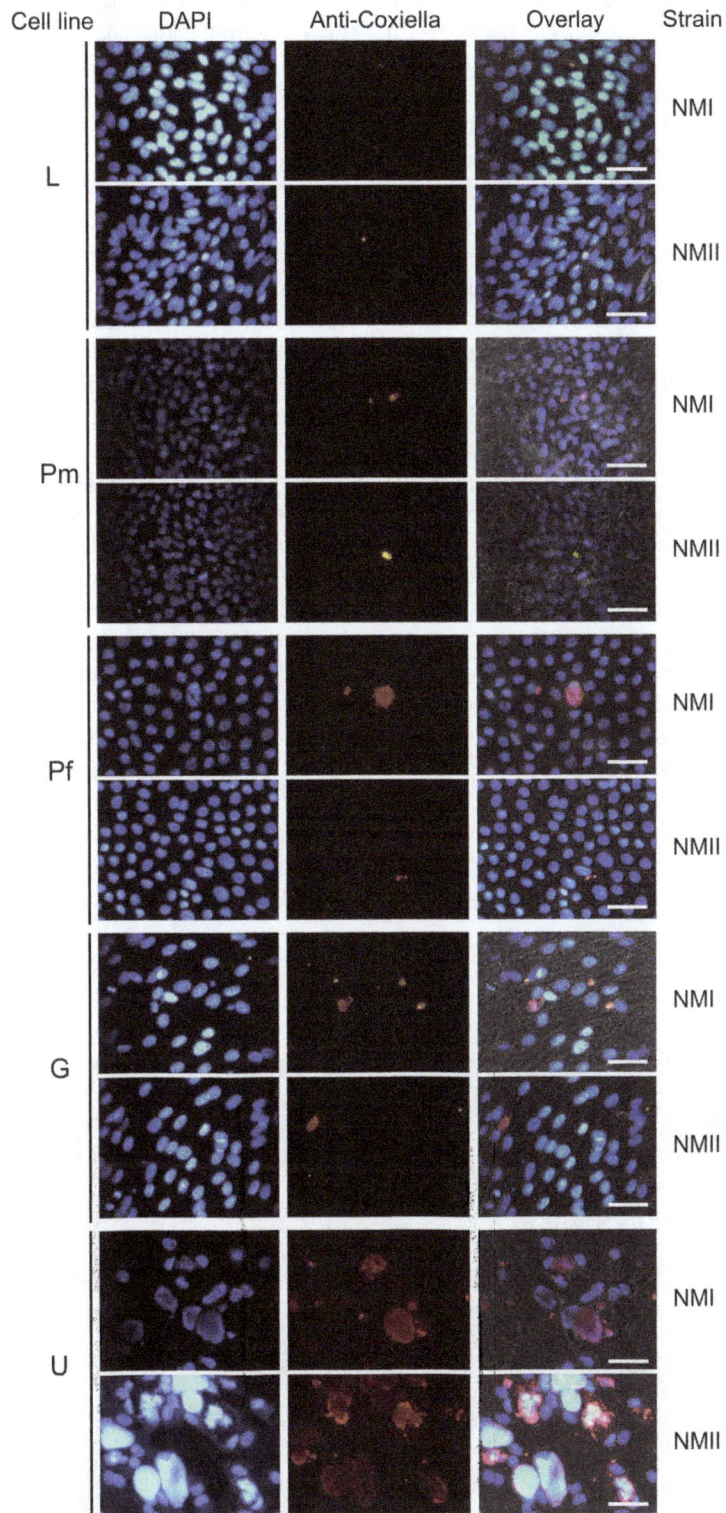

Figure 3 Infection of bovine epithelial cells with *C. burnetii*. Fluorescence microscopy images showing bovine epithelial cells infected with *C. burnetii*-strains NMI and NMII. Nuclei were stained with DAPI (blue), bacteria were detected with an Anti-Coxiella-Alexa Fluor® 594 labeled antibody combination (red). Microscopic pictures were taken 7 days after inoculation. White scale bars represent 50 µm length. Pictures are representative of three independent experiments.

LCV and SCV in the extracellular space originated from the described CCV. Some CCV were densely packed with *C. burnetii*. Most of them were mainly filled with LCV, but in a few CCV both LCV and SCV were present. Small amounts of cellular debris were regularly admixed with *C. burnetii*. Intestinal epithelial cells were characterized by numerous, sometimes large phagolysosomes. Small numbers of LCV and SCV were present in very few of these phagolysosomes only (Figure 6). They were obscured by the large amounts of cellular debris. No extracellular *C. burnetii* were detected.

Epithelial cells infected with NMI or NMII retained their typical cell morphology after 7 days of infection and displayed no signs of cell death processes, e.g., disrupted cell membrane or fragmented nuclei. These observations could be confirmed by cell vitality assays. Independent of the *C. burnetii* strain, infection neither affected metabolic activity nor cytoplasmic membrane integrity of any of the epithelial cell lines after 1 and 7 days of inoculation compared to uninfected control cells (data not shown).

CR3 and $\alpha_v\beta_3$ surface expression does not correlate with epithelial susceptibility to *C. burnetii* invasion

Uptake of NMI is mediated by leukocyte response integrin (LRI $\alpha_v\beta_3$) whereas the avirulent *C. burnetii* enters host cells through the combination of $\alpha_v\beta_3$ and CR3 (complement receptor 3) [21]. To investigate whether differences in the susceptibility of bovine epithelial cells to *C. burnetii* invasion can be explained by varying cell

surface expression pattern of these antigens, we applied flow cytometry analysis on fetal placental, intestinal and udder epithelial cells (Figure 7). All cells of the cell lines studied expressed $\alpha_v\beta_3$. While fetal placental and intestinal epithelial cells expressed the integrin in comparable densities (as deduced from the distribution of fluorescence signals for the detection of the antigens), udder epithelial cells exhibited an enhanced $\alpha_v\beta_3$ expression. Expression of CR3 was barely detectable on all cell lines. Expression pattern of these molecules therefore neither correlate with the enhanced susceptibility of intestinal epithelial cells for *C. burnetii* invasion nor with the fact that udder epithelial cells particularly supported *C. burnetii* replication rather than invasion.

C. burnetii infection failed to induce a consistent inflammatory response in bovine epithelial cells

We previously showed that *C. burnetii* induces a short-lasting but pronounced pro-inflammatory cytokine response in bovine macrophages in the early phase of infection [13]. Stimulation of udder epithelial cells with *E. coli* LPS resulted in a significant increase in mRNAs specific for IL-1β, IL-6 and TNF-α, confirming the general ability of the cell line to respond to microbe-associated molecular patterns (Figure 8). Responses peaked at day 1 or day 2 and either declined upon prolonged stimulation (IL-1β, TNF-α) or remained elevated (IL-6). By stark contrast and despite the development of prominent CCVs in the udder epithelial cell line (see above), infection with

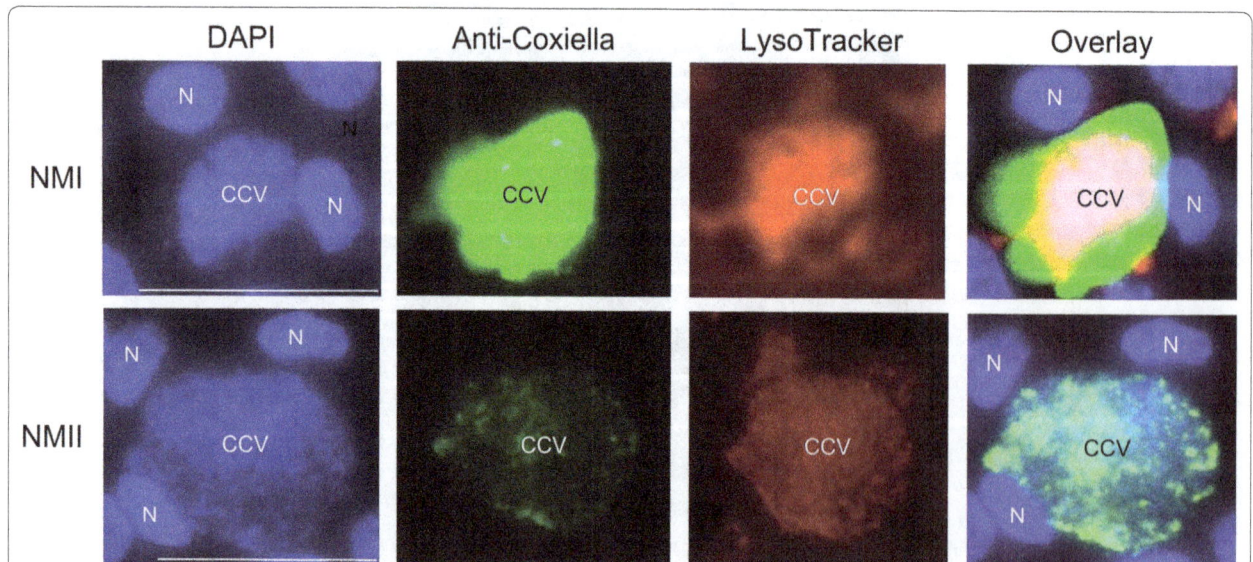

Figure 4 Accumulation of LysoTracker red into *C. burnetii* containing vacuoles. Bovine epithelial cells were infected with NMI and NMII for 7 days at 37 °C (strategy B₃). Afterwards, cells were incubated for 2 h with LysoTracker red and additionally labeled with Anti-Coxiella antibody and DAPI and viewed by fluorescence microscopy. CCV identified by detection of *C. burnetii* (green) in vacuoles presents as acidified compartment (red) of the cell. N marks the nucleus labeled with DAPI (blue). White scale bars represent 50 µm length.

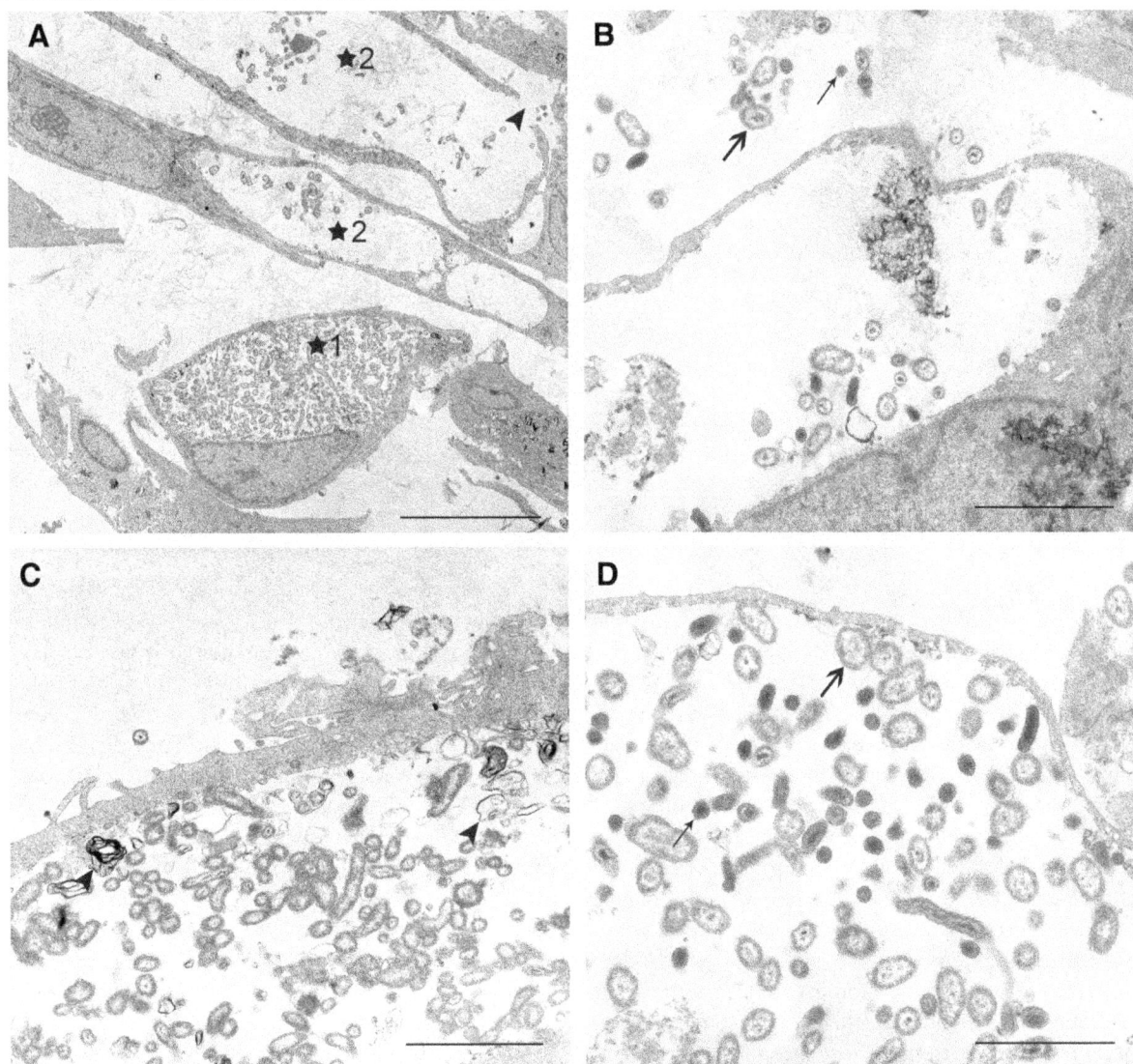

Figure 5 *C. burnetii* NMI and NMII in udder epithelial cells. A CCV in udder cells filled with numerous (*1) or few (*2) *C. burnetii*. Note ruptured CCV (arrowhead). 7 days pi NMII. Bar = 8.0 µm. **B** Extracellular LCV (thick arrow) and SCV (thin arrow) adjacent to a large CCV. 7 days pi. NMI. Bar = 2.3 µm. **C** CCV containing predominantly LCV and small amounts of cellular debris (arrowheads). 7 days pi. NMII. Bar = 2.3 µm. **D** CCV filled with both LCV (thick arrow, exampl.) and SCV (thin arrow, exampl.). 7 days pi. NMII. Bar = 1.7 µm.

neither NMI nor NMII induced an up-regulation of the transcription of the respective cytokines after 1 day and after 7 days of infection. Lung, placental and gut epithelial cells responded to stimulation with *E. coli* LPS with gradual increases of cytokine mRNA expression over a time period of 7 days (data not shown) but also poorly responded to infection with NMI and NMII at 1 day pi (Figure 9). Only gut epithelial cells specifically reacted to NMI infection with a significant upregulation of IL-1β, lung epithelial cells with a specific downregulation of IL-6 whereas infection with NMII resulted in a distinct up-regulation of TNF-α in lung epithelial cells.

Discussion

The bovine epithelial cell lines utilized in this study were selected as surrogates of certain steps in the infection path *C. burnetii* follows inside a mammalian host. The lung represents the entry site for the pathogen to establish the infection with alveolar macrophages considered to play a key role [22]. Placenta, gut and udder are known replication sites immediately prior to transmission events [2]. Here we demonstrated that *C. burnetii* invaded and replicated in bovine epithelial cells from the different organs without destroying the cell integrity or inducing a substantial immune response. Although the *C. burnetii*

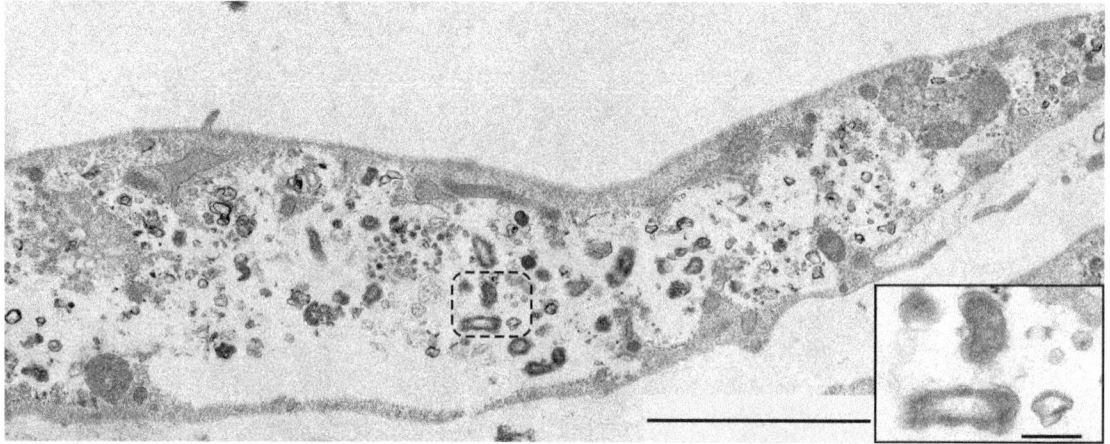

Figure 6 ***C. burnetii* NMI in intestinal epithelial cells.** A large phagolysosome replaces most of the cytoplasm. It contains large amounts of cellular debris and few *C. burnetii* (inside hatched line, example). The area indicated by the hatched line is shown as inset. It contains LCV with the characteristic gram-negative cell wall. 7 days pi. NM1. Bar = 3.0 μm, bar inset = 300 nm.

strain NMI is considered more "virulent" than NMII as deduced from cell culture and rodent experiments, the invasiveness and replication efficacy in the bovine cell lines was similar. Epithelial cells from different organs differed in the individual kinetics of two steps in the cellular infection process. Udder epithelial cells were most effective in propagating *C. burnetii* mainly because of particularly supporting replication after bacterial invasion. Intestinal epithelial cells, by contrast, particularly supported bacterial invasion. The comparably higher replication efficacy detected for the latter cells when applying experimental strategy A as compared to strategy B points to ongoing invasion events even after 24 h of incubation which had paralleled bacterial replication. The interaction pattern with *C. burnetii* of these two cell types represented the extremes displayed by the cell lines under consideration with the suitability of lung, maternal and fetal epithelial cells to act as *C. burnetii* host cells ranging in-between.

Inoculation of bovine mammary gland epithelial cell cultures yielded the highest amounts of *C. burnetii* compared to cultures of epithelial cells from lung, gut and placenta after an incubation time of up to 7 days. Previous histological investigations of tissues from infected cattle primarily detected the pathogen in mammary gland epithelial cells (reviewed in [23]). Tropism for udder tissues in bovines seems to provide the basis for the high numbers of *C. burnetii* shed by milk in this species [9, 24, 25]. It is considered that consumption of dairy products poses a low risk for Q fever infections in humans [26] even though Benson et al. [27] had found that most bulk tank milk samples contained viable Coxiella organisms

and human consumption of *C. burnetii*-containing milk leads to a rise in specific serum antibody titers in absence of clinical disease. A high bacterial load in raw milk was also described by Enright et al. [28], who observed up to 10 000 infective doses of *C. burnetii* per mL of milk from infected dairy cows. Similar bacterial load was observed by Schaal [29] after quantitative analysis of Coxiella containing milk. High numbers of *C. burnetii* in milk at least contribute to spreading of the agent within cattle herds. Newborn calves fed *C. burnetii*-containing milk excrete the bacteria in their feces and urine into the environment [3]. Therefore a dairy herd showing no symptoms of Coxiellosis could still be a *C. burnetii* reservoir for transmission via the tick-independent infection cycle [24].

Typical *C. burnetii* containing structures (CCV) were observed in udder and intestinal epithelial cells by transmission electron microscopy. Mature CCV were seen at 7 days pi in udder cells. Findings are comparable to findings in Vero cells [30, 31]. This indicates that both NMI and NMII undergo a complete replication cycle in these udder epithelial cells. The formation of large CCV requires protein secretion by *C. burnetii* [32] and depends on the actin cytoskeleton of the infected cells [33].

Small ruminants, like goats and sheep, shed *C. burnetii* more frequently via birth products [34] which contain huge numbers of bacteria and are the main source of environmental contamination and subsequent aerogenic transmission to humans. In ovine placentas, van Moll et al. [34] found Coxiella organisms in huge amounts in trophoblast cells which were embedded in acutely inflamed tissue. By contrast, bovine placentas generally contain few or moderate numbers of cells staining

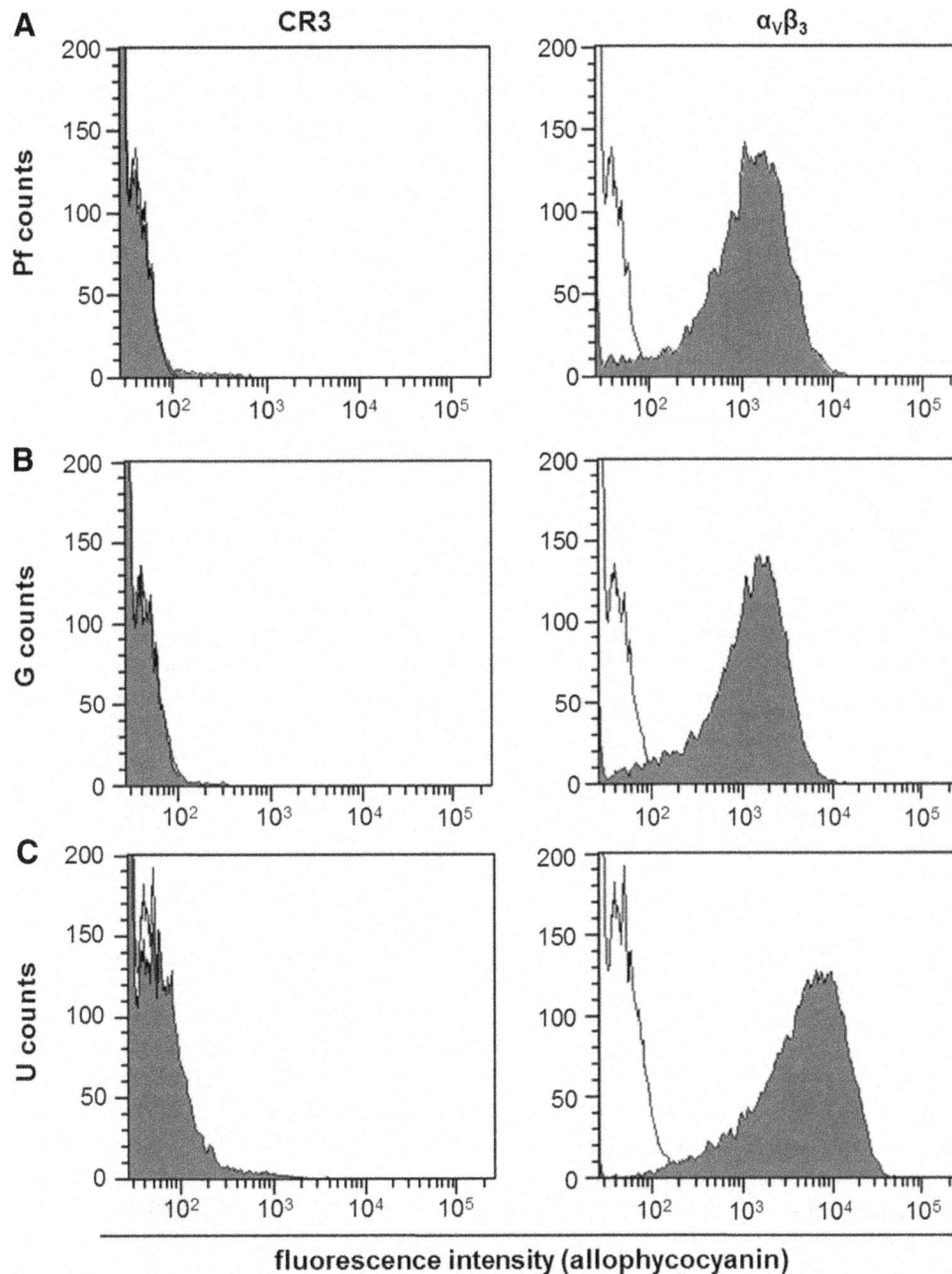

Figure 7 Determination of receptor distribution on bovine epithelial cells. Uninfected epithelial cell (Pf [panel **A**], G [**B**], U [**C**]) were analyzed by flow cytometry for expression of CR3 and $\alpha_V\beta_3$ on their surface. Grey shaded curves depict detection of the respective antigens and black lines represent secondary antibody control (representative results of two technical replicates in two independent experiments).

positive with Coxiella-specific antibodies and with rarely detectable Coxiella-like organisms. Our results of infection experiments with bovine fetal and maternal placental epithelial cell lines are in line with these ex vivo observations and imply that the many tissue-specific properties the placental cell lines have retained also comprise determinants of permissiveness for *C. burnetii* infection [35, 36].

Numbers of *C. burnetii* in the feces of infected small ruminants exceed numbers in bovine feces pointing to another possible shedding route at least in sheep and goats [9]. Feces of aborting ewes contain up to 10^7 GE of Coxiella per gram [37]. Our in vitro study showed that epithelial cells other than mammary gland epithelium also were capable of internalizing *C. burnetii* but there was little further propagation of bacterial numbers within

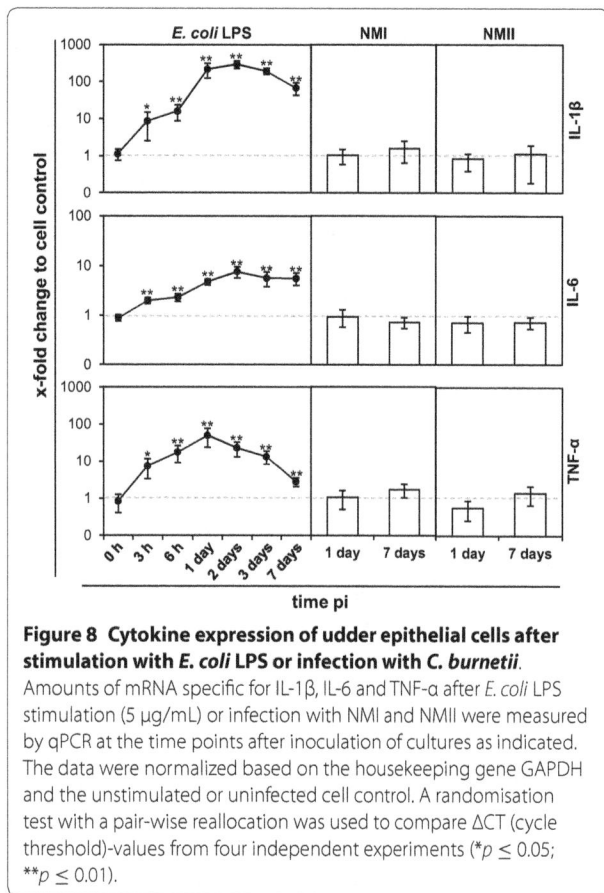

Figure 8 Cytokine expression of udder epithelial cells after stimulation with *E. coli* LPS or infection with *C. burnetii*. Amounts of mRNA specific for IL-1β, IL-6 and TNF-α after *E. coli* LPS stimulation (5 µg/mL) or infection with NMI and NMII were measured by qPCR at the time points after inoculation of cultures as indicated. The data were normalized based on the housekeeping gene GAPDH and the unstimulated or uninfected cell control. A randomisation test with a pair-wise reallocation was used to compare ΔCT (cycle threshold)-values from four independent experiments ($*p \leq 0.05$; $**p \leq 0.01$).

the cells. In organs implicated in *C. burnetii* shedding by cattle, these cells apparently represent rather unsuitable target cells which may be the in vitro correlate of the comparably low numbers of *C. burnetii* detected in the feces and birth fluids of bovines [9, 10].

At the entry site, lung epithelial cells are the first contact of Coxiella when entering the host organism after aerial transmission. It may be argued, that significant replication is not necessary at the entry site but the bacteria just cross the epithelial barrier to reach phagocytosing cells. Calverley et al. [38] concluded that recruited monocytes play an important role in the infection process because they control the distribution of bacteria from the lung. Additionally, resident alveolar immune cells were shown in a mouse model to possess a high susceptibility to Coxiella infection [38] and human and bovine alveolar macrophages can be infected with *C. burnetii* in vitro [13, 39]. There is cumulating evidence, therefore, that lung epithelial cells, being less susceptible to *C. burnetii* infection ([1], this study), do not act as replication sites for the bacteria and as such are poorly implicated in *C. burnetii* transmission between animals and in persistence in different hosts.

Bovine epithelial cells from different tissues varied in their susceptibility to *C. burnetii* invasion and support of replication with little correlation between the two properties as udder epithelial cells particularly supported *C. burnetii* replication whereas intestinal epithelial cells displayed an enhanced susceptibility for *C. burnetii* invasion. Invasion of *C. burnetii* into cells is reported to be influenced by the biochemical composition of the LPS [40]. In a variety of cells, *C. burnetii* strains with phase I and phase II LPS exhibit a different uptake kinetic in that a virulent phase I strain attached slower than the avirulent strain because of the mechanisms these organisms utilize to enter the host cells. Coxiella uses specific eukaryotic receptors such as integrins on macrophages and monocytes to adhere and invade [21]. *C. burnetii* phase I particles bind the leukocyte response integrin ($\alpha_v\beta_3$), whereas the avirulent *C. burnetii* additionally deploy complement receptor 3 (CR3) [21]. Bovine udder epithelial cells exhibited an enhanced $\alpha_v\beta_3$ expression whereas CR3 was essentially absent from the surface of all cell lines studied. Martinez et al. already described the first *C. burnetii* protein involved in host cell invasion [41]. OmpA is a surface protein of Coxiella that increased the internalization within non-phagocytic cells without necessity of Coxiella-specific receptors. Further investigations are required to assess the role of the adhesin OmpA and $\alpha_v\beta_3$ for bacterial attachment, invasion and cellular activation in bovine epithelial cells.

Coxiella organisms can activate immune cells in a strain-dependent manner. Especially avirulent strains promote a higher pro-inflammatory cytokine production compared to virulent strains [39] which may be linked to LPS phase-related differences in attachment of the bacteria [42]. We observed a general failure to induce immune responses which particularly holds for udder epithelial cells independent of the phase-type of the NM variant and the day post-infection. Enterobacterial LPS is a very potent stimulant for immune reactions via pattern recognition receptors (PRRs) [43] and was included as positive control in our studies. LPS-stimulated udder epithelial cells showed an upregulation of pro-inflammatory cytokines. The failure of *C. burnetii* to initiate epithelial immune responses does not result from a process actively steered by a metabolically active pathogen, because infection studies with heat-inactivated NMI and NMII yielded similar results (data not shown). Invasive bacteria normally induce a rapid pro-inflammatory cytokine production as part of the defense mechanisms of the host. Different from bovine epithelial cells, attachment to or invasion of *C. burnetii* into macrophages stimulate a pro-inflammatory immune response to recruit additional immune cells [13, 39]. However, these responses are regulated in a complex manner. Rasmussen et al. [44] described a delay in cytokine expression in *Chlamydia* spp.-infected

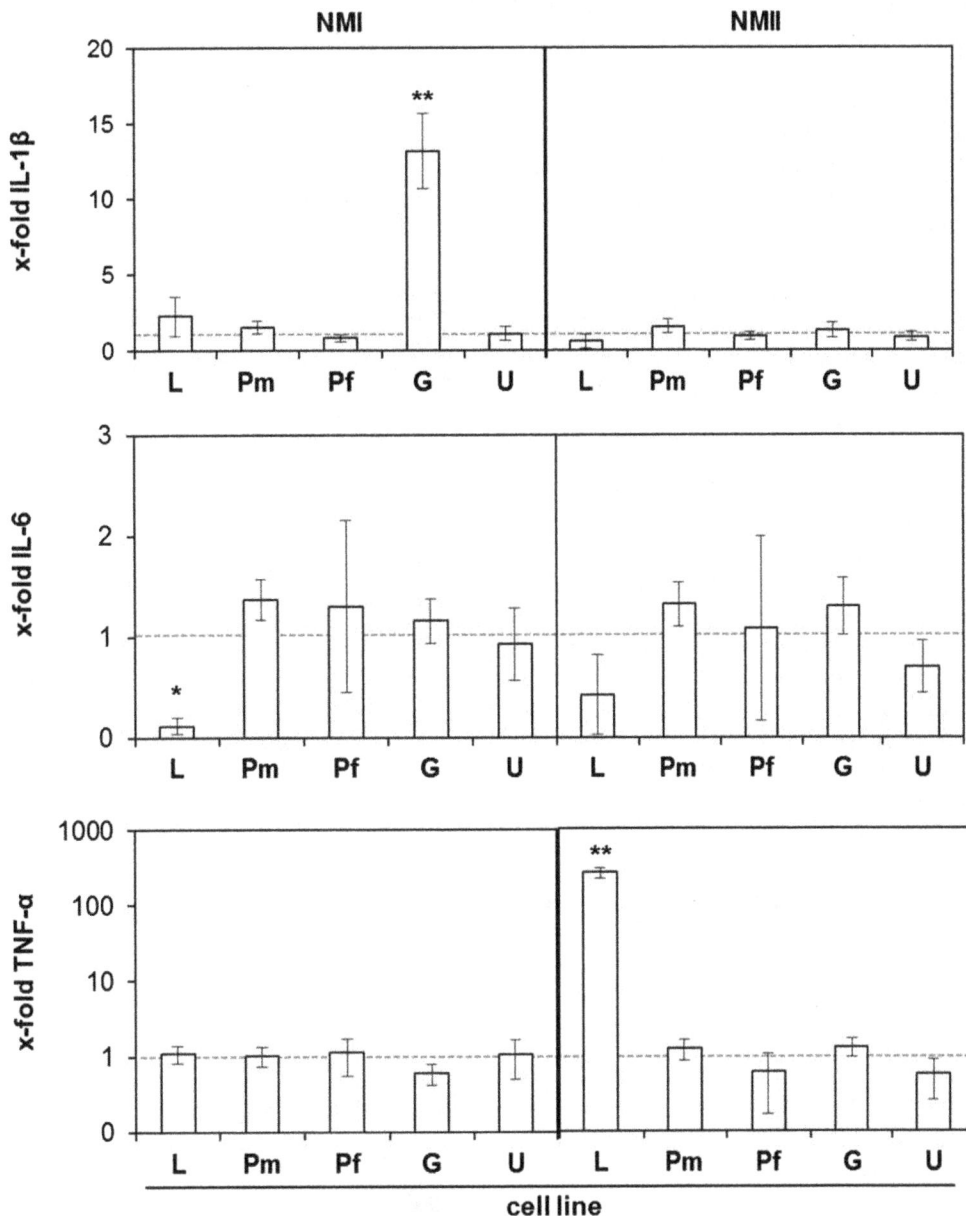

Figure 9 Cytokine expression of epithelial cells after infection with C. burnetii. Amounts of mRNA specific for IL-1β, IL-6 and TNF-α 24 h after infection with NMI and NMII were measured by qPCR. The data were normalized based on the housekeeping gene GAPDH and the uninfected cell control. A randomisation test with a pair-wise reallocation was used to compare ΔCT (cycle threshold)-values from four independent experiments (*$p \leq 0.05$; **$p \leq 0.01$).

cells and that chlamydial invasion alone did not induce an immune response. In human colon epithelial cells, activation of cytokine response upon bacterial invasion is dependent on a special set of signals [45]. The attachment alone did not sufficiently stimulate the immune system for bacterial clearance. Activation of epithelial cells by *Candida albicans*, a common epidermal pathogen, is regulated via two phases of signal pathway activation [46]. On the one hand there is a morphological recognition of the fungus via PRRs and on the other hand a second trigger leads to production of cytokines and further immune reactions inside the host cells. The molecular basis for failure of bovine epithelial cells investigated in our study to initiate inflammatory responses remains to be determined. It can be assumed, though, that this property of *C. burnetii* is instrumental to create a replicative niche in the reservoir host for persistence of the pathogen, similar to what Ben Amara et al. [47] had suggested for human trophoblasts.

The in vitro cell system established and characterized in this study will be useful to further the understanding of the chain of events during the infection process of Coxiella organisms inside the bovine host in respect to epithelial cells as possible target cells. Bovine udder epithelial cells seem to have the highest permissiveness for *C. burnetii* and promote bacterial replication without losing the cell vitality. The udder cell line used was initially isolated from a mammary gland and became permanently cultivable by continuous passaging without deploying artificial transformation. The similarity to primary bovine mammary epithelial cells constitutes a big advantage for further investigations. Even though cell lines assessed in our study significantly varied in their permissiveness, the results strongly imply that *C. burnetii* can make use of epithelial cells beside immune cells as target cells for successful transmission between animals and into the environment as the cells survived the infection for substantial periods of time while helping the pathogen to evade the hosts immune response. For reasons of availability we chose bovine cells and evaluated the invasion and replication of *C. burnetii* by using two biological variants of a commonly used prototype strain. Cattle are not the main source of human infection but may shed *C. burnetii*. The high prevalence of *C. burnetii* genotype ST 20 recently identified in bovine milk in the U.S. [48] points to host species-specific adaptations within of the species of *C. burnetii*. After the proof-of-principle provided in this manuscript, studies are now in progress to assess quantitative differences in the interaction of different Coxiella genotypes with bovine epithelial cells.

Competing interests

The authors declare that they have no competing interests.

Authors' contributions

Design of study and experiments: CM, KS. Generation and characterization of cell lines: PG, PR, NH, CP. Cell infection assays, fluorescence microscopy and real-time PCR: KS, KB. Electron microscopy; ELT. Statistical analysis: KS. Interpretation of data and drafting of the manuscript: KS, KB, ELT, IDJ, CM. All authors read and approved the final manuscript.

Acknowledgements

The authors would like to thank Anja Müller, Anke Hinsching, Lisa Wirker und Wolfram Maginot (Friedrich-Loeffler-Institut, Institute of Molecular Pathogenesis) for their excellent technical assistance.

Funding

The study was financially supported by the European Commission (FP7 programme in the framework of the project "Antigone—ANTIcipating the Global Onset of Novel Epidemics", Project Number 278976). The funding body had no role in the design of the study and collection, analysis, and interpretation of data and in writing the manuscript.

Author details

[1] Institute of Molecular Pathogenesis, Friedrich-Loeffler-Institut (FLI), Naumburger Strasse 96a, 07743 Jena, Germany. [2] ISP, INRA, Université Tours, UMR 1282, 37380 Nouzilly, France. [3] Department of Anatomy, University of Veterinary Medicine Hannover, Bischofsholer Damm 15, 30173 Hannover, Germany. [4] Research Group Microbial Immunology, Leibniz Institute for Natural Product Research and Infection Biology/Hans Knoell Institute, Beutenbergstrasse 11a, 07745 Jena, Germany.

References

1. Maurin M, Raoult D (1999) Q fever. Clin Microbiol Rev 12:518–553
2. Arricau-Bouvery N, Rodolakis A (2005) Is Q fever an emerging or re-emerging zoonosis? Vet Res 36:327–349
3. Lang GH (1990) Coxiellosis (Q fever) in animals. In: Marrie TJ (ed) Q fever: the disease, vol 1. CRC Press, New York
4. Berri M, Souriau A, Crosby M, Crochet D, Lechopier P, Rodolakis A (2001) Relationships between the shedding of *Coxiella burnetii*, clinical signs and serological responses of 34 sheep. Vet Rec 148:502–505
5. Tissot-Dupont H, Amadei MA, Nezri M, Raoult D (2004) Wind in November, Q fever in December. Emerg Infect Dis 10:1264–1269
6. van der Hoek W, Morroy G, Renders NHM, Wever PC, Hermans MHA, Leenders ACAP, Schneeberger PM (2012) Epidemic Q fever in humans in the Netherlands. Adv Exp Med Biol 984:329–364
7. Sánchez J, Souriau A, Buendía AJ, Arricau-Bouvery N, Martínez CM, Salinas J, Rodolakis A, Navarro JA (2006) Experimental *Coxiella burnetii* infection in pregnant goats: a histopathological and immunohistochemical study. J Comp Pathol 135:108–115
8. Roest HJ, van Gelderen B, Dinkla A, Frangoulidis D, van Zijderveld F, Rebel J, van Keulen L (2012) Q fever in pregnant goats: pathogenesis and excretion of *Coxiella burnetii*. PLoS One 7:e48949
9. Rodolakis A, Berri M, Héchard C, Caudron C, Souriau A, Bodier CC, Blanchard B, Camuset P, Devillechaise P, Natorp JC, Vadet JP, Arricau-Bouvery N (2007) Comparison of *Coxiella burnetii* shedding in milk of dairy bovine, caprine, and ovine herds. J Dairy Sci 90:5352–5360
10. Guatteo R, Beaudeau F, Joly A, Seegers H (2007) *Coxiella burnetii* shedding by dairy cows. Vet Res 38:12
11. Valergakis GE, Russell C, Grogono-Thomas R, Bradley AJ, Eisler MC (2012) *Coxiella burnetii* in bulk tank milk of dairy cattle in south-west England. Vet Rec 171:156
12. Muskens J, van Engelen E, van Maanen C, Bartels C, Lam TJGM (2011) Prevalence of *Coxiella burnetii* infection in Dutch dairy herds based on testing bulk tank milk and individual samples by PCR and ELISA. Vet Rec 168:79
13. Sobotta K, Hillarius K, Mager M, Kerner K, Heydel C, Menge C (2016) *Coxiella burnetii* infects primary bovine macrophages and limits their host cell response. Infect Immun 84:1722–1734
14. Elliott A, Schoenlaub L, Freches D, Mitchell W, Zhang G (2015) Neutrophils play an important role in protective immunity against *Coxiella burnetii* infection. Infect Immun 83:3104–3113
15. Khavkin T, Tabibzadeh SS (1988) Histologic, immunofluorescence, and electron microscopic study of infectious process in mouse lung after intranasal challenge with *Coxiella burnetii*. Infect Immun 56:1792–1799
16. Toman R, Škultéty L (1996) Structural study on a lipopolysaccharide from *Coxiella burnetii* strain Nine Mile in avirulent phase II. Carbohydr Res 283:175–185
17. Roussel P, Cunha P, Porcherie A, Petzl W, Gilbert FB, Riollet C, Zerbe H, Rainard P, Germon P (2015) Investigating the contribution of IL-17A and IL-17F to the host response during *Escherichia coli* mastitis. Vet Res 46:56
18. Goellner S, Schubert E, Liebler-Tenorio E, Hotzel H, Saluz HP, Sachse K (2006) Transcriptional response patterns of *Chlamydophila psittaci* in different in vitro models of persistent infection. Infect Immun 74:4801–4808
19. Klee SR, Tyczka J, Ellerbrok H, Franz T, Linke S, Baljer G, Appel B (2006) Highly sensitive real-time PCR for specific detection and quantification of *Coxiella burnetii*. BMC Microbiol 6:2
20. Pfaffl MW, Horgan GW, Dempfle L (2002) Relative expression software tool (REST©) for group-wise comparison and statistical analysis of relative expression results in real-time PCR. Nucleic Acids Res 30:e36
21. Capo C, Lindberg FP, Meconi S, Zaffran Y, Tardei G, Brown EJ, Raoult D, Mege JL (1999) Subversion of monocyte functions by *Coxiella burnetii*: impairment of the cross-talk between ανβ3 integrin and CR3. J Immunol 163:6078–6085
22. Voth DE, Howe D, Heinzen RA (2007) *Coxiella burnetii* inhibits apoptosis in human THP-1 cells and monkey primary alveolar macrophages. Infect Immun 75:4263–4271
23. Agerholm JS (2013) *Coxiella burnetii* associated reproductive disorders in domestic animals—a critical review. Acta Vet Scand 55:13
24. Aitken DID, Bögel DK, Cracea PDE, Edlinger E, Houwers DD, Krauss PDH, Rády DM, Rehácek DJ, Schiefer PDHG, Kazán DJ, Schmeer DN, Tarasevich PDIV, Tringali PDG (1987) Q fever in Europe: current aspects of aetiology, epidemiology, human infection, diagnosis and therapy. Infection 15:323–327

25. Biberstein EL, Behymer DE, Bushnell R, Crenshaw G, Riemann HP, Franti CE (1974) A survey of Q fever (*Coxiella burnetii*) in California dairy cows. Am J Vet Res 35:1577–1582

26. Gale P, Kelly L, Mearns R, Duggan J, Snary EL (2015) Q fever through consumption of unpasteurised milk and milk products—a risk profile and exposure assessment. J Appl Microbiol 118:1083–1095

27. Benson WW, Brock DW, Mather J (1963) Serologic analysis of a penitentiary group using raw milk from a Q fever infected herd. Public Health Rep 78:707–710

28. Enright JB, Sadler WW, Thomas RC (1957) Pasteurization of milk containing the organism of Q fever. Am J Public Health Nations Health 47:695–700

29. Schaal EH (1982) Udder colonization with *Coxiella burnetii* in cattle Q fever. Dtsch Tierarztl Wochenschr 89:411–414 (in German)

30. Coleman SA, Fischer ER, Howe D, Mead DJ, Heinzen RA (2004) Temporal analysis of *Coxiella burnetii* morphological differentiation. J Bacteriol 186:7344–7352

31. van Schaik EJ, Chen C, Mertens K, Weber MM, Samuel JE (2013) Molecular pathogenesis of the obligate intracellular bacterium *Coxiella burnetii*. Nat Rev Microbiol 11:561–573

32. Howe D, Melnicáková J, Barák I, Heinzen RA (2003) Maturation of the *Coxiella burnetii* parasitophorous vacuole requires bacterial protein synthesis but not replication. Cell Microbiol 5:469–480

33. Aguilera M, Salinas R, Rosales E, Carminati S, Colombo MI, Berón W (2009) Actin dynamics and Rho GTPases regulate the size and formation of parasitophorous vacuoles containing *Coxiella burnetii*. Infect Immun 77:4609–4620

34. van Moll P, Baumgärtner W, Eskens U, Hänichen T (1993) Immunocytochemical demonstration of *Coxiella burnetii* antigen in the fetal placenta of naturally infected sheep and cattle. J Comp Pathol 109:295–301

35. Bridger PS, Menge C, Leiser R, Tinneberg HR, Pfarrer CD (2007) Bovine caruncular epithelial cell line (BCEC-1) isolated from the placenta forms a functional epithelial barrier in a polarised cell culture model. Placenta 28:1110–1117

36. Hambruch N, Haeger JD, Dilly M, Pfarrer C (2010) EGF stimulates proliferation in the bovine placental trophoblast cell line F3 via Ras and MAPK. Placenta 31:67–74

37. Joulié A, Laroucau K, Bailly X, Prigent M, Gasqui P, Lepetitcolin E, Blanchard B, Rousset E, Sidi-Boumedine K, Jourdain E (2015) *Coxiella burnetii* circulation in a naturally infected flock of dairy sheep: shedding dynamics, environmental contamination, and genotype diversity. Appl Environ Microbiol 81:7253–7260

38. Calverley M, Erickson S, Read AJ, Harmsen AG (2012) Resident alveolar macrophages are susceptible to and permissive of *Coxiella burnetii* infection. PLoS One 7:e51941

39. Graham JG, MacDonald LJ, Hussain SK, Sharma UM, Kurten RC, Voth DE (2013) Virulent *Coxiella burnetii* pathotypes productively infect primary human alveolar macrophages. Cell Microbiol 15:1012–1025

40. Baca OG, Klassen DA, Aragon AS (1993) Entry of *Coxiella burnetii* into host cells. Acta Virol 37:143–155

41. Martinez E, Cantet F, Fava L, Norville I, Bonazzi M (2014) Identification of OmpA, a *Coxiella burnetii* protein involved in host cell invasion, by multiphenotypic high-content screening. PLoS Pathog 10:e1004013

42. Dellacasagrande J, Ghigo E, Machergui-El S, Hammami Toman R, Raoult D, Capo C, Mege JL (2000) αvβ3 integrin and bacterial lipopolysaccharide are involved in *Coxiella burnetii*-stimulated production of tumor necrosis factor by human monocytes. Infect Immun 68:5673–5678

43. Zamboni DS, Campos MA, Torrecilhas ACT, Kiss K, Samuel JE, Golenbock DT, Lauw FN, Roy CR, Almeida IC, Gazzinelli RT (2004) Stimulation of toll-like receptor 2 by *Coxiella burnetii* is required for macrophage production of pro-inflammatory cytokines and resistance to infection. J Biol Chem 279:54405–54415

44. Rasmussen SJ, Eckmann L, Quayle AJ, Shen L, Zhang YX, Anderson DJ, Fierer J, Stephens RS, Kagnoff MF (1997) Secretion of proinflammatory cytokines by epithelial cells in response to Chlamydia infection suggests a central role for epithelial cells in chlamydial pathogenesis. J Clin Invest 99:77–87

45. Jung HC, Eckmann L, Yang SK, Panja A, Fierer J, Morzycka-Wroblewska E, Kagnoff MF (1995) A distinct array of proinflammatory cytokines is expressed in human colon epithelial cells in response to bacterial invasion. J Clin Invest 95:55–65

46. Moyes DL, Richardson JP, Naglik JR (2015) *Candida albicans*-epithelial interactions and pathogenicity mechanisms: scratching the surface. Virulence 6:338–346

47. Ben Amara A, Ghigo E, Le Priol Y, Lépolard C, Salcedo SP, Lemichez E, Bretelle F, Capo C, Mege JL (2010) *Coxiella burnetii*, the agent of Q fever, replicates within trophoblasts and induces a unique transcriptional response. PLoS One 5:e15315

48. Pearson T, Hornstra HM, Hilsabeck R, Gates LT, Olivas SM, Birdsell DM, Hall CM, German S, Cook JM, Seymour ML, Priestley RA, Kondas AV, Clark Friedman CL, Price EP, Schupp JM, Liu CM, Price LB, Massung RF, Kersh GJ, Keim P (2014) High prevalence and two dominant host-specific genotypes of *Coxiella burnetii* in U.S. milk. BMC Microbiol 14:41

4

Fecal shedding and tissue infections demonstrate transmission of *Mycobacterium avium* subsp. *paratuberculosis* in group-housed dairy calves

Caroline S. Corbett, Jeroen De Buck, Karin Orsel and Herman W. Barkema[*]

Abstract

Current Johne's disease control programs primarily focus on decreasing transmission of *Mycobacterium avium* subsp. *paratuberculosis* (MAP) from infectious adult cows to susceptible calves. However, potential transmission between calves is largely overlooked. The objective was to determine the extent of MAP infection in calves contact-exposed to infectious penmates. Thirty-two newborn Holstein–Friesian calves were grouped into 7 experimental groups of 4, consisting of 2 inoculated (IN) calves, and 2 contact-exposed (CE) calves, and 1 control pen with 4 non-exposed calves. Calves were group housed for 3 months, with fecal samples were collected 3 times per week, blood and environmental samples weekly, and tissue samples at the end of the trial. The IN calves exited the trial after 3 months of group housing, whereas CE calves were individually housed for an additional 3 months before euthanasia. Control calves were group-housed for the entire trial. All CE and IN calves had MAP-positive fecal samples during the period of group housing; however, fecal shedding had ceased at time of individual housing. All IN calves had MAP-positive tissue samples at necropsy, and 7 (50%) of the CE had positive tissue samples. None of the calves had a humoral immune response, whereas INF-γ responses were detected in all IN calves and 5 (36%) CE calves. In conclusion, new MAP infections occurred due to exposure of infectious penmates to contact calves. Therefore, calf-to-calf transmission is a potential route of uncontrolled transmission on cattle farms.

Introduction

Johne's disease (JD) is a chronic, progressive, inflammatory disease in the small intestine of ruminants caused by *Mycobacterium avium* subspecies *paratuberculosis* (MAP). It is well established that MAP infection is widespread in cattle and causes substantial economic losses to dairy producers worldwide [1–3]. Clinical stages of disease cause severe diarrhea and shedding of bacteria into the environment; however, subclinical animals also contribute to the infectious load in the environment and economic losses incurred by the producer, due to reduced milk yield, increased risk of culling and decreased slaughter value [4, 5].

Although vaccines for use in cattle have been developed [6, 7], these vaccines only prevent clinical signs of JD, and there is currently no vaccine available for cattle to prevent infection or shedding of MAP. Therefore, control programs are based on decreasing both the number of new MAP introductions into negative herds and within-herd transmission [2, 3, 8]. The primary route of infection is fecal-oral through ingestion of milk, feed, or water contaminated by infectious animals shedding MAP bacteria in their feces [5, 9, 10]. The assumptions that cows are infectious, calves are susceptible, and calves do not shed until later in life has led to the focus of most control programs interrupting direct and indirect contact of fecal material from infectious adult cows to susceptible young stock [11, 12]. Although the association between JD control programs, management practices, and MAP infections on farms has been

*Correspondence: barkema@ucalgary.ca
Department of Production Animal Health, Faculty of Veterinary Medicine, University of Calgary, Calgary, AB, Canada

well established [2, 12–14], the potential risk of calf–calf transmission is largely overlooked. However, calves can begin shedding as early as 1 month after inoculation [15], calves up to at least 12 months of age are susceptible to MAP infection [16, 17], and a relatively high proportion of young stock on infected farms are shedding MAP in their feces [18, 19]. Although most calves are separated from their dams shortly after birth to prevent transmission, fecal-oral transmission may still be possible during those first hours to days in the calving pen, or even prenatally via intra-uterine transmission [20, 21]. Therefore, group-housing of calves (even though they are isolated from adult cows) may not be an effective practice to eliminate the spread of MAP or prevent new infections.

Recent infection trials have yielded new knowledge that calves inoculated with MAP at an earlier age had more severe tissue lesions [16], and increased fecal shedding was associated with increased numbers of MAP-positive tissue samples [15]. The ability of calves to both infect and become infected has led to several transmission and modelling studies to determine the role of calf-to-calf transmission in causing new infections on farm. However, there have been inconsistent findings regarding the role of calf transmission and its importance for control [17, 22–24]. Furthermore, the extent of infection, subclinical infections, or the ability to suppress an infection, and detecting the signs of infection, all vary depending on several factors, including inoculation dose, immune capabilities, frequency of sampling and individual variability [23, 25, 26]. Therefore, there is a need for an experimental study to examine the extent of infection due to calf-to-calf transmission.

The objective was to determine extent and magnitude of MAP infection in contact-exposed calves resulting from transmission of MAP from inoculated pen-mates, based on fecal shedding and positive tissue samples due to 3 months of group housing.

Materials and methods

Calves

Thirty-two newborn Holstein–Friesian bull calves were purchased from 13 Alberta (Canada) dairy farms selected based on annual testing as part of the Alberta Johne's Disease Initiative [27] and participation in the JD herd health status program in Alberta. All farms had tested negative for at least 4 years using 6 environmental samples and 1 of the following: bacteriological culture of 60 individual fecal samples tested as pooled samples into groups of 5, individual milk ELISA of the whole milking herd, or serum ELISA of the entire herd.

Nutrition, health and husbandry

All calves were collected immediately after birth (to prevent contamination from fecal material on farm or ingesting colostrum), and transported to the research facility. Nutrition was similar to that described by Mortier et al. [16]. In short, calves were fed 6 L (in 2-L portions) of high-quality colostrum within the first 8 h after birth. Colostrum was collected from 4 of the 13 farms that had tested negative consistently for ≥ 4 years. Starting the 2nd day of their life, calves were fed milk replacer, followed by calf starter (without antimicrobials) and high-quality hay. Calves were gradually weaned by 8 week of age, and had ad libitum access to water and hay (supplemented with concentrates).

Calves were housed in a biosecurity Level 2 facility. The facility included 15 custom-built housing units with waterproof liners to contain all bedding and fecal material. Group-housing pens were 10 × 10 feet and 6 feet tall (3.05 × 3.05 × 1.82 m). Each housing unit consisted of a marked-off area containing the pen, 2 pairs of boots, 2 pairs of coveralls and gloves dedicated specifically for use in the pen within the unit. All personnel were trained to monitor health daily, and to observe strict biosafety and isolation protocols to prevent transmission of MAP between pens by any vectors, e.g. buckets, scoops for feed, personnel, etc. All protocols and the experimental design were approved by the University of Calgary Veterinary Sciences Animal Care Committee (protocol AC14-0168).

Study design

Calves were assigned to pens based on time of birth and entry into the research facility. The first 14 calves were designated to be inoculated animals (IN), with 2 calves in each of the 7 experimental pens. The next 14 calves to enter the barn were assigned as contact-exposed (CE) and individually housed temporarily in separate pens from the IN calves. The last 4 calves to enter the barn were designated as the control group, and placed together in the control pen. At 2 weeks of age, the IN calves in each pen were inoculated over 2 consecutive days. After 2 weeks (to allow the inoculum to pass through the calves), pens were relined with new liners and bedded with fresh shavings and straw. Calves designated as CE had to reach a minimum of 1 week of age with no health complications to ensure that they could drink from a bucket without assistance, and that only healthy calves were added to the study. When both CE calves entering the same pen reached a minimum 1 week of age, they were placed into the clean, re-lined experimental pen with the IN calves. Four calves (2 IN and 2 CE) were then group-housed for 3 months following the first day of group housing. The IN calves were euthanized and necropsied after 3 months of group housing. The CE calves were then individually housed in relined and clean pens for an additional 3 months. All 4 control calves were group housed (1 pen) for the entirety of the study.

Inoculum

The inoculum was a virulent MAP cattle type strain from a clinical JD case in Alberta (Cow 69) [16]. In short, a culture was prepared in 7H9/mycobactin/OADC liquid broth, from a first passage frozen stock and quantified using a combination of optical density (OD) at 600 nm, the wet weight method, and qPCR, as described [28]. Once culture grew to a concentration of 5×10^8 CFU/mL, 1 mL aliquots were frozen at −80 °C until 1 week prior to inoculation. Before each inoculation, 1 tube was thawed and suspended in 50 mL 7H9 broth for 1 week, during which time inoculum was tested for contamination. 2.5×10^8 CFU's was quantified using the wet weight method, diluted in 20 mL of broth, placed in a 20-mL syringe and transported to the research facility. Calves were allowed to suckle the syringe containing the inoculum and it was expelled at the root of the tongue (on 2 consecutive days).

Fecal sampling and culture

Fecal samples were collected daily for 14 days following inoculation of IN calves to ensure viability of the inoculum, and monitor passive shedding. As of 14 days after inoculation, shedding was attributed to active MAP infection. For the remainder of the trial, fecal samples from each calf were collected three times/week during group housing for all calves. Following group housing, when calves were housed individually, fecal samples were collected weekly from CE calves for the remainder of the trial. Samples were stored at 4 °C until processing, which occurred within 7 days after collection.

All samples were processed using a modified TREK ESP II culture media (TREK para-JEM®; TREK Diagnostic Systems, Cleveland, OH, USA) with subsequent F57-specific qPCR, as described [15]. Briefly, 2 g of fecal sample was thoroughly mixed with 30 mL of distilled water and left to settle for 30 min. Then, 5 mL of supernatant was transferred to 25 mL of a 0.9% hexadecylpyridinium chloride (HPC) half-strength brain heart infusion (BHI) solution for decontamination. Samples were then incubated for 24 h at 37 °C, followed by centrifugation at $3000 \times g$ for 20 min, and the pellet re-suspended in a mixture of antibiotic solution (AS; para-Jem®), water, and full strength BHI. Tubes were incubated again for 24 h at 37 °C and then 1 mL was added to liquid culture medium in TREK para-JEM® culture bottles (TREK Diagnostic

Systems, Cleveland, OH, USA) and incubated at 37 °C for 49 days.

Environmental sampling and culture

Environmental samples were collected once per week from each pen for the duration of the trial. Samples were collected from 5 locations within the pen, and mixed together, resulting in 1 composite sample from each pen. Samples were collected from the surface of the bed pack (individual piles of feces were avoided). Samples were stored at 4 °C until processing, and were subjected to the same protocol (described above) as fecal samples.

Necropsies and tissue cultures

The IN calves were euthanized after 3 months of group housing at 4 months of age by intravenous injection of barbiturate (Euthanyl Forte®, DIN 00241326, Bimeda-MTC Animal Health Inc., Cambridge, ON, Canada), whereas CE were euthanized at 6 months of age, after an additional 3 months of individual housing. Control calves were euthanized last, after all other animals had exited the trial. Necropsies were performed immediately after euthanasia. No other ruminants were examined in the pathology room during necropsies, and the pathology room and tables were thoroughly cleaned and disinfected before and after each necropsy. Thirteen tissue samples were collected from each calf, including two sections of the duodenum, the ileum (including ileal-cecal valve), three sections of jejunum, and spleen. All associated lymph nodes with each gastrointestinal tract section were also collected, as well as the inguinal lymph nodes. Sample locations were marked and isolated with zip ties prior to collection (to prevent movement of intestinal contents). A new set of disinfected instruments and a new pair of gloves was used for collection of each new sample to prevent cross contamination, and PBS was used to rinse fecal content from intestinal tissues.

Samples were transported to the laboratory, and processed immediately on the same day using a modified version of a previous protocol [16]. Briefly, 2.5 g of tissue was dissociated using gentleMACS M tubes (Miltenyi Biotech Inc, Auburn, CA, USA) in 10 mL 0.5% triton x-100 PBS solution. Samples were then transferred to a falcon tube and centrifuged at $4700 \times g$ for 15 min and the pellet re-suspended in 25 mL of 0.75% HPC, ½ strength BHI, 4-mm sterile glass beads and vortexed vigorously for 1–2 min. Samples were then incubated at 37 °C for 3 h, before centrifugation at $4700 \times g$ for 15 min. The pellet was then re-suspended in 3 mL of antibiotic brew (paraJEM®) and incubated overnight, and 1 mL added to paraJEM® culture bottles and incubated at 37 °C for 49 days.

Fecal shedding and tissue infections demonstrate transmission of Mycobacterium avium...

53

qPCR procedure

Following liquid culture of fecal and tissue samples, DNA was extracted as described [29]. A duplex qPCR targeting the MAP-specific F57 region and an internal amplification control (IAC) was performed, with primers, probes, and IAC sequences identical to those described [30]. Amplification conditions for qPCR were as follows: 50 °C for 2 min, 95 °C for 20 s to allow for initial denaturation, then 42 cycles of 95 °C for 30 s and 59 °C for 30 s. Samples were considered positive when the cycle threshold (CT) value was < 40.

Blood sampling, IFN-γ release assay and ELISA

Blood samples were collected weekly from the jugular vein of all calves, alternating between sides. Whole blood was transported to the lab in heated coolers with hot water bottles (25–35 °C), and processed within 2 h for detection of IFN-γ release, as described [31]. Briefly, each sample of whole blood was treated with 100 µL avium Purified Protein Derivative (aPPD; 0.3 mg/mL; Canadian Food Inspection Agency, Ottawa, ON, Canada), 100 µL of pokeweed mitogen (positive stimulation control; 0.3 mg/mL; Sigma-Aldrich Canada Co., Oakville, ON, Canada), and 100 µL sterile PBS (negative stimulation control). Following overnight incubation at 37 °C, serum was collected after centrifugation and stored at −20 °C until all samples were collected and assayed using the sandwich ELISA BOVIGAM® (Prionics, La Vista, NE, USA). Inclusion criteria and interpretation of the IFN-γ release assay were as described [15, 32]. Consequently, observations were excluded from analysis if negative assay controls were < 0.25, the difference between the positive and negative assay controls was < 0.45 or there was a difference of < 0.20 between the negative stimulation and negative assay control. These criteria resulted in only 12 samples being excluded from the study. The % IFN-γ was calculated as follows [31, 32]:

$$\left[(\text{PPD Johnin} - \text{negative assay control}) / \right.$$
$$\left. (\text{positive} - \text{negative assay control}) \right] \times 100.$$

Serum was collected for antibody testing following centrifugation and stored at −20 °C until antibody ELISA testing was performed, based on manufacturer's directions (IDEXX Laboratories Inc.), with analysis as described [33]. Briefly, sample results were expressed as a proportion of the positive control corrected for the negative control (S/P ratio), and a ratio ≥ 60 was considered positive.

Data and statistical analyses

All statistical analyses were performed using STATA 11.2 (StataCorp LP, College Station, TX, USA). For all analyses, $P < 0.05$ was considered significant.

To define shedding events, isolated fecal culture-positive samples (sample collected week prior and subsequent week were negative), and groups of positive samples in which a positive sample was immediately followed by a subsequent positive fecal sample(s), were categorized as a single shedding event. Difference in mean number of fecal positive samples and shedding events, and length of shedding period between IN and CE calves was evaluated using a Student's t test. The average length of events for IN and CE calves was calculated separately. Calves were also separated into fecal shedding categories based on the number of positive samples during group housing, where: 1 = calves with 0–4 positive fecal samples; 2 = calves with 5–9 positive fecal samples; 3 = calves 10–14 positive fecal samples; and 4 = calves with ≥ 15 positive fecal samples of all 38 samples collected during group housing.

The INF-γ results were dichotomized using a cutoff of 100% IFN-γ by calculating the average of presumed negative calves (control calves) + 1.96 the standard deviation [34]. All samples with a value of % IFN-γ exceeding 100, immediately followed by a sample below 100% IFN-γ, were considered false-positive spikes and removed from analysis (28 samples were excluded).

Differences in fecal shedding category, tissue culture and IFN-γ results between IN and CE calves, as well as the association between having at least 1 positive IFN-γ sample and having at least 1 tissue-positive sample, were evaluated using a Fisher's Exact test.

Results

Tissue culture

All IN calves had at least 3 MAP-positive tissue cultures (range 3–11), whereas 7 (50%) of the CE calves had at least 1 MAP-positive tissue culture, but no more than 2 positive tissue samples (Table 1; Figure 1; $p < 0.001$). None of the control calves had positive tissue cultures.

All tissue locations were positive in at least 2 IN calves. No location was MAP culture-positive in all calves; however, lymph nodes associated with the jejunum were most frequently MAP-positive, especially among tissue-positive CE calves (Figure 1).

Immune responses

For all calves, all samples were antibody ELISA-negative, except for 2 pre-infection samples of Calves 15 and 16 that tested positive on 1 occasion before testing negative for the remainder of the study, and this may be due to the transfer of maternal antibodies absorbed from colostrum intake.

All IN calves had at least 5 positive IFN-γ responses, whereas 5 (36%) CE calves had at least 1 positive IFN-γ response (Figure 2). Additionally, 1 control calf (C29) had 2 positive INF-γ samples at 2 consecutive time points (35

Table 1 Number of *Mycobacterium avium* subspecies *paratuberculosis* fecal culture and tissue culture-positive calves in the 3 experimental groups

Calf status	Fecal culture[a]				Tissue culture[b]			
	1	2	3	4	0	1	2	3
Inoculated (n = 14)	0	1	3	10	0	1	4	9
Contact-exposed (n = 14)	3	10	1	0	7	7	0	0
Control (n = 4)	4	0	0	0	4	0	0	0

[a] 1, calves with 0–4 fecal culture positive samples; 2, calves with 5–9 fecal culture-positive samples; 3, calves with 10–14 culture-positive samples; and 4, calves with ≥ 15 fecal culture-positive samples.

[b] 0, calves with 0 tissue culture-positive samples; 1, calves with 1–3 tissue culture-positive samples; 2, calves with 4–6 tissue culture-positive samples; and 3, calves with > 6 tissue culture-positive samples.

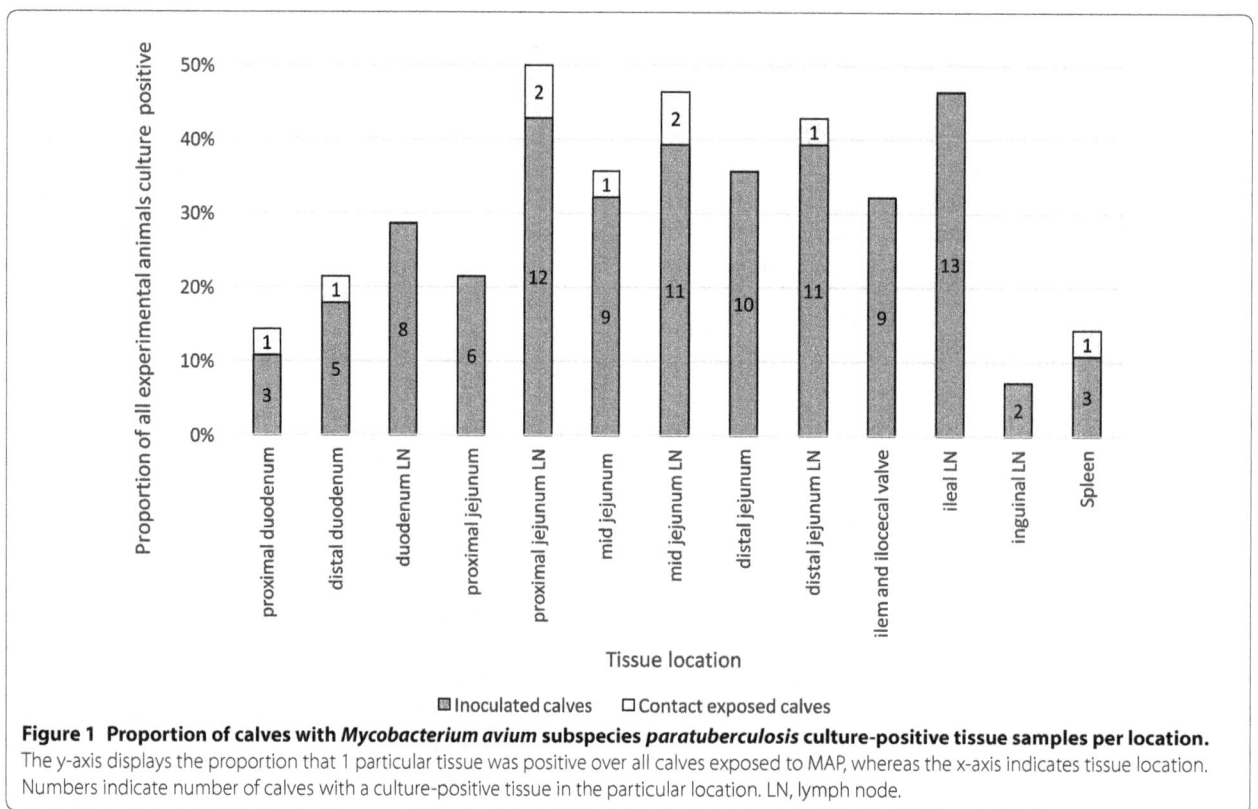

Figure 1 Proportion of calves with *Mycobacterium avium* subspecies *paratuberculosis* culture-positive tissue samples per location. The y-axis displays the proportion that 1 particular tissue was positive over all calves exposed to MAP, whereas the x-axis indicates tissue location. Numbers indicate number of calves with a culture-positive tissue in the particular location. LN, lymph node.

and 42 days after beginning of group housing) during the experimental trial.

The IN calves started to have positive INF-γ samples on average 55 days after inoculation (41 days after the start of group housing), with the earliest and latest being 33 and 73 days after inoculation, respectively. Eight (64%) of the IN calves had their first INF-γ response on or after 56 days following inoculation and the average interval after the start of group housing for the CE calves to have an INF-γ response was 45 days, with the earliest being the day of exposure, and the latest day 89 of group housing ($p = 0.32$); however, 3 (60%) of these CE calves had

positive INF-γ response on or before 33 days after the start of group housing.

Among CE calves, the tissue sample outcome was not associated with the INF-γ result ($p = 0.58$).

Fecal shedding of MAP

No calves fecally shed MAP prior to exposure (inoculation for IN, and group housing for CE). Positive fecal samples were detected consistently in all IN animals for at least 7 days after inoculation (14 days before group housing), and as many as 10 days. The first positive fecal sample collected from a CE calf occurred 5 days after

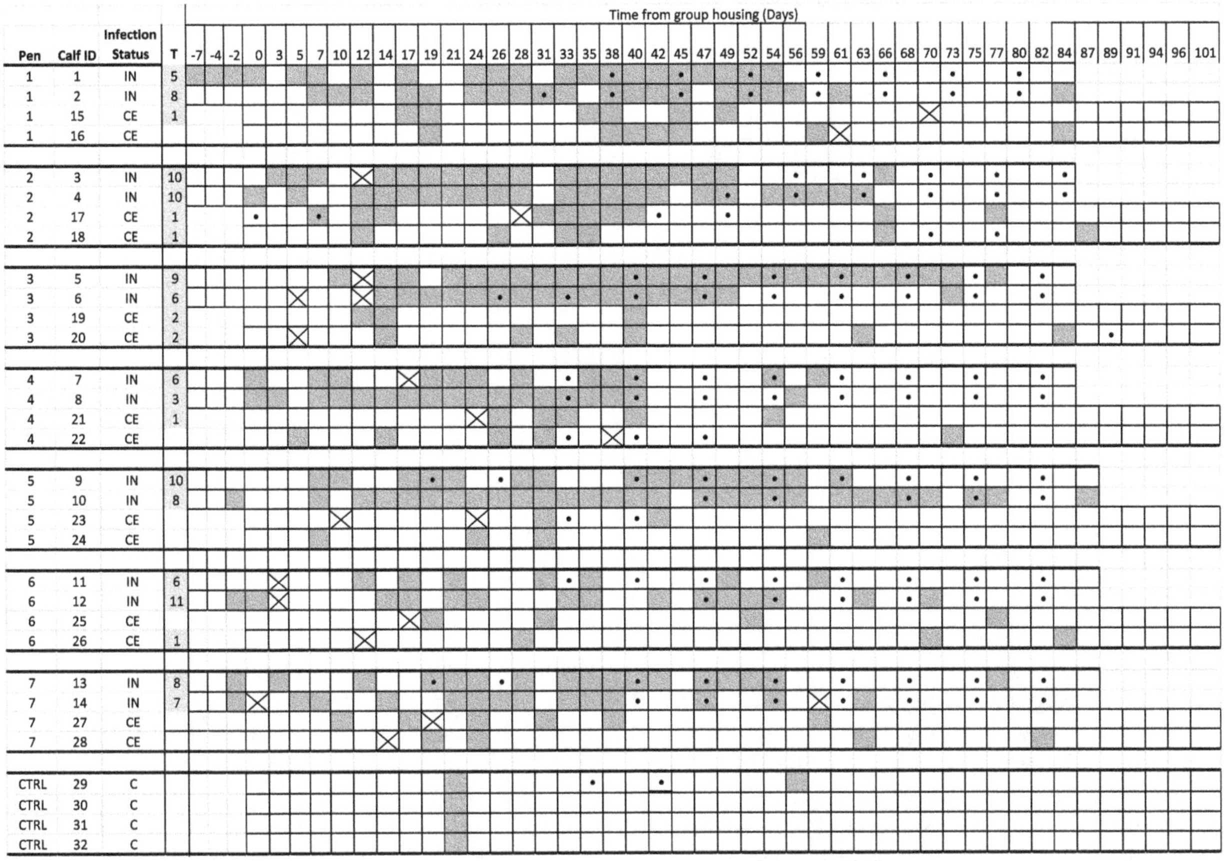

Figure 2 *Mycobacterium avium* subspecies *paratuberculosis* **fecal culture, tissue culture and INF-γ results for individual calves per pen.** A solid dark grey box indicates a positive fecal culture by F57-specific qPCR, a white box indicates a negative culture sample and box with a cross indicates a missing sample. "T" indicates the culture results for tissue samples, boxes shaded light grey indicate positive samples, and number of samples out of 13 that tested positive. Dots indicate blood samples that tested positive for IFN-γ (based on 100% INF-γ cut-off).

the start of group housing, whereas the latest first shedding event was detected 31 days after the start of group housing (Figure 2). All IN and CE calves had at least 2 positive fecal samples during the 3 months of group housing (Figure 2); however, all fecal samples from CE calves were negative after group housing ended and they were housed individually (Figure 2). Fecal samples from control calves were culture-negative for all time points, except for day 21 after the start of group housing at which time all calves had a positive sample (Figure 2), whereas Calf 29 also had 1 additional positive sample on day 56.

Mean number of shedding events was 5.6 (95% CI 4.6–6.7) and 4.1 (95% CI 3.4–4.9) in IN and CE calves, respectively ($p = 0.02$). Mean number of positive samples was 17.6 (95% CI 14.4–20.9) and 5.1 (95% CI 3.9–6.2) in IN and CE calves, respectively ($p < 0.001$). Thirteen (93%) of the IN calves were categorized into Groups 3 and 4, whereas 13 (93%) CE calves were categorized

into Groups 1 and 2 (Table 1). Average length of a shedding event among the IN calves was 7.5 days, ranging from 2 to 54 days, whereas an average shedding event of CE calves lasted 2.9 days, ranging from 2 to 9 days ($p = 0.001$; Figure 2).

Environmental culture

All experimental pens had at least 2 MAP culture-positive environmental samples with a maximum of 7 of the weekly 12 samples collected during group housing (Table 2). The earliest environmental samples were culture-positive was 3 days after the start of group housing, and the latest first positive sample was collected 28 days after the start of group housing. The control pen had no environmental culture-positive samples. There were no significant correlations between positive environmental samples and shedding in all calves ($p = 0.47$), among CE shedding ($p = 0.30$), IN shedding ($p = 0.41$), or positive tissue samples ($p = 0.49$).

Table 2 *Mycobacterium avium* subspecies *paratuberculosis* environmental sampling results for all pens during group housing

Group housing (week)	Pen ID								Total
	1	2	3	4	5	6	7	Controls	
1	−	+	−	+	+	+	−	−	4
2	−	−	+	−	−	−	−	−	1
3	−	−	−	+	+	−	+	−	3
4	+	+	−	−	−	−	+	−	3
5	+	+	+	+	−	+	+	−	6
6	+	+	+	−	−	−	+	−	4
7	+	+	+	−	−	+	+	−	5
8	+	−	+	−	−	−	+	−	3
9	−	−	+	−	−	+	+	−	3
10	−	−	−	−	−	−	−	−	0
11	−	−	−	−	−	−	−	−	0
12	−	−	−	−	−	−	−	−	0
Total	5	5	6	3	2	4	7	0	32

Discussion

In 5 of the 7 experimental pens, at least 1 CE calf had MAP-positive tissue samples, indicating infection caused by exposure to IN animals in the group pen. In total, 50% of CE calves had MAP-positive tissue samples, 5 (36%) had a positive INF-γ response, and all CE calves shed MAP during group housing. However, there was no association between INF-γ, or MAP-positive tissue results among CE calves. The majority of MAP-positive tissue samples from all calves were isolated from the ileum, jejunum, and adjacent lymph nodes, consistent with other studies [16, 35–37].

A low to moderate inoculation dose was chosen to be representative of natural exposure [35, 38, 39]; however, the inoculation protocol will likely have led to a difference in MAP dose between IN and CE calves, as IN calves were artificially infected. Because CE calves were infected by exposure to a contaminated environment and infectious animals, the dose and number of exposure events among CE calves cannot be directly determined. A higher inoculation dose results in a higher number of MAP-positive tissues, and was likely the origin of differences between IN and CE calves in number of positive tissue samples detected [15, 16, 35, 39]. Although there is little known regarding mechanisms of MAP shedding, it is generally agreed that shedding occurs as a result of MAP excretion towards the intestinal lumen [40]. As the majority of positive tissue samples in CE calves were located in the LN associated with the jejunum, jejunal and ileal tissue samples were mostly negative in CE calves, this may explain cessation of shedding following individual housing, as MAP was not detected where

shedding is hypothesized to occur [40]. Additionally, CE calves had considerably fewer positive tissue samples than IN calves, and an increased number of culture-positive tissue samples has been associated with an increased frequency of MAP shedding [15]; therefore, the extent of infection among the CE calves may have been less than the IN calves, leading to less frequent fecal shedding.

All calves had MAP-positive fecal samples during group housing, indicating exposure and risk for infection to all CE calves. Although all CE and IN calves had positive fecal samples, it is possible that a proportion of these samples were not due to active shedding of MAP caused by an infection, but rather the result of passive shedding from exposure to the contaminated environment. It was reported that a higher prevalence of MAP caused more passive shedding events, due to increased environmental contamination [41]. Shedding ceased when CE calves were individually housed in a clean environment; and this may indicate that the shedding detected in group housing was due to passive shedding caused by ingestion of contaminated feces in the environment [26]. However, the decrease in frequency of sampling at that time may have also accounted for this lack of positive fecal samples, due to the frequency of intermittent shedding detected during group housing. It is noteworthy that decreases in calf fecal shedding at 4 months, and as early as 2 months, were reported in experimental trials [15, 22, 23, 37, 42], making it impossible to resolve the nature of this shedding.

Both IN and CE calves shed intermittently in our study, which was detected due to frequent fecal sampling. Others have reported intermittent shedding; however, the interval between positive samples largely depended on the interval between samplings [15, 43]. In the current study, positive fecal samples were followed by negative fecal samples for anywhere from 2 days to 5 weeks before another positive sample was detected. These findings may have large implications for sampling calves on farm and/or incorporating calf sampling into control programs, as calves may shed MAP 1 day, yet cease to be positive on following days/weeks. This creates narrow intervals for detection of potentially infectious young stock that may introduce new infections to pen-mates.

In addition to fecal testing for diagnosis, immune responses are also used to diagnose infected animals [44]. All calves were ELISA-negative for the duration of the experimental trial. This was not surprising, as the main limitation of the antibody ELISA is the ability to detect early stages of infection due to the humoral response being related to the severity of infection [9, 45, 46]. Additionally, the earliest that infection trials with similar doses detected positive antibody responses was 4 months after exposure [28, 33, 37, 47, 48]. The INF-γ immune response is generally a more sensitive indication of early infection or indication that an animal has been exposed to MAP [9, 46]; however, concerns regarding interpretation of the test [32, 49], as well as high individual variability [31] indicate the need for guarded interpretation and further optimization. Among IN calves, consecutive INF-γ positive samples began as early as 43 days after inoculation, and consecutive positive samples continued for all IN calves until euthanasia. Interestingly, of those CE calves with an INF-γ response, it was first detectable at 33 days of group housing (first exposure) or sooner (Calf 17), which indicates that they had a quicker cellular immune response than in IN calves (55 days). It has been reported that a lower dose of antigen may lead to a faster, more effective response [50]. Furthermore, a lower dose of MAP given over a longer interval (trickle dose) may lead to an earlier cellular immune response [28]; however, further research is needed.

All 4 control calves had a positive fecal sample 21 days after the start of group housing, and 1 calf had an additional positive fecal sample on day 56, as well as 2 positive INF-γ samples. It is not unusual to detect positive INF-γ samples among non-infected control calves [51]. All control calves were MAP tissue culture-negative. Despite the 5 positive fecal samples collected from calves in the control pen, all environmental samples collected for the duration of the study were negative. Although the CT threshold is high, resulting in a high specificity of fecal culture to identify true negative samples, control fecal samples collected on day 21 all had CT values well below the cut-off. Perhaps passive shedding of MAP on d 21 resulted from transmission (via an object or air) from an experimental pen in the barn, or samples were contaminated on the day of sampling. However, this was unlikely due to the stringent protocols and strict biosecurity measures in place. It is unlikely that any control calves became infected, based on negative results for tissues, fecal and environmental samples during the trial, and it is possible these samples became positive during processing in the laboratory, as all control animals tested positive on the same day.

In conclusion, this study provided strong evidence that CE calves can become infected with MAP, and are at risk for transmission from infectious calves in group pens. It was noteworthy that 50% of CE calves had MAP-positive tissue results after 3 months of group housing, 5 (36%) had evidence of a cellular immune response, and all had MAP-positive fecal samples (indicating shedding of bacteria). Transmission among group-housed calves is currently largely overlooked in current control programs, but based on evidence from the current study, calf-to-calf transmission may be a source of new infections within a herd. Although there are still important knowledge gaps in the field regarding pathogenesis, progression, and recovery among infected animals, potential transmission among group-housed calves should be considered in JD control and prevention programs.

Abbreviations

CE: contact-exposed; BHI: brain heart infusion; HPC: hexadecylpyridinium chloride; IN: inoculated; LN: lymph node; JD: Johne's disease; MAP: *Mycobacterium avium* subspecies *paratuberculosis*.

Competing interests

The authors declare that they have no competing interests.

Authors' contributions

Designed and conducted the experiment: CSC, JDB, KO, HWB. Developed and conducted inoculum preparation and the inoculation procedure, collected and analysed fecal and blood samples, performed necropsies: CSC. Animal management, health and welfare: CSC, JDB, KO, HWB. Analysis of data: CSC, JDB, HWB. Drafted the manuscript: CSC, JDB, HWB. All authors read and approved the final manuscript.

Acknowledgements

This work was supported by the Natural Sciences and Engineering Research Council of Canada (NSERC) Industrial Research Chair in Infectious Diseases of Dairy Cattle. The NSERC Industrial Research Chair in Infectious Diseases of Dairy Cattle is supported by NSERC; Alberta Milk; Dairy Farmers of Canada; Dairy Farmers of Manitoba; Westgen Endowment Fund; BC Dairy; CanWest DHI; and Canadian Dairy Network. The authors thank Dr John Kastelic for editing the manuscript. In addition, the authors thank Charlotte Pickel, Amanda Mirto, Uliana Kanevets, Indiana Best, Laura Cain, Domonique Carson, Casey Jacobs, and Aaron Lucko for technical assistance and the University of Calgary Veterinary Sciences Research Station staff for animal care assistance. Funding was provided by Canadian Network for Research and Innovation in Machining Technology, Natural Sciences and Engineering Research Council of Canada (Grant No. IRCPJ 463100-13).

References

1. Wolf R, Clement F, Barkema HW, Orsel K (2014) Economic evaluation of participation in a voluntary Johne's disease prevention and control program from a farmer's perspective-The Alberta Johne's Disease Initiative. J Dairy Sci 97:2822–2834

2. McKenna SL, Keefe GP, Tiwari A, VanLeeuwen JA, Barkema HW (2006) Johne's disease in Canada Part II: disease impacts, risk factors, and control programs for dairy producers. Can Vet J 47:1089–1099

3. Cho J, Tauer LW, Schukken YH, Smith RL, Lu Z, Gröhn YT (2013) Cost-effective control strategies for Johne's disease in dairy herds. Can J Agric Econ 61:583–608

4. Smith RL, Grohn YT, Pradhan AK, Whitlock RH, Van Kessel JS, Smith JM, Wolfgang DR, Schukken YH (2016) The effects of progressing and non-progressing Mycobacterium avium ssp. paratuberculosis infection on milk production in dairy cows. J Dairy Sci 99:1383–1390

5. Tiwari A, VanLeeuwen JA, McKenna SL, Keefe GP, Barkema HW (2006) Johne's disease in Canada Part I: clinical symptoms, pathophysioology, diagnosis, and prevalence in dairy herds. Can Vet J 47:874–882

6. Koets A, Hoek A, Langelaar M, Overdijk M, Santema W, Franken P, Eden W, Rutten V (2006) Mycobacterial 70 kD heat-shock protein is an effective subunit vaccine against bovine paratuberculosis. Vaccine 24:2550–2559

7. Kalis CH, Hesselink JW, Barkema HW, Collins MT (2001) Use of long-term vaccination with a killed vaccine to prevent fecal shedding of Mycobacterium avium subsp. paratuberculosis in dairy herds. Am J Vet Res 62:270–274

8. Collins MT, Eggleston V, Manning EJ (2010) Successful control of Johne's disease in nine dairy herds: results of a six-year field trial. J Dairy Sci 93:1638–1643

9. Harris NB, Barletta RG (2001) Mycobacterium avium subsp. paratuberculosis in veterinary medicine. Clin Microbiol Rev 14:489–512

10. Slater N, Mitchell RM, Whitlock RH, Fyock T, Pradhan AK, Knupfer E, Schukken YH, Louzoun Y (2016) Impact of the shedding level on transmission of persistent infections in Mycobacterium avium subspecies paratuberculosis (MAP). Vet Res 47:38

11. Garry F (2011) Control of paratuberculosis in dairy herds. Vet Clin North Am Food Anim Pract 27:599–607

12. Whitlock RH (2010) Paratuberculosis control measures in the USA. In: Behr MA, Collins DM (eds) Paratuberculosis: organism, disease, control. CABI, Wallingford

13. Bakker D (2010) Paratuberculosis control measures in Europe. In: Behr MA, Collins DM (eds) Paratubercuosis: organism, disease, control. CABI, Wallingford

14. Sorge US, Lissemore K, Godkin A, Jansen J, Hendrick S, Wells S, Kelton DF (2011) Changes in management practices and apparent prevalence on Canadian dairy farms participating in a voluntary risk assessment-based Johne's disease control program. J Dairy Sci 94:5227–5237

15. Mortier R, Barkema HW, Orsel K, Wolf R, De Buck J (2014) Shedding patterns of dairy calves experimentally infected with Mycobacterium avium subspecies paratuberculosis. Vet Res 45:71

16. Mortier R, Barkema HW, Bystrom J, Illanes O, Orsel K, Wolf R, Atkins G, De Buck J (2013) Evaluation of age-dependent susceptibility in calves infected with two doses of Mycobacterium avium subspecies paratuberculosis using pathology and tissue culture. Vet Res 44:94

17. van Roermund HJ, Bakker D, Willemsen PT, de Jong MC (2007) Horizontal transmission of Mycobacterium avium subsp. paratuberculosis in cattle in an experimental setting: calves can transmit the infection to other calves. Vet Microbiol 122:270–279

18. Wolf R, Orsel K, De Buck J, Barkema HW (2015) Calves shedding Mycobacterium avium subspecies paratuberculosis are common on infected dairy farms. Vet Res 46:71

19. Weber MF, Kogut J, de Bree J, van Schaik G, Nielen M (2010) Age at which dairy cattle become Mycobacterium avium subsp. paratuberculosis faecal culture positive. Prev Vet Med 97:29–36

20. Whittington RJ, Windsor PA (2009) In utero infection of cattle with Mycobacterium avium subsp. paratuberculosis: a critical review and meta-analysis. Vet J 179:60–69

21. Pithua P, Espejo LA, Godden SM, Wells SJ (2013) Is an individual calving pen better than a group calving pen for preventing transmission of Mycobacterium avium subsp. paratuberculosis in calves? Results from a field trial. Res Vet Sci 95:398–404

22. Santema WJ, Poot J, Segers RP, Van den Hoff DJ, Rutten VP, Koets AP (2012) Early infection dynamics after experimental challenge with Mycobacterium avium subspecies paratuberculosis in calves reveal limited calf-to-calf transmission and no impact of Hsp70 vaccination. Vaccine 30:7032–7039

23. Mitchell RM, Medley GF, Collins MT, Schukken YH (2012) A meta-analysis of the effect of dose and age at exposure on shedding of Mycobacterium avium subspecies paratuberculosis (MAP) in experimentally infected calves and cows. Epidemiol Infect 140:231–246

24. Marce C, Ezanno P, Seegers H, Pfeiffer DU, Fourichon C (2011) Predicting fadeout versus persistence of paratuberculosis in a dairy cattle herd for management and control purposes: a modelling study. Vet Res 42:36

25. McNab B, Meek AH, Duncan RJ, Brooks BW, Van Dreumel AA, Martin SW, Nielson KH, Sugden EA, Turcotte C (1991) An evaluation of selected screening tests for bovine paratuberculosis. Can J Vet Res 55:252–259

26. Sweeney RW, Whitlock RH, Hamir AN, Rosenberger AE, Herr SA (1992) Isolation of Mycobacterium paratuberculosis after oral inoculation in uninfected cattle. Am J Vet Res 53:1312–1314

27. Wolf R, Barkema HW, De Buck J, Slomp M, Flaig J, Haupstein D, Pickel C, Orsel K (2014) High herd-level prevalence of Mycobacterium avium subspecies paratuberculosis in Western Canadian dairy farms, based on environmental sampling. J Dairy Sci 97:6250–6259

28. Eisenberg SW, Koets AP, Nielen M, Heederik D, Mortier R, De Buck J, Orsel K (2011) Intestinal infection following aerosol challenge of calves with Mycobacterium avium subspecies paratuberculosis. Vet Res 42:117

29. Forde T, Kutz S, De Buck J, Warren A, Ruckstuhl K, Pybus M, Orsel K (2012) Occurence, diagnosis, and strain typing of Mycobacterium avium subsp. paratuberculosis infection in Rocky Mountain bighorn sheep (Ovis canadensis canadensis) in southwest Alberta. J Wildlife Dis 48:1–11

30. Slana I, Kralik P, Kralova A, Pavlik I (2008) On-farm spread of Mycobacterium avium subsp. paratuberculosis in raw milk studied by IS900 and F57 competitive real time quantitative PCR and culture examination. Int J Food Microbiol 128:250–257

31. Mortier RA, Barkema HW, Wilson TA, Sajobi TT, Wolf R, De Buck J (2014) Dose-dependent interferon-gamma release in dairy calves experimentally infected with Mycobacterium avium subspecies paratuberculosis. Vet Immunol Immunopathol 161:205–210

32. Kalis CHJ, Collins MT, Hesselink JW, Barkema HW (2003) Specificity of two tests for the early diagnosis of bovine paratuberculosis based on cell-mediated immunity: the Johnin skin test and the gamma interferon assay. Vet Microbiol 97:73–86

33. Mortier RA, Barkema HW, Negron ME, Orsel K, Wolf R, De Buck J (2014) Antibody response early after experimental infection with Mycobacterium avium subspecies paratuberculosis in dairy calves. J Dairy Sci 97:5558–5565

34. Jungersen G, Huda A, Hansen JJ, Lind P (2002) Interpretation of the gamma interferon test for diagnosis of subclinical paratuberculosis in cattle. Clin Vaccine Immunol 9:453–460

35. Sweeney RW, Uzonna J, Whitlock RH, Habecker PL, Chilton P, Scott P (2006) Tissue predilection sites and effect of dose on Mycobacterium avium subs. paratuberculosis organism recovery in a short-term bovine experimental oral infection model. Res Vet Sci 80:253–259

36. Arsenault RJ, Maattanen P, Daigle J, Potter A, Griebel P, Napper S (2014) From mouth to macrophage: mechanisms of innate immune subversion by Mycobacterium avium subsp. paratuberculosis. Vet Res 45:54

37. Waters WR, Miller JM, Palmer MV, Stabel JR, Jones DE, Koistinen KA, Steadham EM, Hamilton MJ, Davis WC, Bannantine JP (2003) Early induction of humoral and cellular immune responses during experimental Mycobacterium avium subsp. paratuberculosis infection of calves. Infect Immun 71:5130–5138

38. Mortier RA, Barkema HW, De Buck J (2015) Susceptibility to and diagnosis of Mycobacterium avium subspecies paratuberculosis infection in dairy calves: a review. Prev Vet Med 121:189–198

39. Begg DJ, Whittington RJ (2008) Experimental animal infection models for Johne's disease, an infectious enteropathy caused by Mycobacterium avium subsp. paratuberculosis. Vet J 176:129–145

40. Koets AP, Eda S, Sreevatsan S (2015) The within host dynamics of Mycobacterium avium ssp. paratuberculosis infection in cattle: where time and place matter. Vet Res 46:61

41. Kralik P, Pribylova-Dziedzinska R, Kralova A, Kovarcik K, Slana I (2014) Evidence of passive faecal shedding of Mycobacterium avium subsp. paratuberculosis in a Limousin cattle herd. Vet J 201:91–94

Fecal shedding and tissue infections demonstrate transmission of Mycobacterium avium...

59

42. Subharat S, Shu D, Wedlock DN, Price-Carter M, de Lisle GW, Luo D, Collins DM, Buddle BM (2012) Immune responses associated with progression and control of infection in calves experimentally challenged with *Mycobacterium avium* subsp. *paratuberculosis*. Vet Immunol Immunopathol 149:225–236

43. Munster P, Volkel I, Wemheuer W, Schwarz D, Doring S, Czerny CP (2013) A longitudinal study to characterize the distribution patterns of *Mycobacterium avium* ssp. *paratuberculosis* in semen, blood and faeces of a naturally infected bull by IS 900 semi-nested and quantitative real-time PCR. Transbound Emerg Dis 60:175–187

44. Collins MT (2011) Diagnosis of paratuberculosis. Vet Clin North Am Food Anim Pract 27:581–591

45. Billman-Jacobe H, Carrigan M, Cockram F, Corner LA, Gill IJ, HIll JF, Milner AR, Wood PR (1992) A comparison of the interferon gamma assay with the absorbed ELISA for diagnosis of Johne's disease in cattle. Aus Vet J 69:25–28

46. Dargatz DA, Beverly AB, Barber LK, Sweeney RW, Whitlock RH, Shulaw WP, Jacobson RH, Stabel JR (2001) Evaluation of a commercial ELISA for diagnosis of paratuberculosis in cattle. J Am Vet Med Assoc 218:1163–1166

47. Kawaji S, Nagata R, Whittington RJ, Mori Y (2012) Detection of antibody responses against *Mycobacterium avium* subsp. *paratuberculosis* stress-associated proteins within 30 weeks after infection in cattle. Vet Immunol Immunopathol 150:101–111

48. Bannantine JP, Bayles DO, Waters WR, Palmer MV, Stabel JR, Paustian ML (2008) Early antibody response against *Mycobacterium avium* subspecies *paratuberculosis* antigens in subclinical cattle. Proteome Sci 6:5

49. Whitlock RH, Wells S, Sweeney RW, Van Tiem J (2000) ELISA and fecal culture for paratuberculosis (Johne's disease): sensitivity and specificity of each method. Vet Microbiol 77:387–398

50. Rogers PR, Dubey C, Swain SL (2000) Qualitative changes accompany memory T cell generation: faster, more effective responses at lower doses of antigen. J Immunol 164:2338–2346

51. McDonald WL, Ridge SE, Hope AF, Condron RJ (1999) Evaluation of diagnostic tests for Johne's disease in young cattle. Aus Vet J 77:113–119

5

Concurrent infection with porcine reproductive and respiratory syndrome virus and *Haemophilus parasuis* in two types of porcine macrophages: apoptosis, production of ROS and formation of multinucleated giant cells

Lenka Kavanová[1,2], Katarína Matiašková[1,3], Lenka Levá[1], Hana Štěpánová[1], Kateřina Nedbalcová[1], Ján Matiašovic[1], Martin Faldyna[1] and Jiří Salát[1*]

Abstract

Porcine reproductive and respiratory syndrome (PRRS) is one of the most significant and economically important infectious diseases affecting swine worldwide and can predispose pigs to secondary bacterial infections caused by, e.g. *Haemophilus parasuis*. The aim of the presented study was to compare susceptibility of two different types of macrophages which could be in contact with both pathogens during infection with PRRS virus (PRRSV) and in co-infection with *H. parasuis*. Alveolar macrophages (PAMs) as resident cells provide one of the first lines of defence against microbes invading lung tissue. On the other hand, monocyte derived macrophages (MDMs) represent inflammatory cells accumulating at the site of inflammation. While PAMs were relatively resistant to cytopathogenic effect caused by PRRSV, MDMs were much more sensitive to PRRSV infection. MDMs infected with PRRSV increased expression of pro-apoptotic Bad, Bax and p53 mRNA. Increased mortality of MDMs may be also related to a higher intensity of ROS production after infection with PRRSV. In addition, MDMs (but not PAMs) infected with *H. parasuis* alone formed multinucleated giant cells (MGC); these cells were not observed in MDMs infected with both pathogens. Higher sensitivity of MDMs to PRRSV infection, which is associated with limited MDMs survival and restriction of MGC formation, could contribute to the development of multifactorial respiratory disease of swine.

Introduction

Porcine reproductive and respiratory syndrome (PRRS) is one of the most significant and economically important infectious diseases affecting swine worldwide [1]. The causative agent is porcine reproductive and respiratory syndrome virus (PRRSV). It is an enveloped, positive-stranded RNA virus, belonging to the family *Arteriviridae*. PRRSV is associated with respiratory distress and reproductive failure in swine and poor growth performance in piglets [2].

The PRRSV targets cells of the porcine monocyte/macrophage lineage [3] where CD163 is the essential receptor for the virus infection [4, 5]. PRRSV primarily replicates in differentiated porcine alveolar macrophages (PAMs) [6, 7] but it has been identified in macrophages located in tissues, including lymph nodes, thymus, spleen, Peyer's patches and liver [7, 8]. The expression of CD163 is dependent on the differentiation levels of monocyte lineage cells. Freshly isolated peripheral blood monocytes express extremely low levels of CD163 and are not

*Correspondence: salat@vri.cz
[1] Veterinary Research Institute, Hudcova 296/70, 62100 Brno, Czech Republic
Full list of author information is available at the end of the article

susceptible to PRRSV infection [5] but as monocytes differentiate/age, the expression of CD163 increases and their susceptibility to PRRSV infection is enhanced [9]. Monocyte-derived macrophages (MDMs) [10] can be used as an alternative model for in vitro infection with PRRSV [5, 11, 12].

There are a number of published studies demonstrating that PRRSV induces apoptosis [13–15]. This highly regulated process is modulated by both pro-apoptotic and anti-apoptotic cellular factors. Two distinct pathways of apoptosis have been described: intrinsic and extrinsic apoptosis. Intrinsic apoptosis is initiated as a response to cellular stressors. The protein p53 is activated following DNA damage and triggers apoptosis through transcriptional activation of the Bcl-2 associated (Bax) gene [16]. It is still unclear whether PRRSV can induce apoptosis directly (within infected cells) or indirectly (within bystander cells) [16]. Cell apoptosis was mainly observed in PRRSV-inoculated MARC-145 cells [13, 14, 17, 18] and PAMs [19] but there is little information about mortality and cell apoptosis of PRRSV infected MDMs.

The PRRSV is considered to be one of the key etiological agents in multifactorial respiratory disease of swine. The virus can predispose pigs to infection by bacteria such as *Streptococcus suis*, *Haemophilus parasuis*, *Mycoplasma hyopneumoniae*, *Actinobacillus pleuropneumoniae* and *Salmonella* spp. [20–24]. The additive effect of PRRSV infection and a secondary bacterial infection in the induction of multifactorial respiratory diseases was described in the case of *H. parasuis* [25, 26].

Macrophages play an important role in the first line of defence against invading pathogens where production of reactive oxygen species (ROS) is one of the most important antimicrobial mechanisms. Oxidative stress caused by ROS has been suggested as an apoptosis mediator in virus-infected cells [27]. Increased ROS production was detected in the lungs of PRRSV-challenged pigs [28]. On the other hand, bacteria such as *Haemophilus influenzae* have evolved the OxyR system which coordinates the expression of numerous defensive antioxidants [29, 30].

Information about sensitivity of various types of macrophages to infection with PRRS virus in co-infection with *H. parasuis* is lacking. Viability of cells, virus replication, ROS production and apoptosis of different types of co-infected macrophages in vitro was analysed in this study in order to gain understanding of macrophage interactions with PRRSV and *H. parasuis* in multifactorial respiratory swine disease.

Materials and methods

Virus
The Lelystad strain of PRRSV (CAPM V-490) was obtained from the Collection of Animal Pathogenic Microorganisms (CAPM) at the Veterinary Research Institute (Brno, Czech Republic). The virus was propagated on the MARC-145 cell line and maintained in Dulbecco Modified Eagle's Medium (DMEM) (Invitrogen) supplemented with 10% foetal bovine serum (FBS) (Thermo Scientific), 1% antibiotics (Antibiotic Antimycotic Solution 100×: 10 000 units penicillin, 10 mg streptomycin, and 25 μg amphotericin B per mL; Sigma-Aldrich) at 37 °C and 5% CO_2. The virus was clarified by centrifugation, and its concentration was determined by plaque assay. The concentration of stock virus used in experiments was 5×10^6 plaque forming units per mL.

Bacteria
Haemophilus parasuis serotype 5, strain HP 132 (CAPM 6475) originating from a pig with meningitis was obtained from CAPM. Bacteria were grown on Mueller–Hinton agar broth with yeast extract and 5% sheep blood (LabMediaServis) overnight at 37 °C, and non-confluent growth was harvested and resuspended in calcium–magnesium free Dulbecco's phosphate-buffered saline (D-PBS, Lonza). Bacteria were washed twice with D-PBS and resuspended in D-PBS, with the final concentration adjusted to optical density of 2.5 equivalent to 10^9 CFU/mL, using a turbidimeter (DEN-1 McFarland densitometer, Biosan).

Preparation of MDMs
CD14+ porcine monocytes were isolated from whole blood as described previously [31]. Peripheral blood mononuclear cells (PBMCs) were isolated from heparinized blood by Histopaque-1077 (Sigma-Aldrich) gradient. Monocytes were further enriched to a purity of >95% by positive magnetic bead selection (QuadroMACS™ cell separator, Miltenyi Biotec) using monoclonal antibody directed against CD14 (clone MIL2, AbD Serotec, Oxford, UK, 10 μL per 10^8 cells) and goat anti-mouse IgG microbeads together with LS separation columns (Miltenyi Biotec). The obtained cells were cultured in 24-well plates at a concentration of 5×10^5 cells per well in 1 mL of complete medium (DMEM with 10% FBS and 1% antibiotics) and incubated for 4 days at 37 °C in 5% CO_2 to differentiate into macrophages. The cells for chemiluminescence assay were cultured in Nunc-Immuno™ Micro-Well™ 96-well polystyrene plates (Sigma-Aldrich) at a concentration of 1×10^5 in 250 μL of complete medium and incubated for 4 days at 37 °C in 5% CO_2 to differentiate into macrophages.

Preparation of PAMs
PAMs were collected as described previously [32] by bronchoalveolar lavage from five 6 to 8 week-old pigs from a PRRSV negative herd. The use of animals was

approved by the Ethical committee of Ministry of Agriculture (approval protocol No. MZe 1487) as a part of project Respig (QJ1210120). Briefly, pigs were euthanized with the intravenous injection of the anaesthetic T61 (Intervet International B.V.) based on body weight according to the manufacturer's recommendations (5 mL/50 kg of body weight) and necropsied. The trachea and lungs were immediately removed, and the lungs were flushed with D-PBS. The aliquots with PAMs were frozen in a medium containing 75% RPMI-1640, 20% FBS and 5% dimethylsulphoxide (DMSO) (Sigma-Aldrich) and stored in liquid nitrogen until use. PAMs were thawed in a water bath at 37 °C before each experiment. Cell viability after the freeze/thaw process as determined by trypan blue exclusion was higher than 90%. The cells were washed by DMEM prior to use in the experiments. Porcine alveolar macrophages were placed into 24-well polystyrene culture plates at a concentration of 5×10^5 cells per well in 1 mL of complete medium (DMEM with 10% FBS and 1% antibiotics) and incubated overnight at 37 °C in 5% CO_2.

Flow cytometry

Differentiation of MDMs and differences in the expression of the surface molecule CD163 between MDMs and PAMs were evaluated by flow cytometry. The cells were harvested by 0.2% EDTA in PBS, washed in PBS and labelled with the following unlabelled primary antibodies against surface protein: anti-CD163 (2A10/11, IgG1, Biorad). AlexaFluor 488-conjugated mouse IgG1 or IgG2a isotype-specific goat antisera (Invitrogen) were used as the secondary antibodies. Control samples were stained with secondary antibody only. Flow cytometry was performed using a LSR Fortessa flow cytometer operated by Diva software (Becton–Dickinson). Data are shown as median fluorescence intensity ratio (MFI ratio); MFI ratio = MFI of specific Ab-stained cells + AlexaFluor 488-conjugated mouse IgG1 (CD163)/MFI of control cells stained only with AlexaFluor 488-conjugated mouse IgG1 or IgG2a isotype-specific secondary antibody. The experiment was performed using PAMs/MDMs isolated from four pigs.

Experimental design and sampling

Prepared macrophages were washed with complete medium and infected with PRRSV in multiplicity of infection (MOI) 0.5 at 24 h after seeding (PAMs) or immediately after differentiation (MDMs). The medium from uninfected MARC-145 cells was used as mock-infection, and complete medium alone was used as a control. Twenty-four hours post-infection (PI) with PRRSV, macrophages were washed to remove antibiotics and subsequently infected with *H. parasuis* (MOI 10).

Dulbecco's PBS was used as a control solution in groups without *H. parasuis*. The following groups were included in the trial: (1) PRRSV + *H. parasuis* infected, (2) PRRSV infected, (3) mock + *H. parasuis* infected, (4) mock infected, (5) *H. parasuis* infected, and (6) non-infected control. The culture supernatants were collected at 4 h PI with *H. parasuis*/28 h PI with PRRSV (4/28 h PI) and 24 h PI with *H. parasuis*/48 h PI with PRRSV (24/48 h PI) for the evaluation cell mortality early (4/28 h) or late (24/48 h) after infection with the bacterium/virus. Total RNA was extracted from the harvested cells at the same experimental time points. Five independent experiments including culture duplicates were conducted, using PAMs/MDMs isolated from five pigs.

Cell mortality

Mortality of infected cells was detected using the CytoTox 96 Non-Radioactive Cytotoxicity assay (Promega) following the manufacturer's instructions.

PRRSV and *H. parasuis* quantification

PRRSV replication in PAMs/MDMs was determined by virus titration method. The growth of bacteria was measured by spectrophotometry (A_{600} nm) according to Bello-Ortí et al. [33] and Lichtensteiger and Vimr [34]. Cells were infected with PRRSV at MOI 0.5 and incubated with the virus for 2 h at 37 °C in 5% CO_2. The cells were washed once and the complete medium was added. Twenty-four hours PI with PRRSV were macrophages infected with *H. parasuis* (MOI 10). Cells were frozen at −80 °C at 0, 28, 48, 72, 96 h PI with PRRSV and 4, 24, 48 and 72 h PI with *H. parasuis* for the evaluation of PRRSV titres and bacterial growth. The supernatant was assayed using the standard method on MARC-145 cells. The virus titres were expressed as $TCID_{50}$/mL (50% tissue culture infectious dose per mL) to examine the virus replication in PAMs or MDMs. $TCID_{50}$/mL was calculated by the Spearman & Kärber algorithm as described in Hierholzer and Killington [35]. Cytopathic effect was observed using light microscopy. Microscopy was performed using a microscope Olympus IX51. Supernatant for evaluation of bacteria growth was centrifuged at 6000 *g* for 10 min, the pellets was resuspended in DPBS and absorbance at 600 nm was measured.

Real-time RT-PCR for the detection of apoptosis related genes mRNA

Bad, Bax, p53 and Bcl-2 expression were quantified by real-time RT-PCR. RNA was isolated from harvested PAMs/MDMs using the RNeasy Mini Kit (Qiagen) following manufacturer's instructions. M-MLV reverse transcriptase (Invitrogen) and oligo-dT primers (Generi Biotech) were used for reverse transcription.

Measurements were performed using the QuantiTect SYBR Green PCR Kit (Qiagen) and gene specific primers (Generi Biotech) (Table 1) on a LightCycler 480 II with a 384-well plate block (Roche). Primers were designed using NCBI primer designing tool (http://www.ncbi.nlm.nih.gov/tools/primer-blast/). Hypoxanthine phosphoribosyltransferase (HPRT) was evaluated as the most constitutively expressed gene in our samples using RefFinder tool (http://www.leonxie.com/referencegene.php) and was selected to adjust mRNA measurements. The other tested genes which showed less stabile transcription were: TATA binding protein 1 and hydroxymethylbilane synthase. The threshold cycle values (Ct) of the genes of interest were first normalized to the Ct value of HPRT reference mRNA (ΔCt), and the normalized mRNA levels were calculated as $2^{(-\Delta Ct)}$. The results are presented as mean values of fold increase of the gene of interest.

Fluorescence microscopy

The cells were grown on 24 well-plates as described above. After 4 h and 24 h PI with *H. parasuis*, the cells were fixed with 4% paraformaldehyde, macrophages were labelled with DAPI (nuclear stain) (Sigma-Aldrich) and with Alexa Fluor (AF) 594 conjugated phalloidin (Life Technologies) to visualize the actin cytoskeleton. Microscopy was performed using an epifluorescence inverted microscope Olympus IX51 equipped with a LUCPlanFLN 40 × (NA 0.60) objective using fluorescence mode to detect DAPI and AF-594.

Chemiluminescence assay

Production of reactive oxygen species of experimentally infected PAMs and MDMs was measured using chemiluminescence (CL). The assay was performed in Nunc-Immuno™ MicroWell™ 96-well polystyrene plates (Sigma-Aldrich). Cells were seeded in DMEM with 1% antibiotics and 10% FBS at a concentration of 1×10^5 cells per well. The cells were incubated overnight at

37 °C in 5% CO_2. The medium with non-adherent cells was removed, and cells were infected with PRRSV at MOI 0.5 or the mock infection solution or the control medium was added. Cells were washed with Hanks' balanced salt solution (HBSS, Lonza) 24 h and 48 h PI with PRRSV. Luminol-derivative L-012 (Wako Chemicals GmbH) was added to amplify the CL induced by ROS of stimulated cells. L-012 was diluted in HBSS to the final concentration of 0.15 mmol/L. A suspension of *H. parasuis* (MOI 10) was then added to the cell culture containing luminol L-012, and the plate was centrifuged at 250g for 5 min. The following groups were included: (1) PRRSV + *H. parasuis* infected, (2) PRRSV infected, (3) mock + *H. parasuis* infected, (4) mock infected, (5) *H. parasuis* infected, and (6) non-infected control. Chemiluminescence was measured immediately after adding *H. parasuis* at 37 °C using a multidetection microplate reader Synergy H1 (BioTek) in kinetic mode for 2 h. The results are expressed as integrals of chemiluminescence intensity (per 1×10^5 viable cells) induced in PAMs/MDMs with infection(s), and data are presented as percentage relative to the non-infected control. The viability of cells was measured using the CCK-8 kit (Sigma-Aldrich), following manufacturer's instructions. Five independent experiments including culture triplicates were performed using PAMs/MDMs isolated from five pigs.

Statistical analysis

The normality of data distribution was confirmed by the Shapiro–Wilk's W test, and homogeneity of variances by the Levene's test. Experimental groups were compared with Student's t test (mortality, multinucleated giant cells) or using a non-parametric test for paired samples, (Wilcoxon signed-rank test; flow cytometry, *H. parasuis* growth, expression of apoptosis related genes, chemiluminescence assay). A p value of < 0.05 was considered significant, unless otherwise stated. Data were analysed using Statistica 12 (StatSoft).

Results

Flow cytometry

Peripheral blood monocytes differentiated within 4 days of culture. Differentiation was confirmed by elevated amounts of CD163(+) population from 42.1 ±5.9% to 93.6 ± 7.0% ($p < 0.05$) (Figure 1A) (Additional file 1).

The difference between the two macrophage types was further observed by the flow cytometry analysis (Figure 1). The percentage of CD163 positive cells in MDMs was similar to percentage of positive cells in PAMs (Figure 1A). On the other hand, the expression of CD163 on MDMs was significantly higher ($p < 0.05$) than on PAMs (Figure 1B).

Table 1 Primers used for real time PCR quantification of gene expression.

	Sequence 5'–3'	Reference
Bad-For	CTG GGC TGC ACA GCG TTA T	This study
Bad-Rev	GGC GAG GAA GTC CCT TCT TG	This study
Bcl2-For	AGT ACC TGA ACC GGC ACC TG	This study
Bcl2-Rev	CAG CCA GGA GAA ATC AAA TAG AGG	This study
Bax-For	AAC ATG GAG CTG CAG AGG ATG	This study
Bax-Rev	GTT GCC GTC AGC AAA CAT TTC	This study
HPRT-For	GAG CTA CTG TAA TGA CCA GTC AAC G	[32]
HPRT-Rev	CCA GTG TCA ATT ATA TCT TCA ACA ATC AA	[32]
p53-For	AAA AGA AGA AGC CAC TGG ATG G	This study
p53-Rev	GTC ATT CAG CTC TCG GAA CAT CT	This study

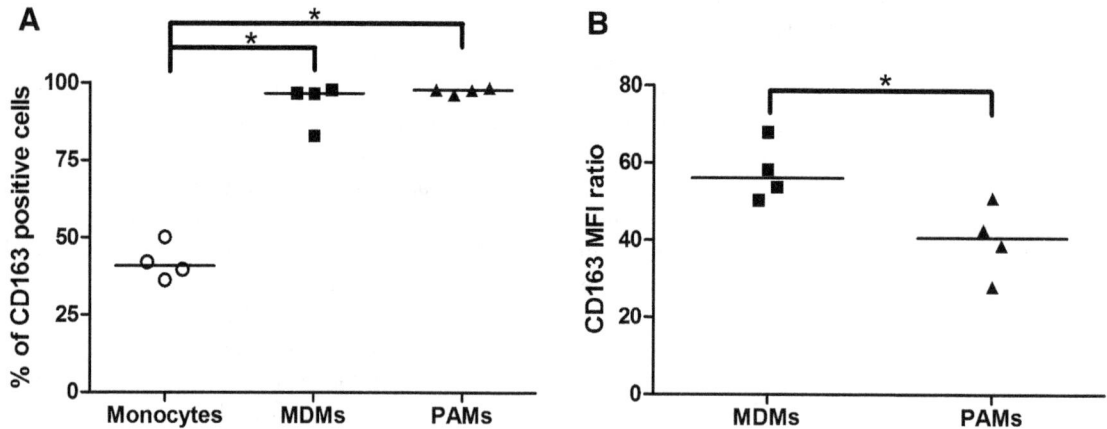

Figure 1 Surface marker CD163 on monocytes, MDMs and PAMs. Percentage of positive cells (**A**) and MFI ratio: the ratio of the MFI of the positive population in a sample to its corresponding isotype control (**B**) was measured by flow cytometry. Data are presented as median of four animals and each dot represents the result of an individual pig. Significant differences between tested groups are denoted by *($p < 0.05$).

Mortality of infected MDMs/PAMs

The average mortality rates of non-infected/mock infected MDMs were 9.1 ± 7.6% and 22.6 ± 18.2% at 4/28 and 24/48 h, respectively. Mortality of the PRRSV infected MDMs was significantly increased to 61.0 ± 14.3% and 70.0 ± 3.7% at 4/28 and 24/48 h PI. The mortality was similar in the *H. parasuis* infected group and in non-infected/mock infected groups (2.2 ± 3.9% and 7.7 ± 11.9% PI with *H. parasuis*) (Figure 2A). *H. parasuis* did not affect mortality of simultaneously infected groups in both types of cells (Figure 2).

Mortality of infected PAMs was published in previous study [26]. Briefly, the mortality of non-infected/mock

infected PAMs was 2.7 ± 0.6% and 9.7 ± 1.5% at 4/28 and 24/48 h PI, respectively. Observed mortality of PRRSV infected PAMs was 3.7 ± 1.5% and 16.7 ± 9.3% at 4/28 and 24/48 h PI, respectively. *H. parasuis* infection was not associated with increased mortality of infected PAMs (3.0 ± 1.0% and 10.0 ± 1.7% at 4/28 and 24/48 h PI with *H. parasuis*) (Figure 2B).

All obtained results of the (3) mock-infected + *H. parasuis* group and the (4) mock infected group did not differ from (5) *H. parasuis* infected group and (6) non-infected control group, respectively. Therefore, only (1) PRRSV + *H. parasuis* infected, (2) PRRSV infected, (3) mock + *H. parasuis* infected, (4) and mock infected groups of PAMs/MDMs were included in the (Figure 2),

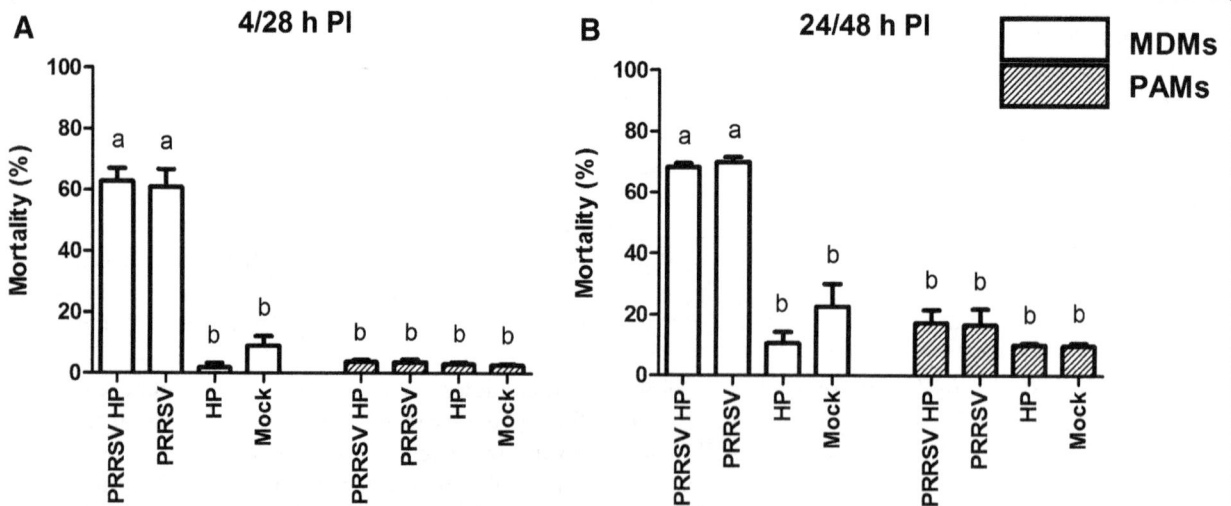

Figure 2 Mortality of macrophages infected with PRRSV and *H. parasuis* (HP). Mortality of MDM and PAMs was measured using CytoTox 96 non-radioactive Cytotoxicity assay at 4/28 h (**A**) and 24/48 h (**B**) PI with PRRSV and *H. parasuis*. Data are the mean ± SEM of three independent experiments. Significant differences between tested groups are denoted by different letters (a, b) ($p < 0.05$).

likewise the results regarding the expression of apoptosis related genes and chemiluminescence assay.

PRRSV replication in MDMs/PAMs

Cell culture medium was collected at 24, 48, 72 and 96 h to determine if elevated mortality of MDMs is related to virus replication. Our results show that PRRSV replicated in a similar pattern in both cell types (Table 2). The highest PRRSV titres were detected in culture supernatants of infected PAMs and MDMs at 24 h PI. Cell viability after PRRSV inoculation was observed by light microscopy. Decline of MDMs viability was observed after 24 h PI with PRRSV, while a decreased number of PAMs was observed after 96 h PI with PRRSV (Figure 3). Replication of virus was not affected by presence of *H. parasuis* (data not shown).

Growth of *H. parasuis*

Haemophilus parasuis growth was determined by spectrophotometry. *H. parasuis* added to the complete medium without antibiotics had absorbance at the background level at all assay times (data not shown). Growth of *H. parasuis* in wells with MDMs was affected by the presence of virus (Figure 4A). In the wells with *H. parasuis* infected MDMs were detected higher amounts of bacteria compared to wells with co-infected MDMs.

Table 2 Viral titres in the supernatant of PRRSV infected cultures from three independent experiments performed in culture triplicates are expressed as $TCID_{50}$/mL.

	Time post infection with PRRSV							
	24 h		48 h		72 h		96 h	
MDMs	3.78×10^5	$+sd\ 2.00 \times 10^5$ $-sd\ 1.31 \times 10^5$	6.31×10^4	$+sd\ 3.15 \times 10^4$ $-sd\ 2.10 \times 10^4$	1.76×10^4	$+sd\ 7.66 \times 10^3$ $-sd\ 5.33 \times 10^3$	1.76×10^4	$+sd\ 1.08 \times 10^4$ $-sd\ 6.68 \times 10^3$
PAMs	3.78×10^5	$+sd\ 2.32 \times 10^5$ $-sd\ 1.44 \times 10^5$	6.31×10^4	$+sd\ 3.88 \times 10^4$ $-sd\ 2.40 \times 10^4$	2.93×10^3	$+sd\ 1.18 \times 10^3$ $-sd\ 8.41 \times 10^2$	1.36×10^3	$+sd\ 7.19 \times 10^2$ $-sd\ 4.70 \times 10^2$

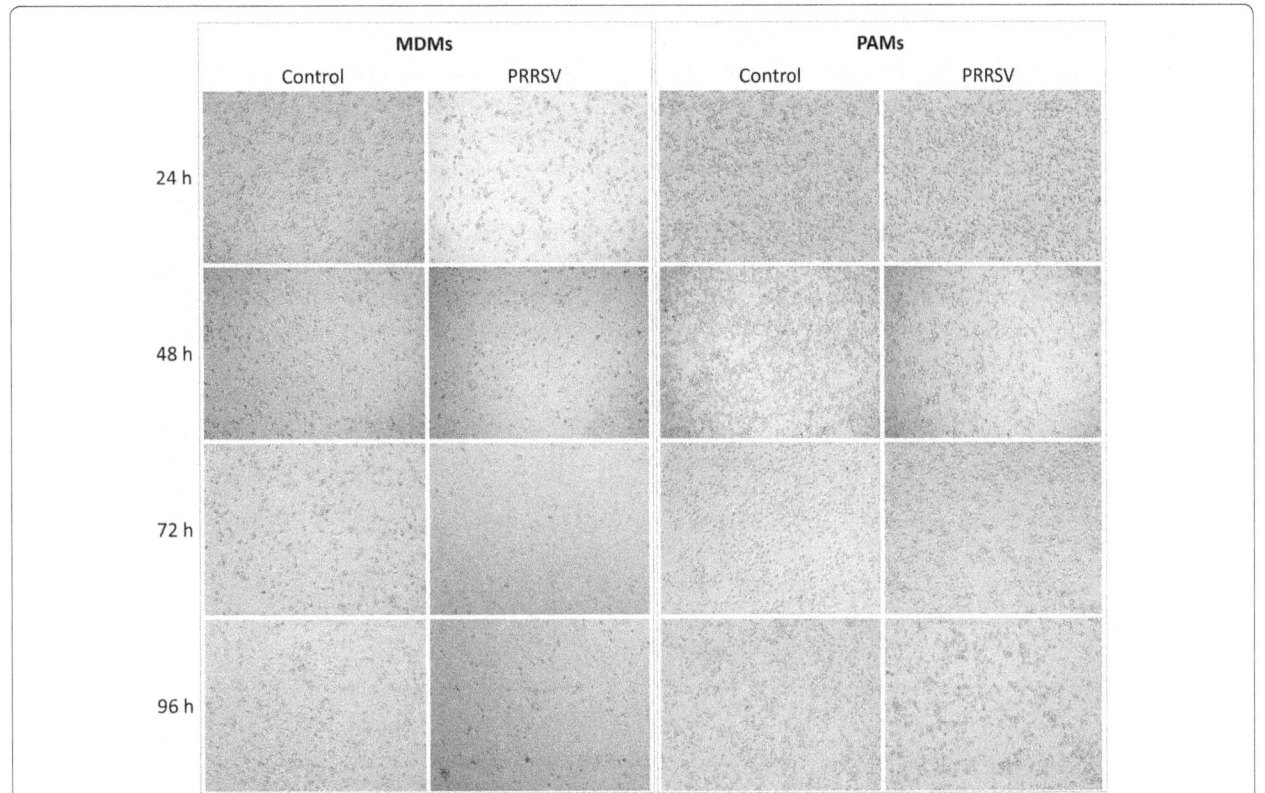

Figure 3 Viability of MDMs and PAMs infected with PRRSV. Cells were infected with PRRSV and observed by light microscopy at 24, 48, 72 and 96 h PI.

On the other hand, the amount of *H. parasuis* in PAMs infected with both pathogens was higher or on the same levels as in PAMs infected only with bacteria (Figure 4B).

Expression of apoptosis related genes

The influence of co-infection with PRRSV and *H. parasuis* on expression of apoptosis related genes was characterized in two types of macrophages. The degree of target gene expression was calculated as fold-expression of the reference gene hypoxanthine phosphoribosyltransferase (HPRT). Apoptosis was analysed using relative quantification of typical pro-apoptotic gene expression markers including Bad, Bax, p53 and anti-apoptotic gene Bcl-2.

MDMs

Haemophilus parasuis only and PRRSV only infected MDMs showed significant ($p < 0.05$) upregulation of the anti-apoptotic molecule Bcl-2 compared to controls at both assay times (Figure 5A). However, combined infection of MDMs with both pathogens or PRRSV only showed significantly ($p < 0.05$) lower expression of Bcl-2 mRNA in comparison with *H. parasuis* only infected MDMs at 4/28 h PI. On the other hand, simultaneously infected cells showed the highest expression ($p < 0.05$) of Bcl-2 mRNA at 24/48 h PI.

Although in both groups infected with PRRSV a significant increase of the pro-apoptotic molecule p53 mRNA was induced at both assay times (Figure 5B), the concurrent infection triggered a significantly lower response ($p < 0.05$) than in the PRRSV only infected group at 4/28 h PI. Expression of p53 mRNA was significantly downregulated ($p < 0.05$) after infection with *H. parasuis* alone compared to the mock infected group at 4/28 h PI.

The observed expression pattern of Bad mRNA (Figure 5C) was similar to that of p53 at 4/28 h PI, with the significantly decreased ($p < 0.05$) production of mRNA in *H. parasuis* infected MDMs in comparison with mock treated cells. The highest production of Bad mRNA ($p < 0.05$) was detected in PRRSV infected groups at both assay times. *H. parasuis* infection did not change the level of Bad mRNA expression compared to mock infected cells at 24/48 h PI.

Both groups infected with PRRSV, but not with *H. parasuis* alone, showed increased ($p < 0.05$) production of Bax mRNA at 4/28 h PI (Figure 5D). The increased level of Bax mRNA was detected after infections with both pathogens compared to mock infection at 24/48 h PI.

Co-infection of MDMs with both pathogens did not influence the expression of Bad and Bax mRNA at both assay times compared to appropriate control.

PAMs

Haemophilus parasuis infected PAMs induced significantly higher expression of anti-apoptotic Bcl-2 mRNA in comparison with mock infected PAMs at both assay times (Figure 5E). Expression of pro-apoptotic p53 mRNA was unchanged in all infected groups at both assay times (Figure 5F).

Decreased expression of pro-apoptotic Bad mRNA was observed at both assay times (Figure 5G). However, expression of the pro-apoptotic gene for Bax was up-regulated at 4 h PI with *H. parasuis* (Figure 5H).

The results showed that pro-apoptotic genes like Bad and Bax were not overexpressed after infection with PRRSV in PAMs (Figures 5G and H). PRRSV did not influence the level of Bcl-2 mRNA expression compared to mock infected cells (Figure 5E).

Combined infection with both pathogens did not change the levels of mRNA expression of apoptosis related genes compared to appropriate controls.

Multinucleated giant cells

The cells were monitored throughout the experiment by light microscopy. Control MDMs and mock-infected cell did not change their morphology during the experiment.

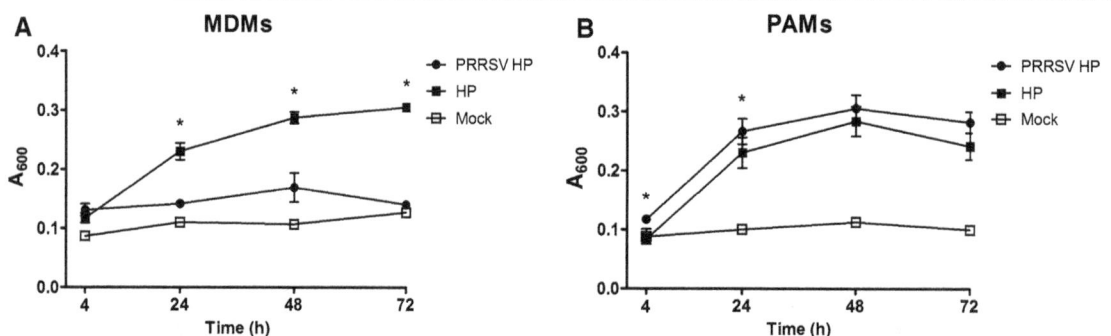

Figure 4 Growth of *H. parasuis* on MDMs (A) or PAMs (B) was measured by spectrophotometry (A_{600} nm). Mock curves serve as a baseline which includes cell debris from cultivated macrophages after freezing and thawing process. Data are presented as mean with SEM of three animals measured in culture duplicates. Significant differences between co-infected cells and cells infected with *H. parasuis* only are denoted by *($p < 0.05$).

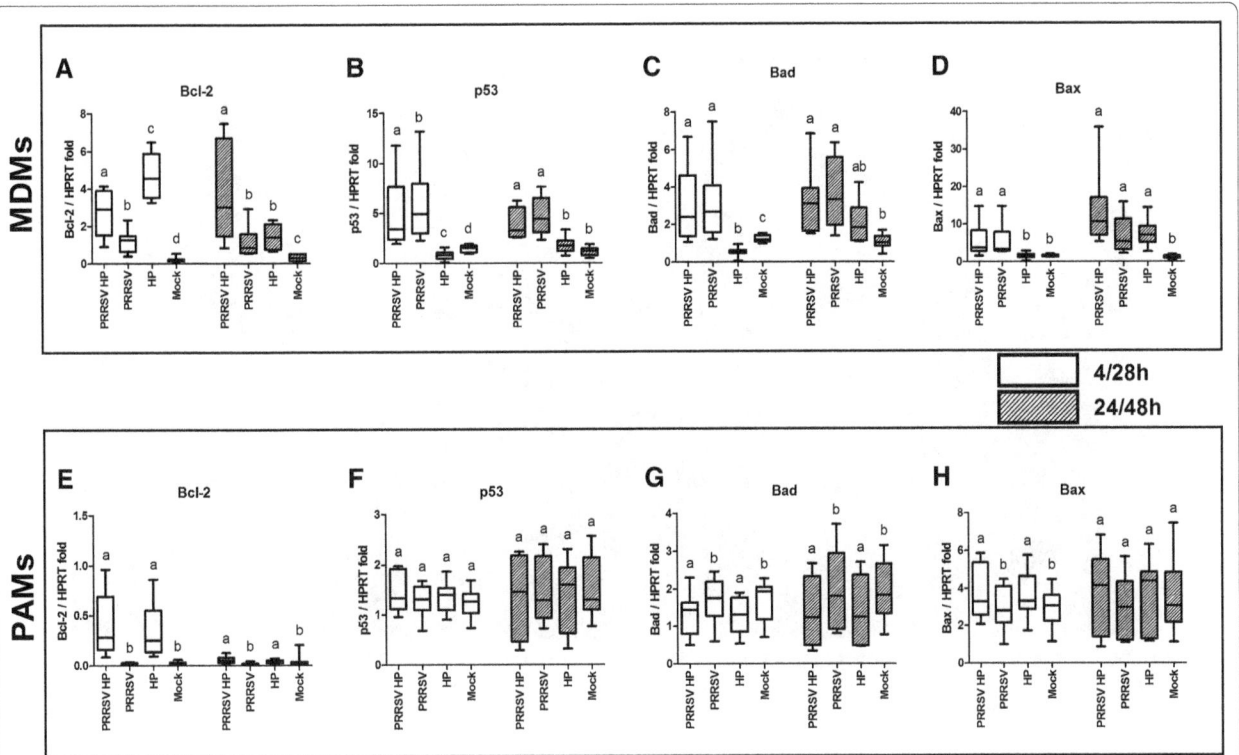

Figure 5 Expression rates of mRNA of selected apoptosis-related genes. Selected anti-apoptotic Bcl-2 (**A**, **E**) and pro-apoptotic p53 (**B**, **F**), Bad (**C**, **G**) and Bax (**D**, **H**) genes were measured by real-time PCR using gene specific primers at 4/28 and 24/48 h PI in MDMs (**A**, **B**, **C**, **D**) or PAMs (**E**, **F**, **G**, **H**). Boxplots indicate the median (middle line), 25th and 75th percentiles (boxes), and maximum and minimum (whiskers) of five independent experiments performed in culture duplicates. The degree of gene expression is displayed as fold change of the housekeeping gene hypoxanthine phosphoribosyltransferase (HPRT) expression. Mock-infected MDMs/PAMs served as controls for PRRSV infection. Significant differences between PRRSV and *H. parasuis* co-infected cells and other tested groups are denoted by different letters (a, b, c, d) ($p < 0.05$).

Excessively large cells were observed by light microscopy in the group of MDMs infected with *H. parasuis* at 24 h PI. Therefore, fluorescence microscopy was used and multinucleated giant cells (MGC) (Figure 6) were detected. The number of MGC induced by the bacterium was determined under a microscope (400 ×). Results showed that the number of nuclei per 100 cells was 102 ± 2.6 in non-infected and 160.2 ± 23.8 in *H. parasuis* infected MDMs ($p < 0.05$). The percentage of MGC induced by *H. parasuis* was $13.6 \pm 2.8\%$. MDMs infected with PRRSV or simultaneously infected with PRRSV and *H. parasuis* did not form MGC. Formation of MGC in PAMs was not observed (101.5 ± 1.2 and 101.3 ± 0.6 nuclei per 100 cells in non-infected and *H. parasuis* infected cells, respectively). Data shown represents means and standard errors of three independent experiments.

Chemiluminescence assay

Comparison of reactive oxygen species production by the co-infected, individually (PRRSV or *H. parasuis*) infected, and mock-infected macrophages is shown in Figure 7.

The highest production of ROS by MDMs was detected in the PRRSV infected group at 24 and 48 h PI (Figure 7A). On the other hand, *H. parasuis* reduced the production of ROS in comparison with relevant control groups at both assay times. MDMs infected with both pathogens showed decreased levels of released ROS in comparison with PRRSV infected groups at both assay times.

The observed ROS production in MDMs after infection with PRRSV and *H. parasuis* was similar to PAMs (Figure 7B). Significantly enhanced ($p < 0.05$) production of ROS was detected in the PRRSV infected group of PAMs at 24 and 48 h PI. Conversely, *H. parasuis* infection significantly reduced ($p < 0.05$) the intensity of the detected CL response compared to the mock-infected group. A significant ($p < 0.05$) reduction in ROS production was also observed in the co-infected group at 24 and 48 h PI compared with PRRSV-only and mock-infected groups.

The highest level of released ROS was observed in MDMs infected with PRRSV at 48 h PI (Figure 7A).

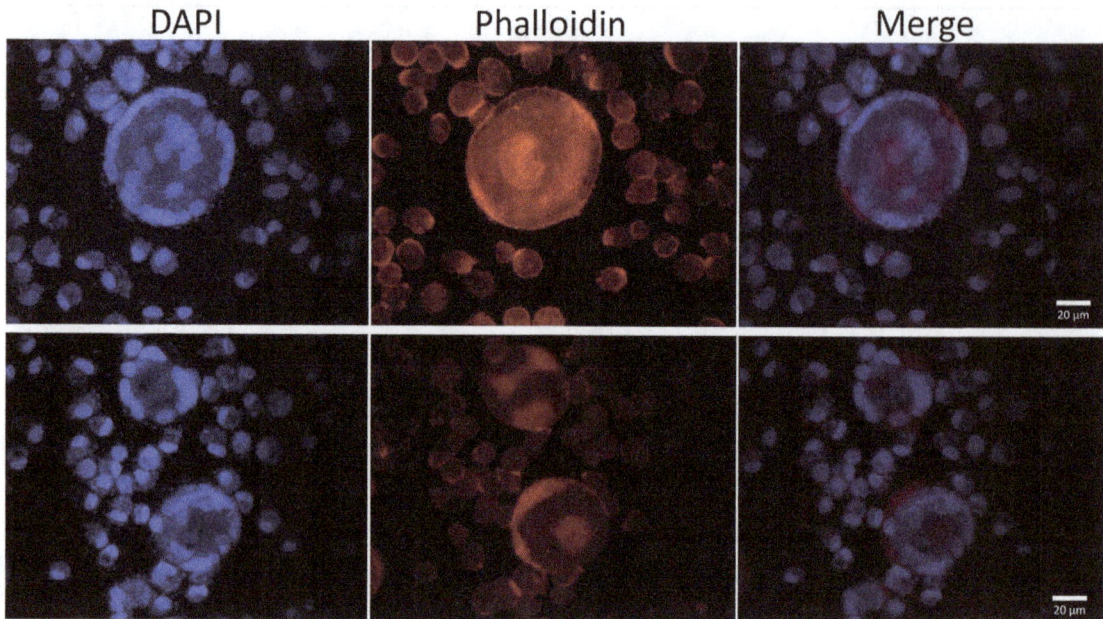

Figure 6 Typical examples of multinucleated giant cells of MDMs infected with *H. parasuis* (24 h PI). MDMs were stained with DAPI to label the nuclei (blue) and with Alexa Fluor 594 conjugate phalloidin to label the cytoskeleton (red).

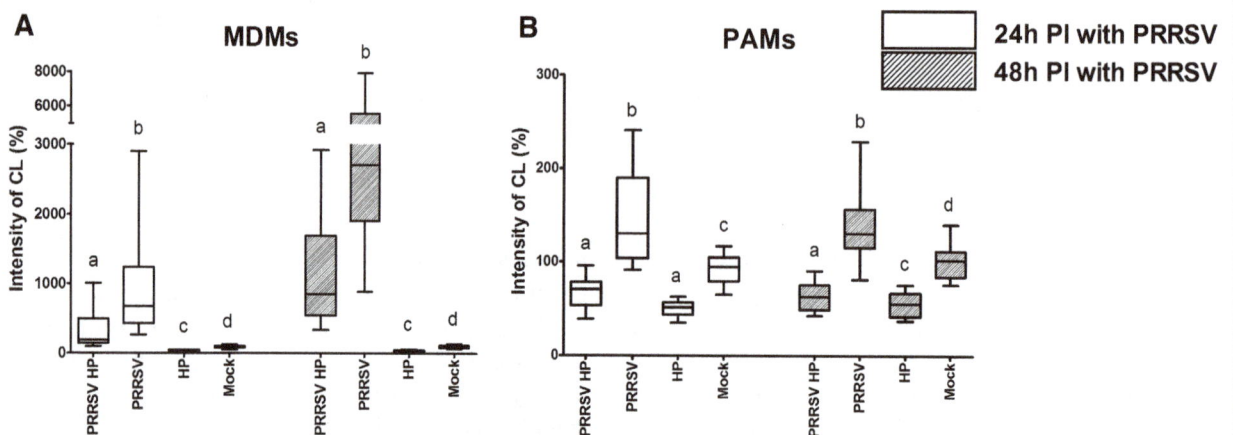

Figure 7 ROS production. ROS produced by MDMs (A) or PAMs (B) were measured by chemiluminescence assay at 24 and 48 h PI with PRRSV. Infection with *H. parasuis* was performed immediately prior to measurement. Data are presented as the percentage of CL levels in non-infected control. Boxplots indicate the median (middle line), 25th and 75th percentiles (boxes), and maximum and minimum (whiskers) of five independent experiments performed in culture triplicates. Significant differences between tested groups are denoted by different letters (a, b, c, d) ($p < 0.05$).

Discussion

PRRSV has a tropism for cells of the monocytic lineage expressing the surface molecule receptor CD163. Alveolar macrophages, as target cells and the primary replication site of PRRSV, have been one of the most widely used porcine cells for in vitro studies of PRRSV pathogenesis [36–38]. The available porcine blood monocytes do not express CD163, or express it at exceedingly low levels.

The expression of CD163 increases with the cultivation of monocytes and this differentiation/aging enhances susceptibility to PRRSV infection [9]. Van Gucht et al. [39] showed that CD14-positive monocytes infiltrate the lungs of pigs after PRRSV infection. Monocytes in the lungs differentiate into CD163-positive macrophages [40]. In most studies, monocytes were cultivated in the presence of M-CSF/GM-CSF [11] or using LM-929 (murine fibroblast cells expressing murine M-CSF and GM-CSF) cell supernatant [9, 10, 41] to prepare MDMs. In the present study, MDMs were prepared without the addition of cytokines, similarly to Vicenova et al. [31] and García-Nicolás et al. [12]. The aim of the presented study was to compare the susceptibility of two different types of macrophages to the infection with PRRS virus and to co-infection with *H. parasuis*. Alveolar macrophages as resident cells provide one of the first lines of defence against microbes invading lung tissue. On the other hand, monocyte derived macrophages represent naive inflammatory cells accumulating at the site of inflammation [39, 40].

Sensitivity of macrophages to infection with PRRSV was the most significant observed difference between PAMs and MDMs. While alveolar macrophages were relatively resistant to cytopathogenic effect caused by PRRSV, monocyte derived macrophages were much more sensitive to PRRSV infection (Figures 2 and 3). A recent study by García-Nicolás et al. [12] showed decreased resistance to PRRSV infection of MDMs non-stimulated by cytokines. In contrast, IFN-γ or IFN-β pre-treated MDMs were protected against cytopathogenic effect caused by different strains of the PRRS virus (including strain Lelystad LVP23) [12].

Different responses of PAMs and MDMs to viral and bacterial infections were also reflected on the expression of pro-apoptotic (Bax, Bad and p53) and anti-apoptotic genes (Bcl-2) (Figure 5). Apoptosis is a strictly regulated mechanism of cell death and is highly modulated by both pro-apoptotic and anti-apoptotic cellular factors [16]. Bax is a pro-apoptotic protein normally occurring in the cytosol which, upon induction of apoptosis, translocates to mitochondria and induces cytochrome c release [42, 43]. In contrast, anti-apoptotic Bcl-2 is an integral membrane protein localized in mitochondria and has been shown to be capable of blocking spontaneous cytochrome c release [44, 45]. The function of another pro-apoptotic protein Bad is supposed to form a heterodimer with Bcl-2, inactivating it and thus allowing Bax triggered apoptosis [46]. The tumour suppressor p53 is activated by external and internal stress signals that promote its nuclear accumulation in an active form and stimulates a wide network of signals that act through two major apoptotic pathways [47, 48]. MDMs infected with PRRSV increased the expression of pro-apoptotic p53, Bad and Bax mRNA (Figures 5B–D). In contrast, expression rates of these genes and Bcl-2 were unchanged in PRRSV infected PAMs (Figures 5E–H). *H. parasuis* infected MDMs downregulated mRNA expression of pro-apoptotic p53 and Bad at 4 h PI (Figures 5B and C). *H. parasuis* as a gram negative bacterium has an outer membrane containing lipopolysaccharides (LPS) and LPS-mediated survival of macrophages has been previously observed by

Lombardo et al. [49]. The expression of these genes may also be associated with a significantly decreased level of ROS production after infection with *H. parasuis* (Figure 7A) as was already described in PAMs [26]. Oxidative stress caused by ROS has been suggested as a mediator of the intrinsic pathway of apoptosis [13, 50]. On the other hand, increased mortality of MDMs may be related to an increased level of ROS production after infection with PRRSV (Figure 7A). These results are related to the data presented by Le and Kleiboeker [13] who demonstrated that oxidative stress caused by ROS production could play a central role in PRRSV-induced apoptosis of MARC-145 cells. In addition, higher expression of the surface molecule CD163 (Figure 1B), which serves as an essential receptor for PRRSV infection [4, 5], could affect the sensitivity of MDMs to PRRSV. Decrease production of ROS by *H. parasuis* and potential antioxidative mechanisms of bacteria was described previously in our study [26]. On the contrary, Fu et al. [51] demonstrated that *H. parasuis* induced ROS production in piglet mononuclear phagocytes after 3 and 6 h incubation with bacteria. This difference could be explained by different type of used cells (monocytes vs macrophages), different strain of *H. parasuis* used (strain SH0165 isolated from lung vs strain HP 132 strain isolated from brain) and different time of exposition to bacteria (0–2 h vs 3–6 h).

We had supposed that higher mortality of MDMs infected with PRRSV would result in decreased replication capabilities of PRRSV and reduced amounts of virus particles released into the culture supernatant compared to PRRSV-infected PAMs. Surprisingly, viral titres detected in MDMs culture supernatant and expressed as $TCID_{50}/mL$ were at similar levels as viral titres detected in the supernatant of PAMs (Table 2). In addition, PRRS virus released from MDMs remained stable over long periods of time, which could be due to the microenvironment created by decaying cells. Alternatively, surviving alveolar macrophages can effectively prevent virus replication and thereupon decrease viral load in the supernatant. Replication of virus was not affected by presence of *H. parasuis* in the case of simultaneously infected cells. On the other hand, the growth of *H. parasuis* was affected by higher mortality of MDMs after infection with PRRSV (Figure 4). Lower multiplication of *H. parasuis* in co-infected cells could be explained by absence of *H. parasuis* essential factor NAD which is produced by living cells [52].

MDMs infected with *H. parasuis* alone, but not in co-infection, formed multinucleated giant cells (Figure 6). These cells originate from fusion of macrophages and have been observed after infection by intracellular pathogens such as *Mycobacterium tuberculosis* [53] and *Burkholderia pseudomallei* [54]. MGCs, also called Langhans giant cells, are frequently present in granulomas with characteristic location of the nuclei at the cell periphery in an arcuate configuration [53]. Yanagishita et al. [55] investigated the possible roles of bacterial endotoxins on macrophage multi-nucleated giant cell formation in a mouse macrophage RAW 246.7 cell line. MGC formation could represent a unique cellular response, which macrophages engage when challenged with bacterial endotoxins [55, 56] or large foreign bodies that cannot be ingested [57]. MDMs when simultaneously infected with PRRSV and *H. parasuis* did not form multinucleated giant cells, which is partly associated with high mortality of MDMs after infection with PRRSV. Infection with PRRSV could therefore facilitate the development of a secondary bacterial infection by avoiding the formation of MGCs by macrophages.

In conclusion, concurrent infection of PAMs or MDMs with PRRSV and *H. parasuis* was performed in vitro and differences dependent on the macrophage type were described. Higher mortality of MDMs infected with PRRSV compared with infected PAMs was observed. MDMs infected with PRRSV also produced higher amounts of ROS and increased the expression of pro-apoptotic genes compared to PAMs. Higher sensitivity of MDMs to PRRSV infection, which is associated with limited MDMs survival and restriction of MGC formation, could contribute to the development of multifactorial respiratory disease of swine.

Competing interests
The authors declare that they have no competing interests.

Authors' contributions
LK, JS and MF designed the study. LK, JS, KM, KN, HS and LL performed the experiments. LK, JS, MF and JM analysed the data. LK performed the statistical analysis. LK and JS wrote the manuscript. MF, HS and JM participated on manuscript preparation. All authors read and approved the final manuscript.

Acknowledgements
The study was supported by project QJ1210120 and RO0615 of the Ministry of Agriculture of the Czech Republic and by project LO1218 with financial support from the Ministry of Education, Youth, and Sports of the Czech Republic under the NPU I program.

Author details
[1] Veterinary Research Institute, Hudcova 296/70, 62100 Brno, Czech Republic. [2] Institute of Experimental Biology, Faculty of Science, Masaryk University, Kotlářská 267/2, 61137 Brno, Czech Republic. [3] University of Veterinary and Pharmaceutical Sciences Brno, Palackého třída 1946/1, 612 42 Brno, Czech Republic.

References
1. Silva-Campa E, Cordoba L, Fraile L, Flores-Mendoza L, Montoya M, Hernández J (2010) European genotype of porcine reproductive and respiratory syndrome (PRRSV) infects monocyte-derived dendritic cells but does not induce Treg cells. Virology 396:264–271

2. Wagner J, Kneucker A, Liebler-Tenorio E, Fachinger V, Glaser M, Pesch S, Murtaugh MP, Reinhold P (2011) Respiratory function and pulmonary lesions in pigs infected with porcine reproductive and respiratory syndrome virus. Vet J 187:310–319
3. Teifke JP, Dauber M, Fichtner D, Lenk M, Polster U, Weiland E, Beyer J (2001) Detection of European porcine reproductive and respiratory syndrome virus in porcine alveolar macrophages by two-colour immunofluorescence and in situ hybridization-immunohistochemistry double labelling. J Comp Pathol 124:238–245
4. Chen Y, Guo R, He S, Zhang X, Xia X, Sun H (2014) Additive inhibition of porcine reproductive and respiratory syndrome virus infection with the soluble sialoadhesin and CD163 receptors. Virus Res 179:85–92
5. Patton JB, Rowland RR, Yoo D, Chang KO (2009) Modulation of CD163 receptor expression and replication of porcine reproductive and respiratory syndrome virus in porcine macrophages. Virus Res 140:161–171
6. Duan X, Nauwynck HJ, Pensaert MB (1997) Virus quantification and identification of cellular targets in the lungs and lymphoid tissues of pigs at different time intervals after inoculation with porcine reproductive and respiratory syndrome virus (PRRSV). Vet Microbiol 56:9–19
7. Rossow KD, Benfield DA, Goyal SM, Nelson EA, Christopher-Hennings J, Collins JE (1996) Chronological immunohistochemical detection and localization of porcine reproductive and respiratory syndrome virus in gnotobiotic pigs. Vet Pathol 33:551–556
8. Lawson SR, Rossow KD, Collins JE, Benfield DA, Rowland RRR (1997) Porcine reproductive and respiratory syndrome virus infection of gnotobiotic pigs: sites of virus replication and co-localization with MAC-387 staining at 21 days post-infection. Virus Res 51:105–113
9. Wang L, Zhang H, Suo X, Zheng S, Feng WH (2011) Increase of CD163 but not sialoadhesin on cultured peripheral blood monocytes is coordinated with enhanced susceptibility to porcine reproductive and respiratory syndrome virus infection. Vet Immunol Immunopathol 141:209–220
10. Chitko-McKown CG, Chapes SK, Miller LC, Riggs PK, Ortega MT, Green BT, McKown RD (2013) Development and characterization of two porcine monocyte-derived macrophage cell lines. Results Immunol 3:26–32
11. Singleton H, Graham SP, Bodman-smith KB, Frossard JP, Steinbach F (2016) Establishing porcine monocyte-derived macrophage and dendritic cell systems for studying the interaction with PRRSV-1. Front Microbiol 7:832
12. García-Nicolás O, Baumann A, Vielle NJ, Gómez-Laguna J, Quereda JJ, Pallarés FJ, Ramis G, Carrasco L, Summerfield A (2014) Virulence and genotype-associated infectivity of interferon-treated macrophages by porcine reproductive and respiratory syndrome viruses. Virus Res 179:204–211
13. Lee SM, Kleiboeker SB (2007) Porcine reproductive and respiratory syndrome virus induces apoptosis through a mitochondria-mediated pathway. Virology 365:419–434
14. Li S, Zhou A, Wang J, Zhang S (2016) Interplay of autophagy and apoptosis during PRRSV infection of Marc145 cell. Infect Genet Evol 39:51–54
15. Suárez P, Diaz-Guerra M, Prieto C, Esteban M, Castro JM, Nieto A, Ortin J (1996) Open reading frame 5 of porcine reproductive and respiratory syndrome virus as a cause of virus-induced apoptosis. J Virol 70:2876–2882
16. Miller LC, Fox JM (2004) Apoptosis and porcine reproductive and respiratory syndrome virus. Vet. Immunol. Immunopathol. 102:131–142
17. Ge M, Zhang Y, Liu Y, Liu T, Zeng F (2016) Propagation of field highly pathogenic porcine reproductive and respiratory syndrome virus in MARC-145 cells is promoted by cell apoptosis. Virus Res 213:322–331
18. Kim TS, Benfield DA, Rowland RR (2002) Porcine reproductive and respiratory syndrome virus-induced cell death exhibits features consistent with a nontypical form of apoptosis. Virus Res 85:133–140
19. Costers S, Lefebvre DJ, Delputte PL, Nauwynck HJ (2008) Porcine reproductive and respiratory syndrome virus modulates apoptosis during replication in alveolar macrophages. Arch Virol 153:1453–1465
20. Pol JM, Van Leengoed LA, Stockhofe N, Kok G, Wensvoort G (1997) Dual infections of PRRSV/influenza or PRRSV/*Actinobacillus pleuropneumoniae* in the respiratory tract. Vet Microbiol 55:259–264
21. Solano GI, Segalés J, Collins JE, Molitor TW, Pijoan C (1997) Porcine reproductive and respiratory syndrome virus (PRRSV) interaction with *Haemophilus parasuis*. Vet Microbiol 55:247–257
22. Thanawongnuwech R, Brown GB, Halbur PG, Roth JA, Royer RL, Thacker BJ (2000) Pathogenesis of porcine reproductive and respiratory syndrome virus-induced increase in susceptibility to *Streptococcus suis* infection. Vet Pathol 37:143–152

23. Thanawongnuwech R, Thacker B, Halbur P, Thacker EL (2004) Increased production of proinflammatory cytokines following infection with porcine reproductive and respiratory syndrome virus and *Mycoplasma hyopneumoniae*. Clin Diagn Lab Immunol 11:901–908

24. Wills RW, Gray JT, Fedorka-Cray PJ, Yoon KJ, Ladely S, Zimmerman JJ (2000) Synergism between porcine reproductive and respiratory syndrome virus (PRRSV) and *Salmonella choleraesuis* in swine. Vet Microbiol 71:177–192

25. Yu J, Wu J, Zhang Y, Guo L, Cong X, Du Y, Li J, Sun W, Shi J, Peng J, Yin F, Wang D, Zhao P, Wang J (2012) Concurrent highly pathogenic porcine reproductive and respiratory syndrome virus infection accelerates *Haemophilus parasuis* infection in conventional pigs. Vet Microbiol 158:316–321

26. Kavanová L, Prodělalová J, Nedbalcová K, Matiašovic J, Volf J, Faldyna M, Salát J (2015) Immune response of porcine alveolar macrophages to a concurrent infection with porcine reproductive and respiratory syndrome virus and *Haemophilus parasuis* in vitro. Vet Microbiol 180:28–35

27. Lowy RJ, Dimitrov DS (1997) Characterization of influenza virus-induced death of J774.1 macrophages. Exp Cell Res 234:249–258

28. Binjawadagi B, Dwivedi V, Manickam C, Torrelles JB, Renukaradhya GJ (2011) Intranasal delivery of an adjuvanted modified live porcine reproductive and respiratory syndrome virus vaccine reduces ROS production. Viral Immunol 24:475–482

29. Eason MM, Fan X (2014) The role and regulation of catalase in respiratory tract opportunistic bacterial pathogens. Microb Pathog 74:50–58

30. Whitby PW, Morton DJ, VanWagoner TM, Seale TW, Cole BK, Mussa HJ, McGhee PA, Bauer CY, Springer JM, Stull TL (2012) *Haemophilus influenzae* OxyR: characterization of its regulation, regulon and role in fitness. PLoS One 7:e50588

31. Vicenova M, Nechvatalova K, Chlebova K, Kucerova Z, Leva L, Stepanova H, Faldyna M (2014) Evaluation of in vitro and in vivo anti-inflammatory activity of biologically active phospholipids with anti-neoplastic potential in porcine model. BMC Complement Altern Med 14:339

32. Zelnickova P, Matiasovic J, Pavlova B, Kudlackova H, Kovaru F, Faldyna M (2008) Quantitative nitric oxide production by rat, bovine and porcine macrophages. Nitric Oxide 19:36–41

33. Bello-Ortí B, Deslandes V, Tremblay YD, Labrie J, Howell KJ, Tucker AW, Maskell DJ, Aragon V, Jacques M (2014) Biofilm formation by virulent and non-virulent strains of *Haemophilus parasuis*. Vet Res 45:104

34. Lichtensteiger CA, Vimr ER (1997) Neuraminidase (sialidase) activity of *Haemophilus parasuis*. FEMS Microbiol Lett 152:269–274

35. Hierholzer JC, Killington RA (1996) Virus isolation and quantitation. In: Mahy BWJ, Kangro HO (eds) Virology methods manual, 1st edn. Academic Press, London, pp 24–32

36. Chang HW, Jeng CR, Liu JJ, Lin TL, Chang CC, Chia MY, Tsai YC, Pang VF (2005) Reduction of porcine reproductive and respiratory syndrome virus (PRRSV) infection in swine alveolar macrophages by porcine circovirus 2 (PCV2)-induced interferon-alpha. Vet Microbiol 108:167–177

37. Song S, Bi J, Wang D, Fang L, Zhang L, Li F, Chen H, Xiao S (2013) Porcine reproductive and respiratory syndrome virus infection activates IL-10 production through NF-κB and p38 MAPK pathways in porcine alveolar macrophages. Dev Comp Immunol 39:265–272

38. Zhang K, Hou Q, Zhong Z, Li X, Chen H, Li W, Wen J, Wang L, Liu W, Zhong F (2013) Porcine reproductive and respiratory syndrome virus activates inflammasomes of porcine alveolar macrophages via its small envelope protein E. Virology 442:156–162

39. Van Gucht S, Labarque G, Van Reeth K (2004) The combination of PRRS virus and bacterial endotoxin as a model for multifactorial respiratory disease in pigs. Vet Immunol Immunopathol 102:165–178

40. Ondrackova P, Leva L, Kucerova Z, Vicenova M, Mensikova M, Faldyna M (2013) Distribution of porcine monocytes in different lymphoid tissues and the lungs during experimental *Actinobacillus pleuropneumoniae* infection and the role of chemokines. Vet Res 44:98

41. Huang C, Zhang Q, Guo XK, Yu ZB, Xu AT, Tang J, Feng WH (2014) Porcine reproductive and respiratory syndrome virus nonstructural protein 4 antagonizes IFNβ expression by targeting the NF-κB essential modulator. J Virol 88:10934–10945

42. Dewson G, Kluck RM (2009) Mechanisms by which Bak and Bax permeabilise mitochondria during apoptosis. J Cell Sci 122:2801–2808

43. Finucane DM, Bossy-Wetzel E, Waterhouse NJ, Cotter TG, Green DR (1999) Bax-induced caspase activation and apoptosis via cytochrome c release from mitochondria is inhibitable by Bcl-xL. J Biol Chem 274:2225–2233

44. Gross A, McDonnell JM, Korsmeyer SJ (1999) BCL-2 family members and the mitochondria in apoptosis. Genes Dev. 13:1899–1911

45. Kluck RM, Bossy-Wetzel E, Green DR, Newmeyer DD (1997) The release of cytochrome c from mitochondria: a primary site for Bcl-2 regulation of apoptosis. Science 275:1132–1136

46. Bogdał MN, Hat B, Kochańczyk M, Lipniacki T (2013) Levels of pro-apoptotic regulator Bad and anti-apoptotic regulator Bcl-xL determine the type of the apoptotic logic gate. BMC Syst Biol 7:67

47. Bellamy CO (1997) P53 and apoptosis. Br Med Bull 53:522–538

48. Haupt S, Berger M, Goldberg Z, Haupt Y (2003) Apoptosis—the p53 network. J Cell Sci 116:4077–4085

49. Lombardo E, Alvarez-Barrientos A, Maroto B, Boscá L, Knaus UG (2007) TLR4-mediated survival of macrophages is MyD88 dependent and requires TNF-α autocrine signalling. J Immunol 178:3731–3739

50. Chen Q, Chai YC, Mazumder S, Jiang C, Macklis R, Chisolm G, Almasan A (2003) The late increase in intracellular free radical oxygen species during apoptosis is associated with cytochrome c release, caspase activation, and mitochondrial dysfunction. Cell Death Differ 10:323–334

51. Fu S, Xu L, Li S, Qiu Y, Liu Y, Wu Z, Ye C, Hou Y, Hu CA (2016) Baicalin suppresses NLRP3 inflammasome and nuclear factor-kappa B (NF-κB) signaling during *Haemophilus parasuis* infection. Vet Res 47:80

52. Biberstein EL, Mini PD, Gills MG (1963) Action of *Haemophilus* cultures on delta-aminolevulinic acid. J Bacteriol 86:814–819

53. Lay G, Poquet Y, Salek-Peyron P, Puissegur MP, Botanch C, Bon H, Levillain F, Duteyrat JL, Emile JF, Altare F (2007) Langhans giant cells from *M. tuberculosis*-induced human granulomas cannot mediate mycobacterial uptake. J Pathol 211:76–85

54. Utaisincharoen P, Arjcharoen S, Limposuwan K, Tungpradabkul S, Sirisinha S (2006) *Burkholderia pseudomallei* RpoS regulates multinucleated giant cell formation and inducible nitric oxide synthase expression in mouse macrophage cell line (RAW 264.7). Microb Pathog 40:184–189

55. Yanagishita T, Watanabe D, Akita Y, Nakano A, Ohshima Y, Tamada Y, Matsumoto Y (2007) Construction of novel in vitro epithelioid cell granuloma model from mouse macrophage cell line. Arch Dermatol Res 299:399–403

56. Puissegur MP, Lay G, Gilleron M, Botella L, Nigou J, Marrakchi H, Mari B, Duteyrat JL, Guerardel Y, Kremer L, Barbry P, Puzo G, Altare F (2007) Mycobacterial lipomannan induces granuloma macrophage fusion via a TLR2-dependent, ADAM9- and beta1 integrin-mediated pathway. J Immunol 178:3161–3169

57. Brodbeck WG, Anderson JM (2009) Giant cell formation and function. Curr Opin Hematol 16:53–57

6

Surface displaying of swine IgG1 Fc enhances baculovirus-vectored vaccine efficacy by facilitating viral complement escape and mammalian cell transduction

Zehui Liu[†], Yangkun Liu[†], Yuanyuan Zhang, Yajuan Yang, Jingjing Ren, Xiaoying Zhang[*] and Enqi Du[*]

Abstract

Baculovirus-mediated gene transfer has been developed as a vaccine design strategy against a number of diseases without apparent viral replication. However, it has been hampered by complement-dependent inactivation, thus hindering the in vivo application of baculovirus. A variety of approaches have been exploited to bypass the complement system in the serum. In this study, we constructed and screened a series of baculovirus vectors displaying complement interfering factors, of which a baculovirus vector displaying swine IgG1 Fc (pFc) showed the highest complement antagonism (75.6%). Flow cytometry analysis of transduced cells demonstrated that the baculovirus display of pFc had a significant increase in transduction efficiency and transgene expression of reporter genes. On this basis, a VSV-G-pseudotyped with swine IgG1 Fc surface displayed baculovirus vector was developed to express the classical swine fever virus (CSFV) E2 gene. The translational enhancers Syn21 and P10UTR were incorporated to improve the antigen expression. The E2 gene was efficiently expressed in both insect and mammalian cells. Pigs immunized with this recombinant baculovirus developed high levels of E2-specific antibody, CSFV-specific neutralizing antibody and IFN-γ-secreting cellular immune responses. These results demonstrate that the strategy of surface-displaying swine IgG1 Fc has a great potential to improve the efficiency of baculovirus-vectored vaccine for CSFV and other swine pathogens.

Introduction

The baculovirus-based protein expression system has been used extensively to produce a variety of heterogenous proteins in insect cells. Recombinant baculoviruses carrying mammalian cell active expression cassettes, BacMam viruses, have been developed as a vaccine strategy against diseases in several animal models. Intramuscular, intraperitoneal or intranasal vaccination with these recombinant baculoviruses is shown to elicit humoral and cellular immune responses against various antigens [1, 2]. As a gene delivery vector, baculovirus offers several advantages over other viral vectors, including a strong

biosafety profile [3, 4], a high capacity for insertion of heterologous DNA, and ease of production. In addition, baculovirus can be used as an adjuvant to stimulate the innate immune system by regulating toll-like receptor 9 (TLR9) and RIG-I-like receptor (RLR) pathways [5]. Therefore, baculovirus is an effective tool for gene delivery.

Baculovirus infects insect cells in nature. The glycoprotein gp64 mediates virus attachment to the cell surface and internalization [6], which comprises an N-terminal signal peptide (SP) and a mature domain that includes the transmembrane domain (TM) and cytoplasmic domain (CTD). After anchoring in insect cells, the gp64 SP directs its transport to the plasma membrane, where gp64 is exhibited on the surface of infected cells as homotrimers. The gp64 CTD interacts with the budding nucleocapsids and directs the incorporation of gp64 into

*Correspondence: zhang.xy@nwsuaf.edu.cn; duenqi227@126.com
[†]Zehui Liu and Yangkun Liu contributed equally to this work
College of Veterinary Medicine, Northwest A&F University, Yangling, Shaanxi 712100, People's Republic of China

the virion [7]. Thus, foreign proteins coupled to gp64 will be routed efficiently to the cell membrane to be displayed on the surface of infected cells and on baculovirus particles. Recombinant baculoviruses made with this surface display technique have been used in a variety of applications, including functional studies of glycoproteins, drug screening and development of vaccine candidates [8, 9].

Although baculovirus does not suffer from pre-existing antibodies in vertebrates, baculovirus-based gene delivery faces two bottlenecks: complement-dependent inactivation and low transduction efficacy targeting immune cells, such as dendritic cells, macrophages, B cells, and T cells. This has thus affected, to a great extent, the efficacy of baculovirus-vectored vaccines [10]. A number of approaches have been applied to bypass the complement using chemical compounds or complement receptors, and surface display of complement inactivators, such as soluble complement receptor type 1 (sCR1), decay acceleration factor (DAF), membrane cofactor protein (MCP), Smallpox inhibitor of complement enzymes (SPICE) and ornithodoros moubata complement inhibitor (OmCI) [11]. A pseudotyped baculovirus replacing gp64 with vesicular stomatitis virus G (VSV-G) protein has shown improved efficiency in transducing various mammalian cells and antagonism against complement-mediated inactivation [3].

Classical swine fever virus (CSFV) is a causative agent of CSF, a highly contagious Class A infectious disease being classified by the World Organization for Animal Health (OIE), leading to great economic losses in the pig industry [12]. The viral E2 glycoprotein is responsible for eliciting neutralizing antibodies in immunized animals and protecting them from lethal dose challenge. This protein also plays multiple roles in the viral life cycle, and mediating viral entry into host cells [13].

At present, the most extensively used CSFV vaccine is a lapinized attenuated vaccine based on the C-strain. Although it can confer complete protection against CSF, this vaccine does not allow differentiating infection in vaccinated animals (DIVA). Other vaccination strategies, such as avirulent and low-pathogenic viral vectored vaccines expressing E2 protein [14–16], still remain biosecurity concerns.

In this study, we aimed to further improve baculovirus-vectored vaccine efficacy. To explore the effects of complement interfering factor OmCI, SPICE, DAF and pFc displayed on the baculoviral envelope for baculovirus-mediated gene delivery, we constructed four recombinant baculoviruses displaying OmCI, SPICE, DAF and pFc, respectively. We hypothesized that by displaying these elements, the in vitro complement antagonism and transgenic expression of these four recombinant baculoviruses would promote as vaccine delivery vectors.

The modified recombinant BacMam carrying CSFV E2 expression cassette under the CMV promoter was tested as a novel CSFV vaccine in generating effective immunity in pigs.

Materials and methods
Virus, plasmids, and cells
The CSFV Shimen and CSFV C strains vaccine was purchased from Jilin Zhengye Biological Products Co., Ltd, Jilin, China. The pFc, SPICE, DAF, OmCI and E2 genes were synthesized by GENEWIZ (Suzhou, China). E. coli SW106 (with multigene baculovirus expression vector AmMultiBac) was obtained from Professor Yao Lunguang of Nanyang Normal University, China. Plasmid pFBDM-VSV-ED-CMV-DsRed (containing the CMV promoter and VSVG-ED), swine intestinal epithelial cells (IEC), porcine kidney cells (PK-15) and Sf-9 insect cells were also maintained in our lab. The IEC and PK-15 cells were cultured in Dulbecco modified Eagle medium (DMEM, HyClone, China) supplemented with 10% heat-inactivated fetal bovine serum (FBS, Gibco, CA, USA), 100 units/mL penicillin and 100 µg/mL streptomycin (Invitrogen), and incubated at 37 °C in a humidified 5% CO_2 atmosphere.

Construction of baculovirus vectors
Six plasmids including pFBDM-VSVG-ED-pFc-CMV-DsRed, pFBDM-VSVG-ED-SPICE-CMV-DsRed, pFBDM-VSVG-ED-DAF-CMV-DsRed, pFBDM-VSVG-ED-OmCI-CMV-DsRed, pFBDM-VSVG-ED-CMV-DsRed and pFBDM-gp64-CMV-DsRed, were constructed by standard methods. A recombinant baculovirus vector vaccine, pFBDM-VSVG-ED-CMV-E2, was constructed to express CSFV E2 gene derived from CSFV strain Shimen (Accession AY775178) under the control of CMV promoter, and pFBDM-VSVG-ED-pFc-CMV-S/P-E2 plasmid was constructed by introducing translational enhancers Syn21 and P10UTR [17], into the above vector (Figure 1). The plasmids were transformed into E.coli SW106 competent cells, and recombinant Bacmid (rBac) DNA, including rBac-VSVG-ED-pFc, rBac-VSVG-ED-SPICE, rBac-VSVG-ED-DAF, rBac-VSVG-ED-OmCI, rBac-VSVG-ED, rBac-gp64, rBac-VSVG-ED-CMV-E2, and rBac-VSVG-ED-CMV-S/P-E2, were amplified by PCR amplification using gene-specific and M13R primers.

Generation and titration of recombinant baculovirus
Sf-9 insect cells were cultured at 27 °C in Sf-900II SFM medium containing 10% FBS (Gibco, CA, USA) and 1% antibiotics (100 U/mL penicillin and 100 µg/mL streptomycin). The cells were transfected with each of the above recombinant Bacmid DNA, and the supernatant were

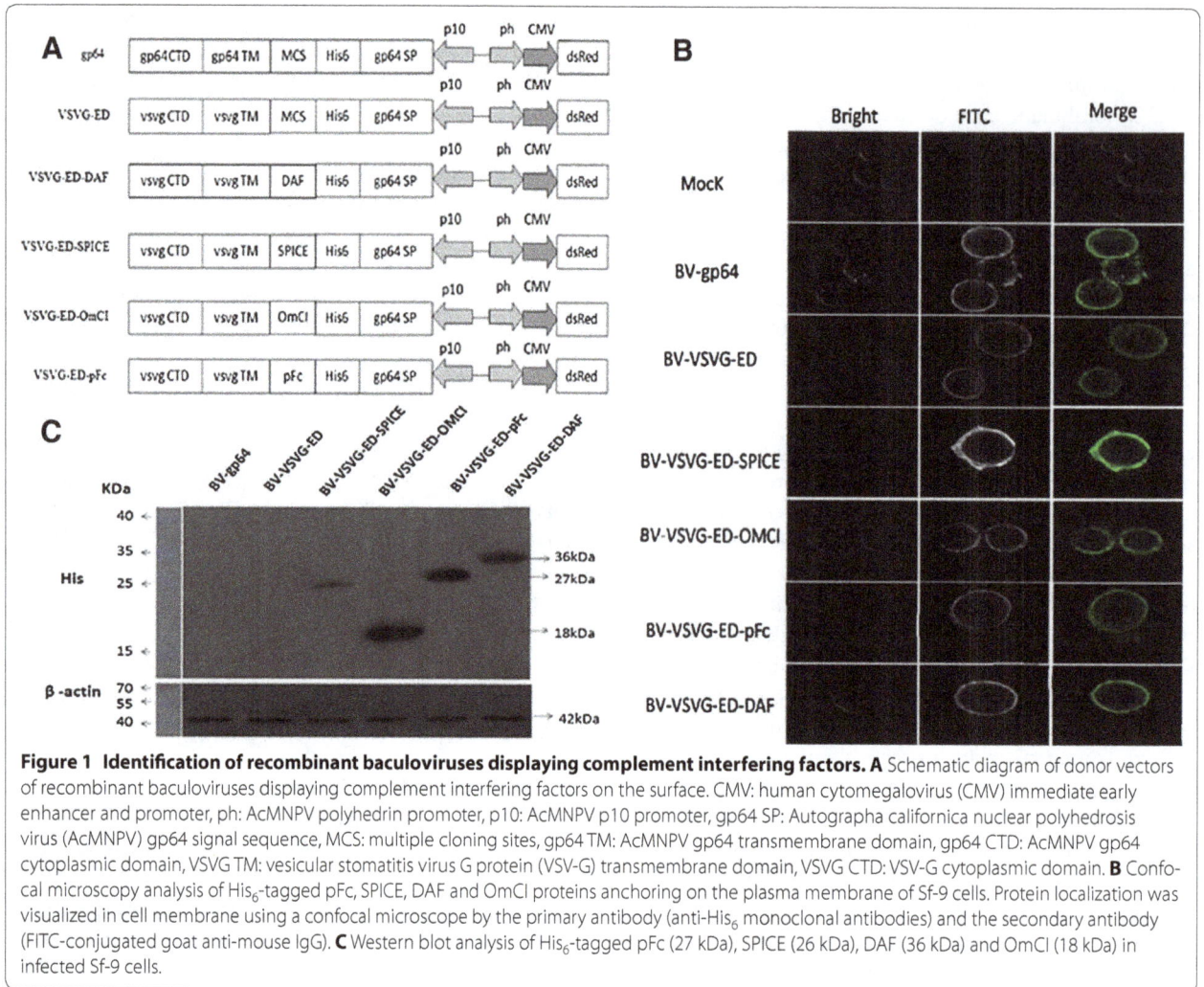

Figure 1 Identification of recombinant baculoviruses displaying complement interfering factors. A Schematic diagram of donor vectors of recombinant baculoviruses displaying complement interfering factors on the surface. CMV: human cytomegalovirus (CMV) immediate early enhancer and promoter, ph: AcMNPV polyhedrin promoter, p10: AcMNPV p10 promoter, gp64 SP: Autographa californica nuclear polyhedrosis virus (AcMNPV) gp64 signal sequence, MCS: multiple cloning sites, gp64 TM: AcMNPV gp64 transmembrane domain, gp64 CTD: AcMNPV gp64 cytoplasmic domain, VSVG TM: vesicular stomatitis virus G protein (VSV-G) transmembrane domain, VSVG CTD: VSV-G cytoplasmic domain. **B** Confocal microscopy analysis of His_6-tagged pFc, SPICE, DAF and OmCI proteins anchoring on the plasma membrane of Sf-9 cells. Protein localization was visualized in cell membrane using a confocal microscope by the primary antibody (anti-His_6 monoclonal antibodies) and the secondary antibody (FITC-conjugated goat anti-mouse IgG). **C** Western blot analysis of His_6-tagged pFc (27 kDa), SPICE (26 kDa), DAF (36 kDa) and OmCI (18 kDa) in infected Sf-9 cells.

collected at 120 h after cultivation. The viruses were passaged in Sf-9 cells to obtain high titer viral stocks. The culture supernatants from infected cells were collected once 90% of the cells had been infected. The recombinant baculovirus genome was extracted and then checked for the presence of the insert by PCR using gene-specific and baculovirus polyhedron-specific primer pairs. The recombinant baculoviruses were named BV-VSVG-ED-pFc, BV-VSVG-ED-SPICE, BV-VSVG-ED-DAF, BV-VSVG-ED-OmCI, BV-VSVG-ED, BV-gp64, BV-VSVG-ED-CMV-E2 and BV-VSVG-ED-pFc-CMV-S/P-E2, respectively. The titer of the baculovirus stocks was measured by end-point dilution assay. Briefly, Sf-9 cells were plated in 96-well plates, and tenfold serial dilutions of the virus stocks were added to the cells. Viruses and cells were allowed to interact for 1 h before the viruses were removed, and the cells were incubated for 8 days and examined for GFP expression. Wells that

appeared green fluorescence were deemed to be baculovirus-positive, otherwise deemed to be baculovirus-negative. Subsequently, the titer for every virus stock was calculated according to the Reed-Muench method.

Western blot analysis of purified recombinant baculoviruses

The virus supernatant was purified by ultracentrifugation as described before [1]. Briefly, cell debris was first removed by centrifugation for 10 min at 2000 rpm. Infected cell supernatant was then layered over 27% sucrose and centrifuged at 24 000 rpm for 75 min in SW28 tubes. The virus pellet was resuspended in phosphate-buffered saline (PBS, pH 7.5) and centrifuged in SW28 tubes at 27 000 rpm for 150 min. The final pellet was resuspended in PBS. The incorporation of His_6-tagged pFc, SPICE, DAF, and OmCI into baculoviruses was probed using mouse anti-His_6 monoclonal antibody (Boster, Wuhan, China). The Sf-9 cells infected with recombinant BV-VSVG-ED-CMV-E2 or BV-VSVG-ED-pFc-CMV-S/P-E2 baculovirus vaccine were analyzed by mouse anti-His$_6$ monoclonal antibody or rabbit anti-CSFV polyclonal antibody, followed by confirmation of the expression of pFc and E2.

Indirect fluorescent assay (IFA)
The IEC cells were collected at 48 h post-transduction, fixed with 4% paraformaldehyde for 20 min at room temperature, and then exposed to rabbit anti-CSFV polyclonal antibody for 1 h at 37 °C. After three washes with PBS, the cells were incubated with Alexa 594-conjugated goat anti-rabbit IgG (Invitrogen, Carlsbad, CA, USA) for 1 h at 37 °C. Fluorescence images were collected using an inverted fluorescence microscope.

Confocal microscopy
The Sf-9 cells were cultured on sterile cover slips and infected at a multiplicity of infection (MOI) of 10. Two days after infection, the cells were fixed by methanol/acetone (1:1) for 5 min at −20 °C, rinsed with PBS, and blocked with 5% skimmed milk for 30 min at 37 °C. The cells were then sequentially incubated with anti-His$_6$ mouse monoclonal antibody and FITC-conjugated goat anti-mouse IgG antibody (Boster, Wuhan, China) for 1 h at 37 °C, and washed for three times with PBS. Protein localization was visualized using a confocal microscope (LSM 510, Zeiss, Thornwood, NY, USA).

Complement antagonism of recombinant baculoviruses
One of the major challenges of baculoviruses as gene transfer vectors is inactivation by serum complement. We therefore tested the survival rate of recombinant baculoviruses in the presence of serum. Briefly, healthy pig serum and mice serum were divided into two parts: one part was heat-inactivated at 56 °C for 30 min, another was left untreated. Recombinant baculoviruses were incubated with inactivated serum and untreated serum, respectively. After 60 min incubation at 37 °C, these recombinant baculoviruses were subjected to titration by end-point dilution assay. The survival rates of baculoviruses were denoted as the percentage of vector survival in the indicated sera compared to the corresponding heat-treated sera [18].

Flow cytometry analysis
The IEC cells were transduced with BV-VSVG-ED-pFc or BV-VSVG-ED at a MOI of 100, and subjected to flow cytometry (FACSCalibur, BD Biosciences, Franklin Lakes, New Jersey) analysis 1 day after transduction. The percentage of cells emitting fluorescence (% dsRed + cells) and mean FI of each sample were measured three times by counting 10 000 cells in each measurement.

Evaluation of recombinant baculovirus vaccines
Complement antagonism of BV-VSVG-ED-CMV-E2 and BV-VSVG-ED-pFc-CMV-E2 was measured as mentioned above. Transduction efficiency of swine cells with recombinant baculovirus vaccines was also a critical checkpoint. A third passage (P3) of baculoviruses (BV-VSVG-ED-CMV-E2 and BV-VSVG-ED-pFc-CMV-S/P-E2) was transduced with swine IEC using an MOI of 100 for 12 h. The media containing the virus was replaced by fresh DMEM, and the cells were incubated for an additional 48 h before being fixed for IFA analysis as described above.

Pig immunization and immune response detection
Four week old pigs (CSFV antigen and antibody negative, provided by China Institute of Veterinary Drug Control) were randomly divided into 4 groups (5 pigs per group). The pigs were intramuscularly immunized with BV-VSVG-ED-CMV-E2 and BV-VSVG-ED-pFc-CMV-S/P-E2 baculoviruses (10^9 PFU), CSFV commercial vaccine C-strain (vaccinated control, 2 mL), and PBS (unvaccinated control), respectively, boosted once at 14 days. The CSFV-specific antibodies were tested in sera collected at 0, 7, 14, 21 and 28 days post-infection (dpi) using commercial ELISA kit (Keqian, Wuhan, China), and IFN-γ was assayed in sera collected at 0, 14 and 28 dpi using a commercial ELISA kit (4A Biotech, Beijing, China). All animal procedures were approved and supervised by the Animal Care Commission of the College of Veterinary Medicine, Northwest Agriculture and Forestry University. Every effort was made to minimize animal pain, suffering and distress and to reduce the number of animals used.

Serum-virus neutralization test (SNT)
Sera collected at 0, 7, 14, 21 and 28 dpi were tested for neutralizing antibodies as previously described [19]. Briefly, serially diluted sera were mixed with an equal volume of 200 TCID$_{50}$ of CSFV Shimen strain, incubated at 37 °C for 1 h, added to PK-15 cells preplated in 96-well culture plates, and cultured for 3 days. The CSFV neutralizing antibody (NAb) titers were determined and expressed as the reciprocal of the highest dilution at which infection of PK-15 cells was inhibited in 50% of the culture wells.

Statistical analysis
All experiments were performed with at least three independent experiments. Statistical significance was determined by the Student t test when two groups were compared, or by one-way analysis of variance (ANOVA), when more than two groups were compared. P value < 0.05 was considered to be statistically significant.

Results

Identification of recombinant baculoviruses displaying complement interfering factors

Recombinant BV-VSVG-ED-pFc, BV-VSVG-ED-SPICE, BV-VSVG-ED-DAF and BV-VSVG-ED-OmCI baculoviruses were constructed by cloning pFc, SPICE, DAF or OmCI containing a N-terminal His_6 and C-terminal VSV-G (Figure 1A). The gp64 signal peptide was aimed at translocating the protein to the insect cell plasma membrane and was cleaved, thus exposing the His_6 tag to the outer surface. To determine whether the complement interfering factors were properly translocated to the cell surface, the baculovirus-infected cells were collected at 2 days after infection, and subjected to IFA. As shown in Figure 1B, the test proteins localized within the plasma membrane, demonstrating that the complement interfering factors were located on the surface of Sf-9 cells. To confirm the expression of His_6-tagged pFc, SPICE, DAF, and OmCI, Sf-9 cells were infected with recombinant BV-VSVG-ED-pFc, BV-VSVG-ED-SPICE, BV-VSVG-ED-DAF and BV-VSVG-ED-OmCI baculoviruses, respectively, harvested at 3 days after infection, and used for detection. Western blot analyses showed that the complement interfering factors were correctly expressed (Figure 1C).

Enhanced complement antagonism and transformation efficiency of recombinant baculoviruses

For application in vivo, recombinant baculoviruses should remain active in the presence of mammal sera. The survival rates of recombinant baculovirus vector were evaluated for complement antagonism. Recombinant BV-VSVG-ED-pFc, BV-VSVG-ED-SPICE, BV-VSVG-ED-DAF, and BV-VSVG-ED-OmCI baculoviruses were treated and titrated as described above. In mouse serum, recombinant baculovirus display of DAF showed a higher complement antagonism activity (90.2%) than recombinant baculovirus display of swine IgG1 Fc (pFc) (65.6%, $P < 0.05$) (Figure 2A). As shown in Figure 2B, in pig serum, recombinant baculovirus display of pFc showed a significantly higher complement antagonism activity (75.6%, $P < 0.05$) than other recombinant baculoviruses. Furthermore, BV-VSVG-ED demonstrated a higher complement antagonism activity ($P < 0.05$) compared with wild type BV-gp64. DsRed expression was analyzed by fluorescence microscopy following transduction of IEC cells with BV-VSVG-ED-pFc or BV-VSVG-ED at an MOI of 100 (Figures 3A and 3B). Transduction efficiency was further quantified by flow cytometry analysis, in which BV-VSVG-ED-pFc demonstrated significantly increased numbers of DsRed positive cells (Figure 3C), and the mean fluorescence intensity (MFI) of DsRed fluorescence was significantly higher with BV-VSVG-ED-pFc than with BV-VSVG-ED (Figure 3D).

In vitro evaluation of BacMam expressing E2 based on swine IgG1 Fc surface display

Recombinant BV-VSVG-ED-CMV-E2 and BV-VSVG-ED-pFc-CMV-S/P-E2 baculoviruses were constructed by replacing dsRed with CSFV E2 gene, and incorporating translational enhancers Syn21 and P10UTR to improve E2 expression (Figure 4A). Sf-9 cells infected with recombinant BV-VSVG-ED-CMV-E2 and BV-

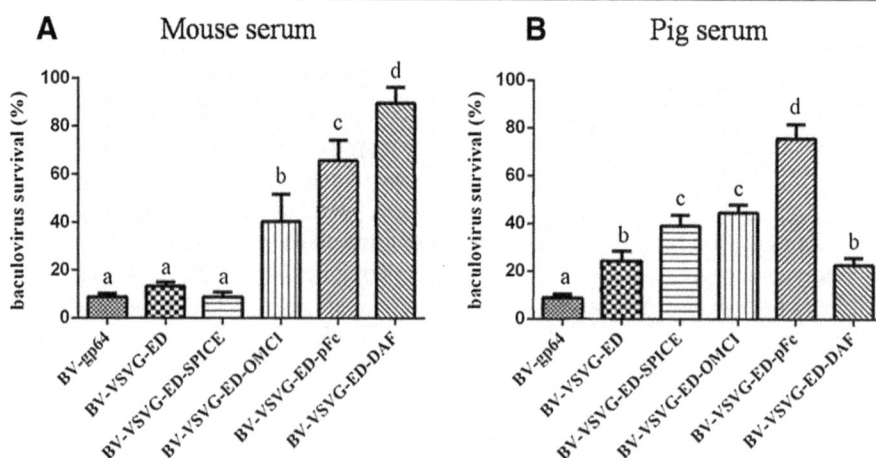

Figure 2 Evaluation of complement antagonism of recombinant baculoviruses displaying complement interfering factors in serum.
A Baculovirus was incubated with 40% mice serum, and then subjected to titration by end-point dilution assays. Bars denote the percentage of vector survival, which was determined as the percentage of virus titer resulting from pre-incubation with untreated compared to heat-treated serum. Bars with different letters were significantly different ($P < 0.05$). **B** Baculovirus vector survival in pig serum tested as above. Bars with different letters were significantly different ($P < 0.05$).

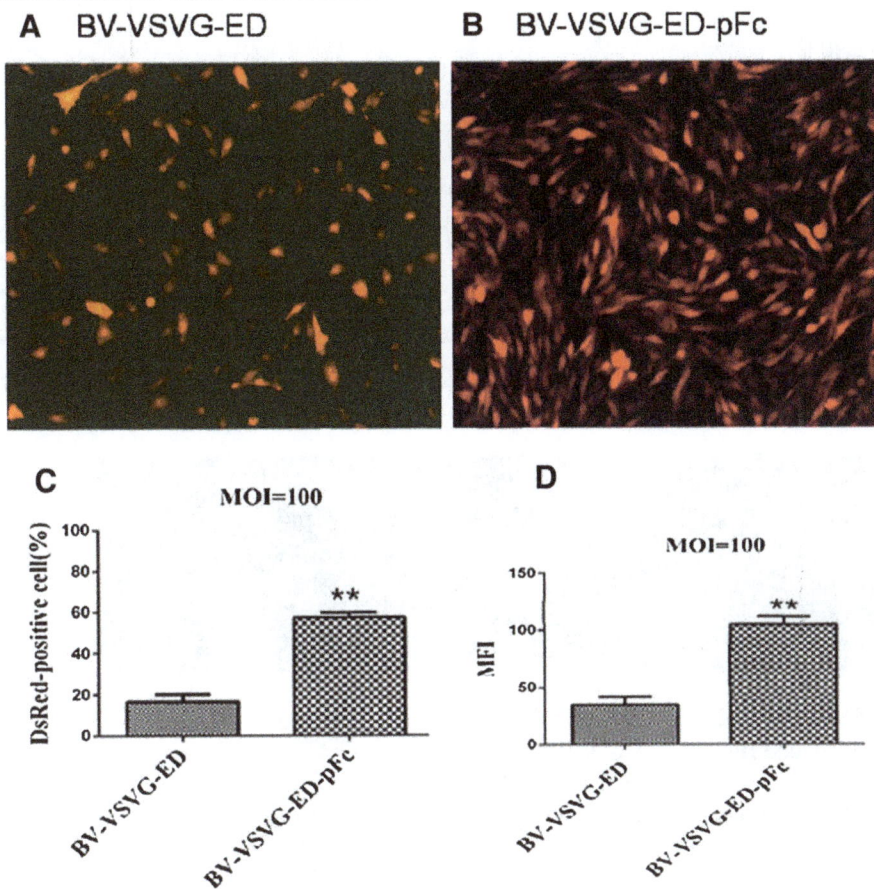

Figure 3 Surface displayed swine IgG1 Fc enhanced baculovirus-mediated DsRed expression. A, **B** Fluorescent microscopic analysis of transduced IEC cells 36 h after transduction (×100). **C**, **D** Flow cytometry analysis of transduced cells. **C** Percentage of DsRed positive cells in IEC. **D** Mean fluorescence intensity (MFI) of DsRed positive IEC cells (**$P < 0.05$).

VSVG-ED-pFc-CMV-S/P-E2 baculoviruses were subject to Western blot analyses (Figure 4B), and it revealed that the E2 and His$_6$-tagged pFc protein were correctly expressed in Sf-9 cells. The results from IFA indicated that IEC cells transduced with BV-VSVG-ED-CMV-E2 and BV-VSVG-ED-pFc-CMV-S/P-E2 developed immunofluorescence signals, confirming the expression of E2 protein in IEC cells. Particularly, BV-VSVG-ED-pFc-CMV-S/P-E2 had higher efficiency of gene transduction compared with BV-VSVG-ED-CMV-E2 (Figure 4C). These data were in agreement with the complement antagonism result of BV-VSVG-ED-CMV-E2 and BV-VSVG-ED-pFc-CMV-S/P-E2, which showed that BV-VSVG-ED-pFc-CMV-S/P-E2 resulted in a significantly higher survival rate than that of BV-VSVG-ED-CMV-E2 (Figure 5) ($P < 0.05$).

Immune responses elicited by BV-VSVG-ED-pFc-CMV-S/P-E2 in pigs

To explore the ability of BV-VSVG-ED-pFc-CMV-S/P-E2 to induce CSFV-specific humoral immune responses, pigs were immunized with this baculovirus, as well as BV-VSVG-ED-CMV-E2, commercial vaccine C-strain, and PBS controls, and detected for E2-specific antibodies by ELISA. All the pigs immunized with BV-VSVG-ED-pFc-CMV-S/P-E2, C-strain vaccine, and BV-VSVG-ED-CMV-E2 developed high levels of antibody, without significant difference. The pigs immunized with PBS only demonstrated a non-specific antibody response below the threshold (Figure 6A).

To detect CSFV-specific NAb titers, SNT was performed at 0, 7, 14, 21 and 28 dpi. The results showed that pigs immunized with the commercial vaccine C-strain developed the highest NAb titers, and those immunized with BV-VSVG-ED-pFc-CMV-S/P-E2 also induced considerable level of Nabs, followed by those immunized with BV-VSVG-ED-CMV-E2. Nevertheless, the pigs immunized with PBS did not develop a detectable NAb titer against CSFV even at 4 weeks following prime immunization (Table 1).

The IFN-γ levels in immunized sera can reflect the immune state of the host. IFN-γ secreted by T-helper

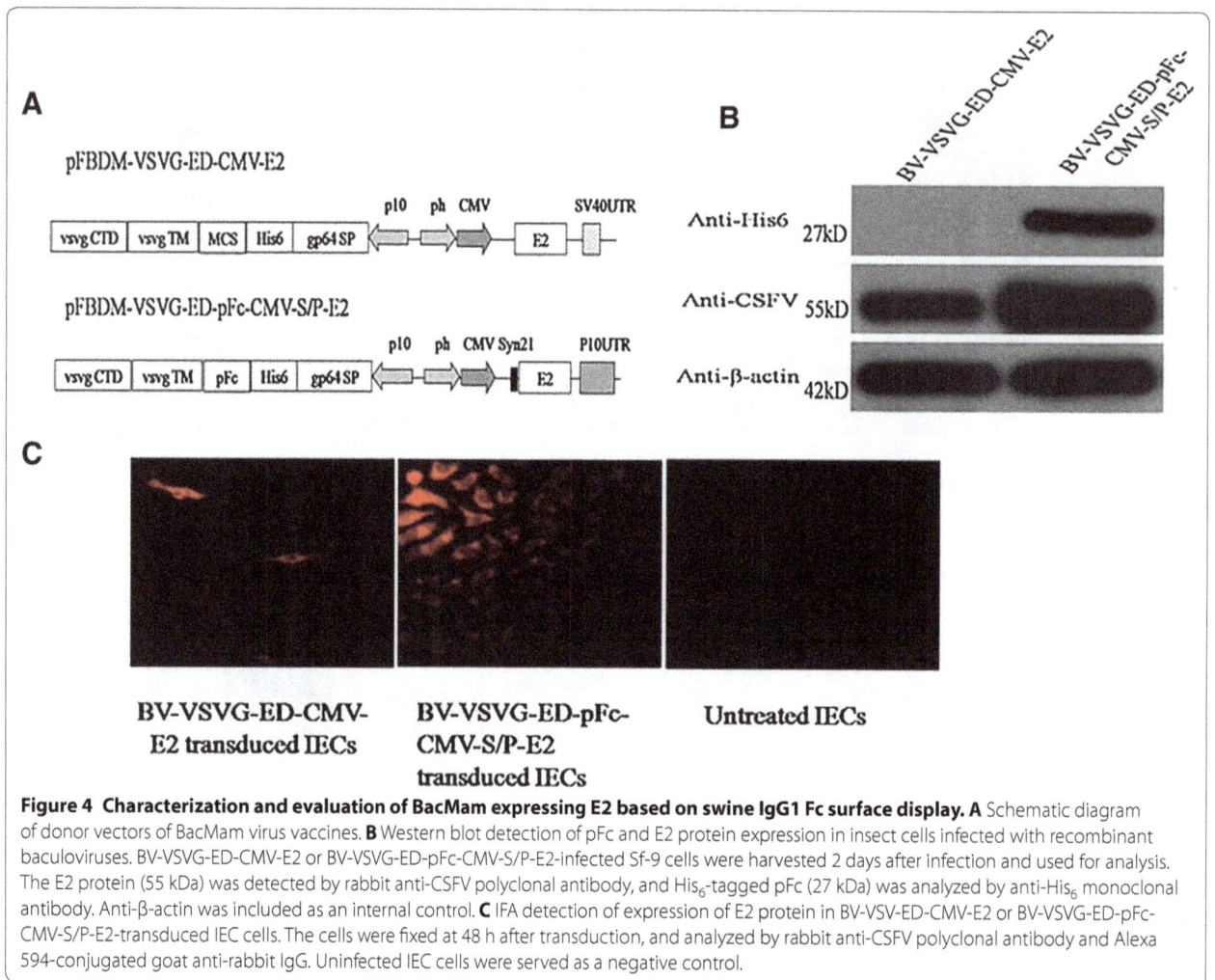

Figure 4 Characterization and evaluation of BacMam expressing E2 based on swine IgG1 Fc surface display. A Schematic diagram of donor vectors of BacMam virus vaccines. **B** Western blot detection of pFc and E2 protein expression in insect cells infected with recombinant baculoviruses. BV-VSVG-ED-CMV-E2 or BV-VSVG-ED-pFc-CMV-S/P-E2-infected Sf-9 cells were harvested 2 days after infection and used for analysis. The E2 protein (55 kDa) was detected by rabbit anti-CSFV polyclonal antibody, and His$_6$-tagged pFc (27 kDa) was analyzed by anti-His$_6$ monoclonal antibody. Anti-β-actin was included as an internal control. **C** IFA detection of expression of E2 protein in BV-VSV-ED-CMV-E2 or BV-VSVG-ED-pFc-CMV-S/P-E2-transduced IEC cells. The cells were fixed at 48 h after transduction, and analyzed by rabbit anti-CSFV polyclonal antibody and Alexa 594-conjugated goat anti-rabbit IgG. Uninfected IEC cells were served as a negative control.

type 1 (Th1) cells plays important roles in regulating the cellular immune response. The serum IFN-γ concentrations (14 and 28 dpi) were a little higher in the group immunized with commercial vaccine C strain than the group immunized with BV-VSVG-ED-pFc-CMV-S/P-E2, but not significantly different. Most notably, the IFN-γ level in the group immunized with BV-VSVG-ED-pFc-CMV-S/P-E2 was significantly higher than that of the group immunized with BV-VSVG-ED-CMV-E2 ($P < 0.05$) (Figure 6B) ($P < 0.05$).

Discussion

Baculoviruses are insect-specific viruses in nature, thus being non-pathogenic for mammals. Baculovirus has been proved to be able to transduce various mammalian cells of human, rodent, porcine, canine, avian, feline and rabbit origins. BacMam viruses are emerging as a gene delivery vector with additional advantages over conventional vectors.

In this study, considering the complement-mediated inactivation of baculovirus, we developed four baculovirus constructs displaying complement interfering factors, and by in vitro evaluation of complement antagonism, the baculovirus displaying pFc achieved a survival rate up to 75.6% in pig serum and 65.6% in mouse serum. Flow cytometry analysis of transduced IEC cells, a cell line with high level expression of Fc receptors, demonstrated that the baculovirus display of pFc showed a significant increase in transduction efficiency (57.5 vs 16.7%) and transgene expression of reporter genes. These results revealed that baculovirus displaying pFc can be used as a promising vaccine delivery vector.

To test the potential of baculovirus displaying pFc as a vaccine delivery vector in vivo, a novel baculovirus vaccine for CSFV was constructed. In terms of optimizing the vaccine constructs, the regulatory elements VSV-G increased antigen presentation, and Syn21 and P10UTR improved antigen expression. Although it did not develop

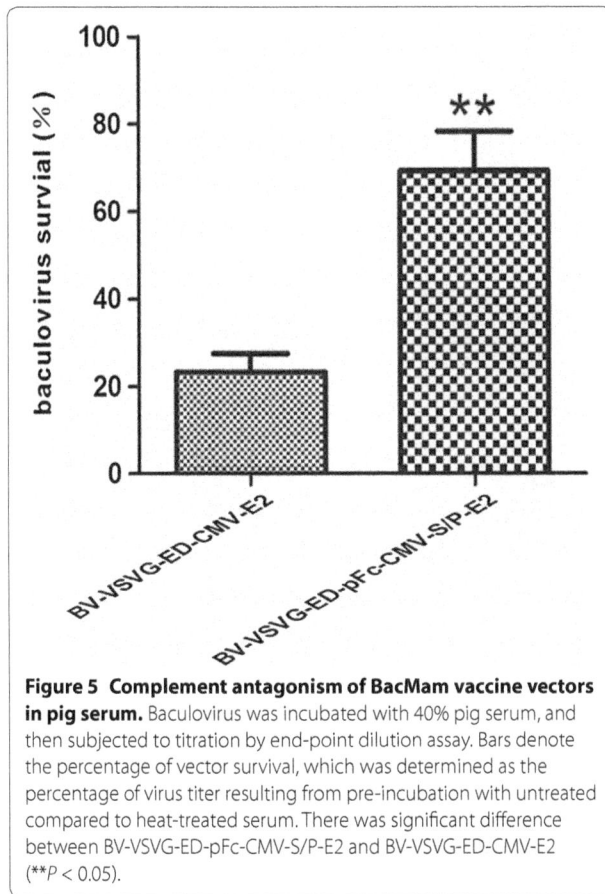

Figure 5 Complement antagonism of BacMam vaccine vectors in pig serum. Baculovirus was incubated with 40% pig serum, and then subjected to titration by end-point dilution assay. Bars denote the percentage of vector survival, which was determined as the percentage of virus titer resulting from pre-incubation with untreated compared to heat-treated serum. There was significant difference between BV-VSVG-ED-pFc-CMV-S/P-E2 and BV-VSVG-ED-CMV-E2 (**$P < 0.05$).

comparative immune response as the commercial vaccine C-strain, this baculovirus vaccine demonstrated a potential for further usage. The high titers of CSFV-specific antibody and neutralizing antibody, and increased levels of IFN-γ secretion indicated that the baculovirus effectively delivered exogenous antigen to the swine cells and stimulated the production of humoral and cellular immune responses. These results suggest a promising vaccine strategy based on the BacMam virus and baculovirus surface display system. It is notable that BV-VSVG-ED-pFc-CMV-S/P-E2 induced stronger CSFV-specific immune response than BV-VSVG-ED-CMV-E2, potentially because it has the translational enhancers Syn21 and P10UTR.

Another important question needing to be addressed is that surface display system-based IgG1 Fc makes a great difference in the efficacy of the BV-VSVG-ED-pFc-CMV-S/P-E2 vaccine. IgG Fc has been intensely investigated as a scaffold for the design of novel therapeutics due to its beneficial biological and pharmacological properties. One of the benefits of Fc-fusion proteins is their interaction with the neonatal Fc receptor (FcRn) on immune cells, thus to increase plasma half-life, and prolong therapeutic activity, providing a new perspective for vaccine development [20, 21]. It has been demonstrated that the Fc part of IgG or IgY (egg yolk antibody) can function as an immunoenhancer [22, 23]. The Fc can also fold in its independent manner and facilitate the stability of the fused proteins. In most cases, the Fc domain forms homodimers with higher affinity for the FcγRs, which enhances binding and the signaling capacity. Takashima et al. demonstrated that pseudorabies virus surface displaying IgG1 Fc gives rise to a better immune efficacy [24]. They also found that vaccination with recombinant cell surface expressing mouse IgG Fc achieves an increase in interleukin, but does not activate the complement classical pathway [25]. Another group has proved that surface display of IgG Fc on baculovirus vectors could enhance the binding to antigen-presenting cells and cell lines expressing Fc receptors [26]. These findings indicate that baculovirus based on IgG Fc surface display can be further explored as a vaccine strategy.

Our study demonstrates that the surface displayed Fc markedly improved the potency of BacMam virus. The molecular mechanism underlying this enhanced efficacy may include the following: (1) prolonging baculovirus-vectored vaccine half-life and promoting effective antigen presentation by interaction with FcRn, (2) using adjuvant function of IgG antibody Fc to activate stronger innate and adaptive immunity by interaction with FcγRs, usually with high level expression in immune cells (dendritic cells, macrophage, and B cells), thus enhancing the signaling capacity for the immune system, and (3) escaping from complement-mediated inactivation in the similar way of Fc-fusion drugs and recombinant cells displaying IgG1 Fc [25, 27–29].

The in vitro studies have proved that baculovirus can bind directly to IgM and C3b in serum, thus activating the classical and alternative pathways [30]. Our previous study has also demonstrated that the complement derived from pig serum inactivated baculovirus by activating the classical and alternative pathways (Additional file 1). Interestingly, we found that BV-VSVG-ED-pFc bound more poorly to IgM in pig serum compared to BV-VSVG-ED, indicating that this surface-displaying swine IgG1 Fc resulted in an increase in complement escape by the classical pathway (Additional file 2). To some extent, this phenomenon was in agreement with previous observations that most Fc-fusion drugs and recombinant cells displaying IgG1 Fc demonstrated remarkable complement antagonism, partially because

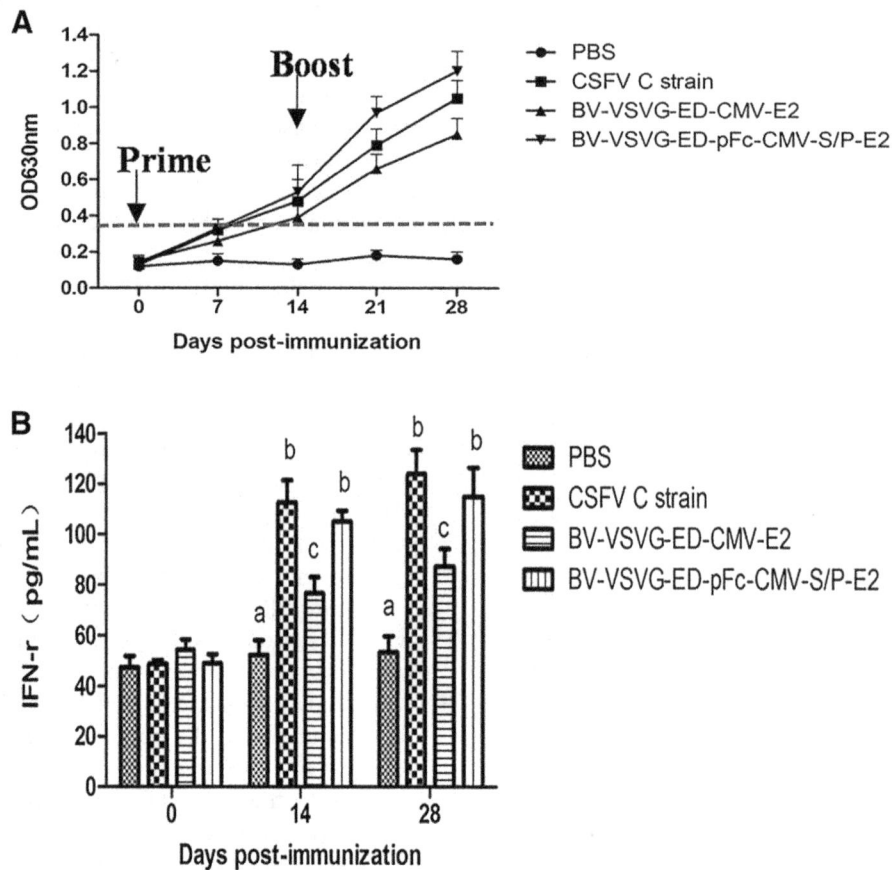

Figure 6 Detection of antibody and cellular immune responses induced by recombinant baculoviruses. A Antibody levels in sera of immunized pigs by indirect ELISA. Four groups of pigs were intramuscularly injected twice with commercial vaccine C-strain, BV-VSVG-ED-pFc-CMV-S/P-E2 or BV-VSVG-ED-CMV-E2 at a 1-week interval. Serum samples from each group were collected weekly and tested. A dashed line indicates the positive cutoff value of ELISA (OD630 nm = 0.35). **B** IFN-γ levels in sera of immunized pigs by ELISA. Serum samples from each group were collected and tested using a commercial ELISA kit (4A Biotech, Beijing, China) for quantitative detection of pig IFN-γ. Bars with different letters were significantly different (P < 0.05).

complement activation depends on the Fab (especially the CH1 domain) and hinge area [31].

In addition to serum complement, baculovirus-specific adaptive immunity also neutralizes the particles and impedes subsequent baculovirus injection in vivo [32]. Given that the BV-VSVG-ED-pFc-CMV-S/P-E2 vaccine was initially tested to evaluate immune responses in pigs with an immune procedure without optimization, though the baculovirus vector surface-displaying pFc potentiated higher level of E2-specific antibody, CSFV neutralizing antibody titer, and IFN-γ than that without pFc surface display, the efficiency of adaptive immune responses was a little lower than the commercial vaccine C-strain. Therefore, it can be improved for better efficacy by using a 3-week immunization interval or adoption of heterologous prime-boost vaccine strategy. Heterologous prime-boost regimens mostly use a viral or DNA vector for priming, followed by a boost with a subunit vaccine. This immunization strategy combines a stronger cellular immune response with a higher antibody response against the vaccine target compared to homologous immunization and can overcome the issue of anti-vector immunity [33].

We aimed to break the bottlenecks limiting baculovirus-based gene delivery for mammals. The swine IgG1 Fc displayed on the BV-VSVG-ED-pFc-CMV-S/P-E2 surface was closely related to the transduction efficiency targeting cells harboring Fc receptors, IEC cells in this study, and it also facilitated baculovirus escape from the complement in pig serum. A more comprehensive understanding of this BacMam based vaccine is essential to improve the immunogenicity of the baculovirus vector. To this end, we are currently focusing on two issues: (1) exploring in more detail the interaction between the baculovirus vector surface-displaying pFc and Fc receptors

Table 1 CSFV-specific neutralizing antibody titers in pigs immunized with BV-VSVG-ED-pFc-CMV-S/P-E2 at different days post-immunization

Groups	Pig No.	Days post-immunization				
		0	7	14	21	28
		NAbs				
A	039	<1	<1	<1	<1	<1
	075	<1	<1	<1	<1	<1
	086	<1	<1	<1	<1	<1
	116	<1	<1	<1	<1	<1
	200	<1	<1	<1	<1	<1
	$\overline{X} \pm S$	<1	<1	<1	<1	<1
B	022	<1	6	16	64	128
	046	<1	8	16	64	128
	105	<1	6	16	64	128
	142	<1	8	24	80	144
	183	<1	8	16	64	108
	$\overline{X} \pm S$	<1	7.2 ± 1.1	17.6 ± 3.6	67.2 ± 7.2	131.5 ± 12.8
C	035	<1	6	8	16	44
	056	<1	8	8	16	64
	073	<1	6	8	32	64
	117	<1	8	12	16	64
	152	<1	4	8	16	64
	$\overline{X} \pm S$	<1	6.4 ± 1.7	8.8 ± 1.8	19.2 ± 7.2	60 ± 8.9
D	026	<1	6	12	48	84
	084	<1	8	16	48	96
	093	<1	6	12	64	96
	128	<1	8	16	48	100
	192	<1	4	16	64	88
	$\overline{X} \pm S$	<1	6.4 ± 1.7	14.4 ± 2.2	54.4 ± 8.8	95.2 ± 6.6

Four groups (n = 5) of 4 week old pigs were immunized with BV-VSVG-ED-pFc-CMV-S/P-E2. Serum were collected at different time after the immunization, and subjected to detection of CSFV-specific neutralizing antibodies (NAbs) by serum-virus neutralization test (SNT). $\overline{X} \pm S$: mean ± standard deviation. Group A-D indicate pigs immunized with PBS, CSFV commercial vaccine C-strain, BV-VSVG-ED-CMV-E2 and BV-VSVG-ED-pFc-CMV-S/P-E2, respectively.

or elements in the pig serum complement system and (2) testing BV-VSVG-ED-pFc-CMV-S/P-E2 in different immunization schedules to induce stronger immune responses.

In summary, this study provides supporting evidence for the use of the BacMam virus as a vaccine delivery vector. This novel VSV-G-pseudotyped baculovirus based on IgG1 Fc surface display offers an alternative strategy for vaccine development for CSFV and other pathogens.

Additional files

Additional file 1. Effect of chelating agents on the survival of baculovirus in pig serum. Baculovirus vectors were pre-incubated with 90% serum for 60 min at 37 ℃ with or without the addition of a chelating agent, 20 mM EDTA, to chelate Ca^{2+} and Mg^{2+}, thereby inhibiting all three complement pathways, or 20 mM EGTA/14 mM $MgCl_2$ to chelate Ca^{2+}, thereby isolating the alternative pathway. The survival of virus was determined by point-end dilution assay on Sf-9 insect cells. Bars denote the percentage of vector survival in the indicated sera referred to the corresponding heat-treated sera. Data represent mean ± standard deviation (SD) of three experiments each of two repeats. Survival in EDTA serum was significantly improved compared with normal serum (P < 0.05).

Additional file 2. Detection of interaction between IgM in pig serum and recombinant baculoviruses by ELISA. 7×10^6 pfu of baculovirus was coated, and then exposed to pig serum, followed by addition of HRP-conjugated goat-anti-swine IgM. Bars denote the OD_{450}. The assay was performed in triplicate and the data are presented as mean ± SD (**P < 0.05).

Competing interests
The authors declare that they have no competing interests.

Authors' contributions
ZL and YL designed the study, carried out the experiments, analyzed data and wrote the manuscript. YZ, YY and JR helped perform the experiments. XZ and ED designed the study and draft the manuscript. All authors read and approved the final manuscript.

Acknowledgements

This work was supported by grants from Agriculture-related Special Fund for 13th Five Year Plan (2016YFD0500306), the National Natural Science Foundation of China (Grant Number 31572556), Open Foundation of State Key Laboratory of Pathogen and Biosecurity (SKLPBS1522) and the Key Construction Program (Grant Number 2015SD0018) of International Cooperation Base in S&T, Shaanxi Province, China.

References

1. Facciabene A, Aurisicchio L, La Monica N (2004) Baculovirus vectors elicit antigen-specific immune responses in mice. J Virol 78:8663–8672

2. Liu X, Li K, Song J, Liang C, Wang X, Chen X (2006) Efficient and stable gene expression in rabbit intervertebral disc cells transduced with a recombinant baculovirus vector. Spine 31:732–735

3. Kost TA, Condreay JP, Jarvis DL (2005) Baculovirus as versatile vectors for protein expression in insect and mammalian cells. Nat Biotech 23:567–575

4. Wang KC, Wu JC, Chung YC, Ho YC, Chang MD, Hu YC (2005) Baculovirus as a highly efficient gene delivery vector for the expression of hepatitis delta virus antigens in mammalian cells. Biotech Bioeng 89:464–473

5. Felberbaum RS (2015) The baculovirus expression vector system: a commercial manufacturing platform for viral vaccines and gene therapy vectors. Biotech J 10:702–714

6. Hefferon KL, Oomens AG, Monsma SA, Finnerty CM, Blissard GW (1999) Host cell receptor binding by baculovirus GP64 and kinetics of virion entry. Virology 258:455–468

7. Oomens AG, Blissard GW (1999) Requirement for GP64 to drive efficient budding of Autographa californica multicapsid nucleopolyhedrovirus. Virology 254:297–314

8. Makela AR, Oker-Blom C (2008) The baculovirus display technology — an evolving instrument for molecular screening and drug delivery. Comb Chem High Throughput Screen 11:86–98

9. Kaba SA, Hemmes JC, van Lent JW, Vlak JM, Nene V, Musoke AJ, van Oers MM (2003) Baculovirus surface display of *Theileria parva* p67 antigen preserves the conformation of sporozoite-neutralizing epitopes. Prot Eng 16:73–78

10. Kitajima M, Hamazaki H, Miyano-Kurosaki N, Takaku H (2006) Characterization of baculovirus Autographa californica multiple nuclear polyhedrosis virus infection in mammalian cells. Biochem Biophys Res Commun 343:378–384

11. Kaikkonen MU, Yla-Herttuala S, Airenne KJ (2011) How to avoid complement attack in baculovirus-mediated gene delivery. J Invertebr Pathol 107(Suppl):S71–S79

12. Ji W, Guo Z, Ding NZ, He CQ (2015) Studying classical swine fever virus: making the best of a bad virus. Virus Res 197:35–47

13. van Rijn PA, Bossers A, Wensvoort G, Moormann RJ (1996) Classical swine fever virus (CSFV) envelope glycoprotein E2 containing one structural antigenic unit protects pigs from lethal CSFV challenge. J Gen Virol 77:2737–2745

14. Voigt H, Merant C, Wienhold D, Braun A, Hutet E, Le Potier MF, Saalmüller A, Pfaff E, Büttner M (2007) Efficient priming against classical swine fever with a safe glycoprotein E2 expressing Orf virus recombinant (ORFV VrV-E2). Vaccine 25:5915–5926

15. Sun Y, Liu DF, Wang YF, Liang BB, Cheng D, Li N, Qi QF, Zhu QH, Qiu HJ (2010) Generation and efficacy evaluation of a recombinant adenovirus expressing the E2 protein of classical swine fever virus. Res Vet Sci 88:77–82

16. Sun Y, Tian DY, Li S, Meng QL, Zhao BB, Li Y, Li D, Ling LJ, Liao YJ, Qiu HJ (2013) Comprehensive evaluation of the adenovirus/alphavirus-replicon chimeric vector-based vaccine rAdV-SFV-E2 against classical swine fever. Vaccine 31:538–544

17. Liu Y, Zhang Y, Yao L, Hao H, Fu X, Yang Z, Du E (2015) Enhanced production of porcine circovirus type 2 (PCV2) virus-like particles in Sf9 cells by translational enhancers. Biotechnol Lett 37:1765–1771

18. Hofmann C, Strauss M (1998) Baculovirus-mediated gene transfer in the presence of human serum or blood facilitated by inhibition of the complement system. Gene Ther 5:531–536

19. Buonavoglia C, Falcone E, Pestalozza S, Di Trani L, D'Amore E (1989) A rapid serum neutralization test in microplates for the detection of antibodies to hog cholera virus. J Virol Methods 23:77–79

20. Butler JE, Wertz N, Deschacht N, Kacskovics I (2009) Porcine IgG: structure, genetics, and evolution. Immunogenetics 61:209–230

21. Jiang X, Hu J, Thirumalai D, Zhang X (2016) Immunoglobulin transporting receptors are potential targets for the immunity enhancement and generation of mammary gland bioreactor. Front Immunol 7:214

22. Getahun A, Heyman B (2006) How antibodies act as natural adjuvants. Immunol Lett 104:38–45

23. Levin D, Golding B, Strome SE, Sauna ZE (2015) Fc fusion as a platform technology: potential for modulating immunogenicity. Trends Biotechnol 33:27–34

24. Takashima Y, Tsukamoto M, Ota H, Matsumoto Y, Hayashi Y, Otsuka H (2005) Immunization with pseudorabies virus harboring Fc domain of IgG makes a contribution to protection of mice from lethal challenge. Vaccine 23:3775–3782

25. Batanova TA, Ota H, Kitoh K, Matsumoto Y, Hayashi Y, Takashima Y (2006) Cell surface expression of a chimeric protein containing mouse immunoglobulin G1 Fc domain and its immunological property. J Vet Med Sci 68:87–90

26. Martyn JC, Cardin AJ, Wines BD, Cendron A, Li S, Mackenzie J, Powell M, Gowans EJ (2009) Surface display of IgG Fc on baculovirus vectors enhances binding to antigen-presenting cells and cell lines expressing Fc receptors. Arch Virol 154:1129–1138

27. Michaelsen TE, Sandlie I, Bratlie DB, Sandin RH, Ihle O (2009) Structural difference in the complement activation site of human IgG1 and IgG3. Scand J Immunol 70:553–564

28. Mekhaiel DN, Czajkowsky DM, Andersen JT, Shi J, El-Faham M, Doenhoff M, McIntosh RS, Sandlie I, He J, Hu J, Shao Z, Pleass RJ (2011) Polymeric human Fc-fusion proteins with modified effector functions. Sci Rep 1:124

29. Czajkowsky DM, Hu J, Shao Z, Pleass RJ (2012) Fc-fusion proteins: new developments and future perspectives. EMBO Mol Med 4:1015–1028

30. Georgopoulos LJ, Elgue G, Sanchez J, Dussupt V, Magotti P, Lambris JD, Tötterman TH, Maitland NJ, Nilsson B (2009) Preclinical evaluation of innate immunity to baculovirus gene therapy vectors in whole human blood. Mol Immunol 46:2911–2917

31. Gaboriaud C, Juanhuix J, Gruez A, Lacroix M, Darnault C, Pignol D, Verger D, Fontecilla-Camps JC, Arlaud GJ (2003) The crystal structure of the globular head of complement protein C1q provides a basis for its versatile recognition properties. J Biol Chem 278:46974–46982

32. Luo WY, Lin SY, Lo KW, Lu CH, Hung CL, Chen CY, Chang CC, Hu YC (2013) Adaptive immune responses elicited by baculovirus and impacts on subsequent transgene expression in vivo. J Virol 87:4965–4973

33. Kardani K, Bolhassani A, Shahbazi S (2016) Prime-boost vaccine strategy against viral infections: mechanisms and benefits. Vaccine 34:413–423

7

Cytokine response to the RSV antigen delivered by dendritic cell-directed vaccination in congenic chicken lines

Jitka Mucksová[1], Jiří Plachý[2], Ondřej Staněk[3], Jiří Hejnar[2], Jiří Kalina[1], Barbora Benešová[1] and Pavel Trefil[1]*

Abstract

Systems of antigen delivery into antigen-presenting cells represent an important novel strategy in chicken vaccine development. In this study, we verified the ability of Rous sarcoma virus (RSV) antigens fused with streptavidin to be targeted by specific biotinylated monoclonal antibody (anti-CD205) into dendritic cells and induce virus-specific protective immunity. The method was tested in four congenic lines of chickens that are either resistant or susceptible to the progressive growth of RSV-induced tumors. Our analyses confirmed that the biot-anti-CD205-SA-FITC complex was internalized by chicken splenocytes. In the cytokine expression profile, several significant differences were evident between RSV-challenged progressor and regressor chicken lines. A significant up-regulation of IL-2, IL-12, IL-15, and IL-18 expression was detected in immunized chickens of both regressor and progressor groups. Of these cytokines, IL-2 and IL-12 were most up-regulated 14 days post-challenge (dpc), while IL-15 and IL-18 were most up-regulated at 28 dpc. On the contrary, IL-10 expression was significantly down-regulated in all immunized groups of progressor chickens at 14 dpc. We detected significant up-regulation of IL-17 in the group of immunized progressors. LITAF down-regulation with iNOS up-regulation was especially observed in the progressor group of immunized chickens that developed large tumors. Based on the increased expression of cytokines specific for activated dendritic cells, we conclude that our system is able to induce partial stimulation of specific cell types involved in cell-mediated immunity.

Introduction

Generation of de novo adaptive responses, including responses to vaccines, is primarily elicited by dendritic cells (DC), specialized leukocytes adapted for antigen capture, processing and presentation to T lymphocytes. Knowledge of these cells in a target species is therefore crucial in finding the most effective means of vaccination. The key role of T cell-mediated responses to cancer has been established in several models [1]. The antitumor immune response relies on DC, which act as professional antigen-presenting cells (APC). Altered DC function is common in tumors producing soluble factors—cytokines—with immunosuppressive activity [2,

3]. DC express, among other, the CD205 (Ly75, DEC205) molecule that functions as an endocytic receptor involved in the uptake of extracellular antigens. In the chicken, the presence of this molecule was also confirmed, along with its endocytic properties [4]. Importantly, DC could be targeted with antigen-conjugated monoclonal antibodies specific for CD205, which are then efficiently internalized, processed in the endosomal compartment, and presented to both major histocompatibility complex I (MHC I) and MHC II molecules [5].

In this study, we used a monoclonal antibody (anti-CD205) for direct antigen delivery. This strategy of activating different DC populations by direct in vivo targeting of their surface receptors has been pioneered by Steinman and Nussenzweig, who used antigen coupling to antibodies to target receptors on DC surfaces [6–8]. We used genetic fusion of the antigen with streptavidin (SA), which in its tetrameric form binds a biotinylated

*Correspondence: pavel.trefil@bri.cz
[1] BIOPHARM, Research Institute of Biopharmacy and Veterinary Drugs, Jílové U Prahy, Czech Republic
Full list of author information is available at the end of the article

antibody targeting a surface receptor on the APC. Thus prepared complexes can deliver immunogens into DC through endocytosis with the selected surface receptor, enabling antigen processing and presentation, and leading to induction of adaptive immunity [9, 10].

We applied this novel vaccination approach to our previously described model system of inbred lines resistant (CB, CB.RI; regressors) or susceptible (CC, CC.RI; progressors) to progressive growth of Rous sarcoma virus (RSV)-induced tumors [2, 3]. RSV harbors the oncogene v-*src*, which is responsible for cell transformation [11]. Previous studies using the model system of Prague congenic lines established a decisive role of the B-F—chicken MHC class I—genes in the ability to regress RSV-induced tumors [12]. The immune-based mechanism of tumor regression in this experimental system has also been demonstrated. Both v-src and RSV envelope (env) proteins serve as antigens in particular chicken lines [13–16]. On the contrary to the MHC of typical mammals, there is only a single dominantly expressed class I molecule in the chicken MHC, which is of crucial importance for the function of particular haplotypes [17, 18]. Dominantly expressed class I (B-F) molecules of the B-F12 and B-F4 haplotypes of congenic lines CB and CC, respectively, have been analyzed in detail as to the binding capacity of predicted peptides derived either from the v-src oncogene or env-encoded protein products of RSV [19–21]. Furthermore, coevolution of the B-F and peptide transporter genes (TAP) within the abovementioned haplotypes has been established [20]. Thus, the ability of certain class I (B-F) molecules to specifically bind the RSV-derived peptides correlates precisely with the outcome of the RSV-induced tumors—regression/progression [19, 22]. The molecular mechanism of B-F (class I) and TAP interaction is well understood [20]. On the contrary, the function of the B-G (class IV) molecules and their possible interaction with the B-F (class I) molecules is still not clear [23], despite a wealth of experimental evidence suggesting the role of the B-G molecules in modulation of some immune based phenomena [24–28].

In this study, we describe a new system of antigen delivery into chicken DC and assess its potential for vaccination of chickens. In order to get some insight into the cellular and molecular mechanisms, we paid particular attention to changes in the cytokine profile after vaccination and immune challenge.

Materials and methods

For preparation of anti-chCD205 and for construction, expression and purification of the recombinant SA-RSV fusion proteins, see Additional files 1, 2, 3.

Experimental animals

All immunization and tumor induction experiments were carried out with the highly inbred chicken lines CB (B12/B12), CB.RI (B12r1/B12r1) and CC (B4/B4), CC.RI (B4r1/B4r1) maintained at the Institute of Molecular Genetics, Prague. Recombinant haplotype B12r1 is composed of B-F12 and B-G4 genes whereas the haplotype B4r1 is reciprocal being composed of B-F4 and B-G12 genes [29]. All chicken lines were free of exogenous avian leukosis viruses. All procedures were conducted in accordance with the EU Directive 2010/63/EU for animal experiments, comply with the ARRIVE guidelines and with the Guide for the Care and Use of Laboratory Animals and were approved by the Animal Care and Use Committee of the Academy of Sciences of the Czech Republic.

Specificity of the monoclonal antibody anti-chCD205 and its internalization

For Western blotting, the recombinant proteins CD205B and CD205F were separated on Tris-Tricine SDS PAGE and transferred to the nitrocellulose membrane (Immobilon-P, GE Healthcare). Membranes were blocked with 5% nonfat milk in PBS containing 0.05% Tween-20 (PBST) for 1 h at room temperature, incubated with primary antibodies in PBST containing 5% nonfat milk for 1 h at room temperature prior to incubation with horseradish peroxidase-conjugated goat anti-mouse antibody (GE Healthcare) diluted in 5% nonfat milk PBST for 1 h at room temperature. Detection was carried out using a SuperSignal West Femto Maximum Sensitivity Substrate chemiluminescence reagent kit (Pierce, Thermo Fisher Scientific).

For the flow cytometry, peripheral blood mononuclear cells (PBMC) were isolated from chicken heparinized blood samples. Pieces of freshly isolated chicken spleen were crushed on a steel sieve. Splenocytes as well as PBMC were washed and centrifuged in a 1.077 density Histopaque gradient (Sigma-Aldrich) to remove nucleated erythrocytes. The monoclonal antibodies against chicken antigens CD4 (MCA2164F, AbDSerotec, USA), CD8a (MCA2166PE, AbDSerotec, USA), Bu1 (8395-08, AV20, Southern Biotech, USA), MHCII (8350-01, 2G11, Southern Biotech, USA), KUL01 (8420-02, Southern Biotech, USA), TCRλδ (CON5-CZ, TCR1, Exbio, Czech Republic), and putative CD11c (clone 8F2, a generous gift from Prof. Kaspers, University of Munich) were used. Conjugated complexes CD205-biot (clone 104-2C4/D8) and SA-FITC (SA1001, Invitrogen, USA) as well as secondary antibodies rabbit anti-mouse IgG-APC (SAB1426, Gentaur), mouse anti-chicken IgG-FITC (clone G-1, Southern Biotech, USA), and goat anti-mouse IgM-PE (sc-3768, SantaCruz Biotech) were employed.

For internalization, chicken spleen cells were incubated at 1×10^6 cells per well at 4 °C with 1.5 µg/mL of antibody against CD205-biot. The cells were then washed and incubated with SA-FITC conjugate for 1 h at 4 °C. After that, the cells were incubated either at 40 or 4 °C for 1 or 2 h. The reduction of mean fluorescence intensity (MFI) of the cell surface-bound anti-chCD205 monoclonal antibody after endocytosis was calculated as $100 - ((\text{MFI biot-mAb} + \text{FITC-SA 40 °C}) - (\text{MFI biot-control Ig} + \text{FITC-SA 4 °C})/(\text{MFI biot-mAb} + \text{FITC-SA 4 °C}) - (\text{MFI biot-control Ig} + \text{FITC-SA 4 °C})) \times 100$. The cells were analyzed using a FacsCalibur device (Becton–Dickinson) and FlowJo software (TreeStar).

Immunization of chickens

Chickens were immunized with a dose of 100 nmol of the mixture of SA-RSV tetramers complexed with 200 nmol anti-CD205 in the presence of 200 µg poly I:C (Sigma Aldrich, P1530) per chicken. The mixture of SA-RSV was composed of equal amounts of tetramers SA-vsrcA; SA-vsrcB; SA-ENVoep; SA-ENVly; SA-POL; SA-GAG—approximately 17 nmol (~4 µg) of each per chicken. The immunization dose was adjusted as described previously [9, 10]. The control group was mock-immunized with 200 µg of poly I:C per chicken.

Chickens were immunized with 0.2 mL of appropriately diluted freshly prepared antigenic solution subcutaneously (sc) into the left wing web (needle 23G × 25 mm). Immunization was repeated three times, first at the age of three weeks and then with two consecutive boosts at 7-day intervals.

RSV challenge, tumor monitoring

The Prague strain of RSV (PR-RSV-C) was used [30] as tumor inducing challenge. Chickens were sc inoculated with a dose of to 100 (CB, CB.RI) or 20 (CC, CC.RI) focus-forming units (FFU) in 0.2 mL of cultivation medium (DMEM) into the outer area of pectoral muscle one week after the last immunization. At the end of the defined experimental period (28–35 days post-challenge, dpc), chickens were sacrificed, tumors were excised and weighed with 0.1 g precision. Tumors were then arbitrarily divided into two groups: small tumors, i.e. tumors up to 5 g (including completely regressed tumors) in the regressor lines CB and CB.RI, and tumors up to 20 g in the progressor lines CC and CC.RI; large tumors, i.e. tumors over 5 g in the CB and CB.RI, and over 20 g in the CC and CC.RI lines.

RNA isolation, reverse transcription

Leukocytes from whole blood were obtained using Histopaque-1077 (Sigma) centrifugation. Total RNA from chicken leukocytes was isolated using Tri Reagent according to the manufacturer's protocol (MRC, USA; Thermo Scientific, USA). RNA integrity number (RIN) was measured using capillary electrophoresis performed in Agilent Bioanalyzer 2100 with RNA 6000 Nano Assay (Agilent Technologies, CA, USA) and was adjusted to be higher than 6.5 in all samples selected for the analyses. RNA samples (400 ng/µL) were reverse transcribed to cDNA using a Transcriptor High Fidelity cDNA Synthesis Kit (Roche) according to the manufacturer's instructions.

Gene expression analysis

Gene expression analysis was performed in BioMark (Fluidigm, CA, USA), which enables a large number of real-time PCR (RT-PCR) reactions in a single run. Before BioMark analysis, the samples were pre-amplified. The RT-PCR reactions were carried out in GE Dynamic Chip 96.96 in a BioMark HD System (Fluidigm). 5 µL of sample premix consisted of 1 µL of 20 × diluted pre-amplified cDNA, 0.25 µL of 20 × DNA Binding Dye Sample Loading Reagent (Fluidigm), 2.5 µL of FastEvaGreen Supermix (Bio-Rad), 0.1 µL of 4 × diluted ROX (Invitrogen, USA) and 1.15 µL of RNase/DNase-free water. Each 5 µL assay premix consisted of 2.5 µL of 10 µM primers and 2.5 µL of DA Assay Loading Reagent (Fluidigm). The conditions of RT-PCR were the following: 95 °C for 3 min, 30 cycles of 95 °C for 5 s, and 60 °C for 20 s. The melting curve analysis was then performed. Primers were designed using Primer3 software or described sequences were used [31, 32] (Additional file 4). The GAPDH and 28S reference genes were selected out of the reference gene candidates by Normfinder (GenEx, Sweden). Each sample was analyzed in three technical replicates. The data were collected using BioMark 3.1.2. Data Collection software and analyzed by Fluidigm Real-Time PCR Analysis Software 4.1.2. (Fluidigm).

The cut-off value for Cq was set at 23 and values higher than that were replaced by the Cq value of 25. A few missing values were replaced by the highest value plus 2, then the data were recalculated into relative quantities and logarithms were applied. Data were normalized with GAPDH. The fold change in expression was calculated using the 2^{-Cq} method for each sample and then expressed as the mean of all fold changes. The control was set as 100% and experimental samples were compared to the control.

In vitro antigen restimulation and Multiplex cytokine assays

Chickens were sc immunized three times at seven day intervals with a dose of 100 nmol of the SA-RSV tetramers (equal amounts of tetramers SA-vsrcA; SA-vsrcB; 50 nmol of each) complexed with 200 nmol biotin-anti-CD205 in the presence of 200 µg poly I:C per chicken.

At day 10 after the last immunization, PBMC were isolated and in vitro restimulated (250 000 cells/well) with SA-vsrcA + SA-vsrcB antigen (10 µg/mL) and free SA (10 µg/mL) as a control. Cells were cultivated at 37 °C in RPMI-1640 (Sigma) supplemented with 10% FBS (Gibco) and 1% Glutamine–Penicillin–Streptomycin (Sigma). 4 days after in vitro restimulation, the v-src-specific interleukin (IL-12, IL-2, IFNγ, IL-10) responses were measured using the Bio-Plex system in the culture supernatants. For each cytokine, the recombinant protein, capture antibody and detection antibody were obtained as complete kit (Kingfisher Biotech, USA; cat.nos. DIY0686C-003 IL-12; DIY0685C-003 IL-2; DIY0684C-003 IFNγ; DIY1118C-003 IL-10).

Culture supernatants from Ag-restimulation assays were collected at the indicated time. Cytokine profiles were then tested using Bio-Plex Pro Assays (BIO-RAD) according to the manufacturer's instructions. Each cytokine was tested in a single bead assay to determine the optimal concentration of antibody detection. The microspheres were multiplexed and optimized for incubation times and Streptavidin-PE reporter signal. All assays were performed with the same matrix as the culture supernatants, calibration curves from recombinant cytokine standards were prepared with threefold dilution steps. Measurements and data analysis of all assays were performed with the Bio-Plex system in combination with the Bio-Plex Manager Software.

Statistical analyses

The weights of individual tumors were compared using ANOVA with Fisher LSD test, Mann–Whitney test and t test. Data of gene expression were prepared in Genex 5.3.7 software (GenEx). The following analysis was done in SAS 9.4 software. Groups were compared by repeated three-way ANOVA. Contrasts were used for detailed comparison. Linear discriminant function analysis based on all analyzed genes was used to show separation of different groups. The cytokine expression profiles of RSV-challenged chicken groups were classified using methods of principal component analysis (PCA) [33] and linear discrimination analysis in XLSTAT software (StatSoft, Czech Republic).

Results
SA-RSV fusion proteins

The complete sequence of the RSV antigens v-src, env, pol and gag were fused to the N- and C-terminus of the tetramerization core of streptavidin. The SA fusion with whole antigens v-src and env did not form stable tetramers due to their size. These two antigens were therefore split into two overlapping parts. In env, the signal, transmembrane and intracellular domain were also excluded

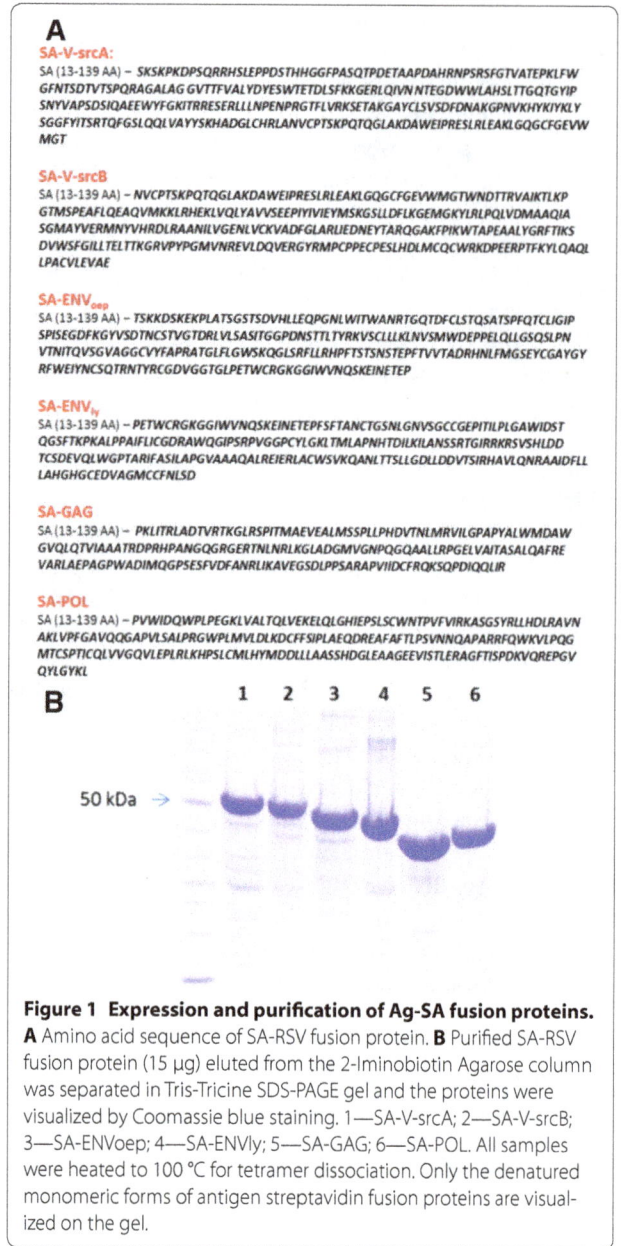

Figure 1 Expression and purification of Ag-SA fusion proteins.
A Amino acid sequence of SA-RSV fusion protein. **B** Purified SA-RSV fusion protein (15 µg) eluted from the 2-Iminobiotin Agarose column was separated in Tris-Tricine SDS-PAGE gel and the proteins were visualized by Coomassie blue staining. 1—SA-V-srcA; 2—SA-V-srcB; 3—SA-ENVoep; 4—SA-ENVIy; 5—SA-GAG; 6—SA-POL. All samples were heated to 100 °C for tetramer dissociation. Only the denatured monomeric forms of antigen streptavidin fusion proteins are visualized on the gel.

(Figure 1A). All fusion proteins were produced in *E. coli* and purified close to homogeneity (Figure 1B). The fusion proteins with antigens fused to the C- terminal part of SA (SA-RSV) were isolated in higher purity and displayed longer stability than the N-terminus fusions (RSV-SA). The SA-RSV tetramers were therefore used for the vaccination study.

Specificity and internalization capacity of the monoclonal antibody anti-chCD205

The specificity of newly prepared anti-chCD205 monoclonal antibodies was tested by ELISA against recombinant antigens CD205B and CD205F (data not shown). The specificity of the positive clones was verified on Western blot, where the recombinant proteins CD205B and CD205F were detected using different clones of monoclonal antibodies (Figure 2A). For the purpose of antigen delivery, it was necessary to select antibodies recognizing natural surface receptor CD205 by flow cytometry on chicken splenocytes and blood cells. Flow cytometry data were gated to exclude cell debris according to the cell granularity and size (SSC/FSC parameters). CD205 was expressed at very low levels on T cell subsets of leukocytes (CD4$^+$, TCRγδ$^+$, and CD8a$^+$) as well as splenocytes. As shown in Figures 2B and C, higher expression levels of CD205 were seen on KUL01$^+$ CD11c$^+$, MHCII$^+$ cells and Bu1$^+$ cells.

FITC-labeled cells incubated at 40 °C showed a substantial decrease of surface fluorescence intensity after 1 and 2 h of incubation, while the cells left incubated at 4 °C showed similar fluorescence to the initial analysis. MFI was reduced reaching 36.4% after 1 h and 26.8% after 2 h of incubation at 40 °C (Figure 2D). This indicates that the biot-anti-CD205-SA-FITC complex was internalized into cells and entered the low pH milieu of the cell endocytic apparatus as FITC dye is pH-sensitive [34].

In vitro antigen restimulation

In order to verify the changed expression of the three major cytokines (IL-2, IL-12 and IFNγ), the in vitro restimulation of PBMC was performed. The levels of three cytokines detected in PBMC culture supernatants (Il-2, IL-12 and IFNγ) were significantly increased in the immunized groups that were restimulated with v-src antigen. On the contrary, the amount of IL-10 was at the same level as in PBMC restimulated with v-src or control antigen or in the group without restimulation respectively (Figure 3).

RSV-induced tumor growth in the high (CB, CB.RI) and low (CC, CC.RI) responder chicken lines

As expected, the general pattern of the response to RSV challenge represented regression of relatively small tumors (≤ 2 g) in the CB and CB.RI lines, while progressive growth of tumors was observed in the CC and CC.RI lines even when challenged with a fivefold lower dose of RSV (Figure 4). The difference in the mean tumor weight 28 dpc between the regressor lines CB and CB.RI and progressor lines CC and CC.RI was highly significant (data not shown). However, on the contrary to expectations, we observed an exacerbating effect of immunization in the CB.RI ($p < 0.01$) and CC ($p < 0.05$) chickens (Figure 4). However, a potential protective effect of immunization can be seen in the CB and CC.RI lines, but these differences were not

significant. Interestingly, the adverse effect of vaccination correlates with the B-G4 allel presented in both CB.R1 and CC chickens. However, a protective effect was seen in the CB (regressors) chicks with MHC-B haplotype composed of its canonical partners the B-F12 and B-G12, and also in the CC.R1 (progressors) chicks with the B-G12 allele present in the recombinant haplotype together with the B-F4—responsible for generally progressor phenotype (for composition of the MHC-B haplotypes see "Materials and methods", and "Discussion").

Comparison of the cytokine profiles in RSV-challenged chickens of different congenic lines

Expression of twenty genes (see Additional file 4) active in chicken blood cells that can influence the process of immune response and consequently the tumor growth were tested. To compare the kinetics of the cytokine profiles in RSV-challenged chickens, we pooled CB and CB.RI lines and CC and CC.RI lines into the groups of regressors and progressors, respectively. The multidimensional information on cytokine gene expression profiles was transformed into a 2-dimensional plot using PCA. Classification of the tested samples based on PCA results was confirmed by discriminant analysis, in which a score of 100% was reached for the confusion matrix. Based on the multidimensional gene expression profile, the samples of all experimental chicken groups were classified into three clusters (Figure 5) at each sampling time. In the group of regressors, the most prominent difference in multidimensional cytokine expression between the immunized and non-immunized groups was detected 14 dpc, while in the group of progressors the most prominent difference was seen 28 dpc. In the non-immunized groups (all times) of regressors there were significant similarities of clusters in comparison to immunized regressor groups. Interestingly, the multidimensional expression profiles in groups at time of challenge and 28 dpc (both non-immunized and immunized) were similar by F1 main component.

When comparing single cytokine expression profiles between progressor and regressor immunized and non-immunized groups, several significant differences were found (see Additional file 5). A significant up-regulation of IL-2, IL-12, IL-15 and IL-18 expression was detected in immunized chickens of both regressor and progressor groups. Of these cytokines, IL-2 and IL-12 expression was most up-regulated 14 dpc, while IL-15 and IL-18 were most up-regulated 28 dpc (Figure 6; IL-12, IL-18). On the contrary, IL-10 expression was significantly down-regulated 14 dpc in all immunized groups of progressor chickens. Interestingly, we detected significant up-regulation of IL-17 in the group of immunized

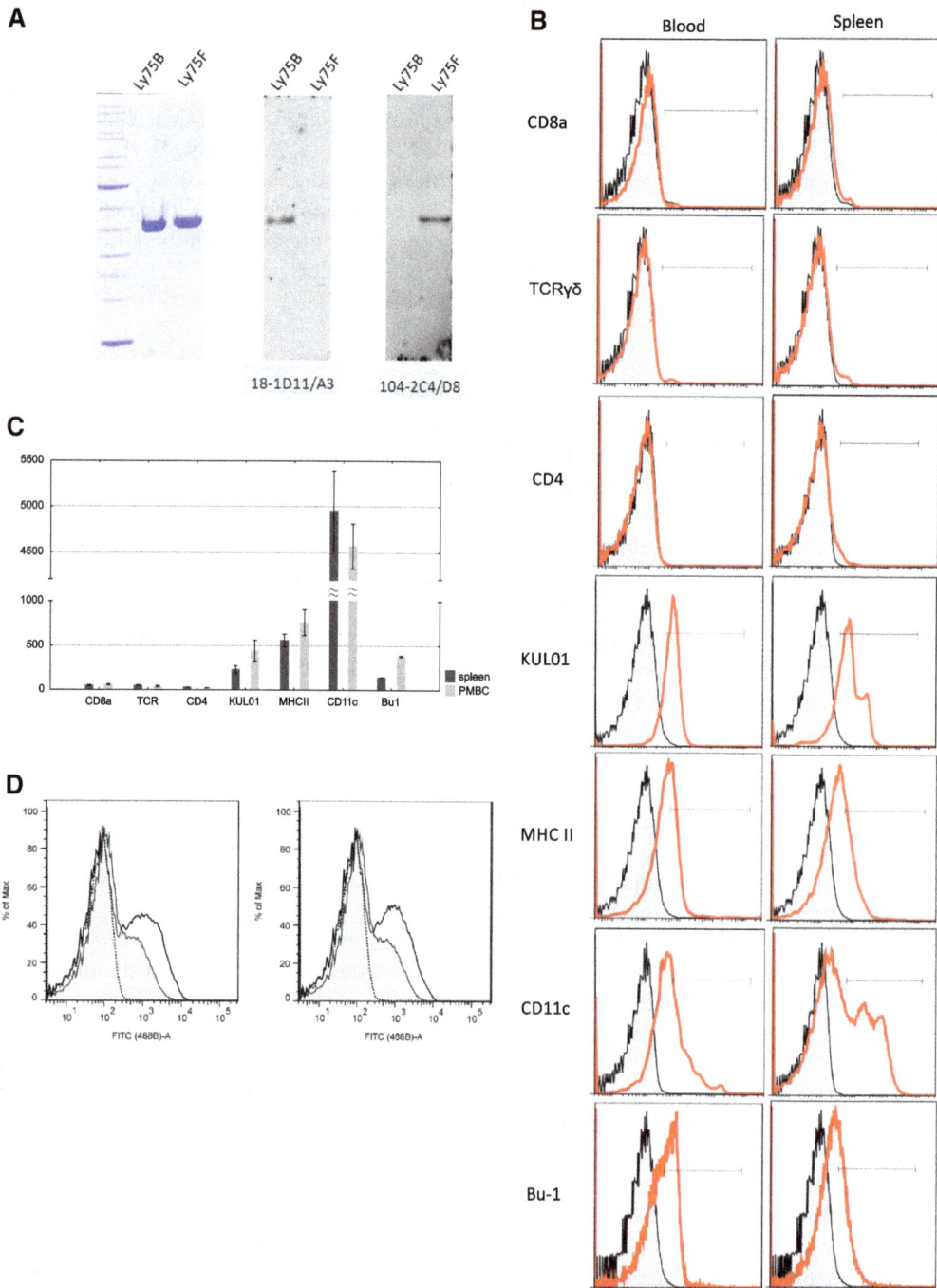

Figure 2 Specific binding of anti-chCD205 and internalization of antigen delivery complex. A The recombinant parts of chicken CD205 receptor used for monoclonal antibody preparation and the monoclonal antibody characterization. The CD205B and CD205F proteins were purified from inclusion bodies on DEAE Sepharose and separated on Tris-Tricine polyacrylamide gel stained by Coomassie blue (left). Monoclonal mouse anti-CD205 antibodies were analyzed using Western blots. Results of two representative detections of monoclonal anti-CD205 specific for CD205B or CD205F are shown. **B** CD205 expression on leukocytes. Splenocytes and peripheral leukocytes were stained with anti-chicken CD205 antibody and antibodies recognizing each of the indicated antigens. Histograms represent the CD205 fluorescence for cells gated for positive expression of the markers indicated at the left. The results of one representative of three experiments are shown. **C** Median fluorescence intensity (MFI) of CD205 stained cells and standard deviation. **D** Internalization of streptavidin-CD205-FITC complex by chicken primary splenocytes one (left) and two (right) hours of incubation in different temperatures. Dotted line plot non-labelled cells (biot—control IgG); Black line plot—FITC labelled cells incubated in 4 °C; Gray line plot—FITC labelled cells incubated in 40 °C.

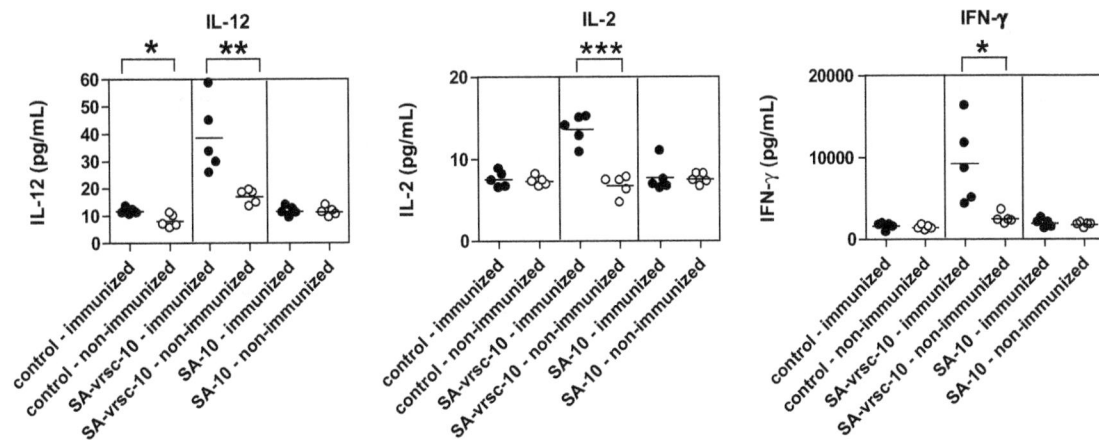

Figure 3 In vitro Ag restimulation. The v-src-specific interleukin (IL-12, IL-2, IFNγ, IL-10) responses were measured in chickens of the CB and CB.RI lines using the Bio-Plex system in the culture supernatants. Horizontal bars indicate the mean values. The results represent at least two independent experiments. Control (n = 5 + 5): non-restimulated control; SA-vsrc-10 (n = 5 + 5): samples restimulated with the mixture of tetramers SA-vsrcA and SA-vsrcB of immunized and non-immunized animals; SA-10 (n = 5 + 5): free SA restimulation control. Statistical significance determined by the Student's t test: *p < 0.05; **p < 0.01; ***p < 0.001.

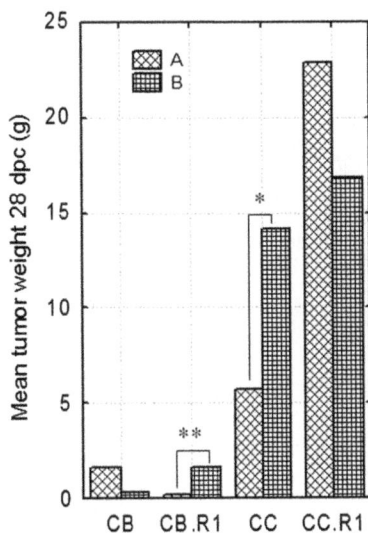

Figure 4 Comparison of tumor size between control and immunized groups of chickens. For statistical analysis, the non-immunized (**A**) and immunized (**B**) chickens of all inbred lines (CB, CB.RI, CC and CC.RI) were considered. Chickens of the regressor lines CB, CB.R1 and the progressor lines CC, CC.R1 were challenged with 100 FFU and 20 FFU of the RSV-PR-C respectively (for details see "Materials and methods"). Each column represents an average tumor size in the group of eight chickens (total number 64 chickens). *p < 0.05 non-parametric test (Mann–Whitney); **p < 0.01 both parametric (t test) and non-parametric test (Mann–Whitney).

progressors and significant up-regulation of MIF and XCL1 in both groups of progressors 14 dpc. Surprisingly, down-regulation of LITAF, a putative chicken analog of TNFα, and up-regulation of iNOS were observed especially in the progressor group of immunized chickens that developed large tumors.

The cytokine pattern correlates with the RSV-induced tumor status (regression/progression)

The PCA method and discrimination analysis were used for classification and discrimination of multimarker gene cytokine expression profiles of experimental chickens. Individual samples were distributed based on the tumor weight.

In the regressor lines, samples taken from chickens with small or large tumors formed distinct compact sets with significantly different expression cytokine profiles (Figure 7A). Analyses of progressor lines also showed significantly different expression profiles (Figure 7B). Among the set of 20 tested genes, 14 genes exhibited altered expression (Additional file 5). Fourteen genes (IL-1, IL-2, MIF, IL-4, IL-12, IL-18, IL-15, TLR7, TRAF5, XCL1, IL-17, TGF-β, iNOS, IFNγ) were found within the progressor lines, whereas six genes (IL-15, IL-18, IL-8, TGF-β, TLR7, iNOS) were found in the regressor lines. For detailed significance of data relations, see Table 1. The remaining marker genes (IFNα, IL-22, IL-13) were excluded from the panel as their expression did not change in response to immunization.

Discussion

In this report, we used a new system of vaccination with antigen delivery into chicken APC. For the first time in the chicken, we verified the ability of fusion complexes of RSV antigens with SA to target specific biotinylated monoclonal antibody. For this purpose, we prepared a

A   **lines CB,CBRI (regressors)**

non-immunized   **immunized**

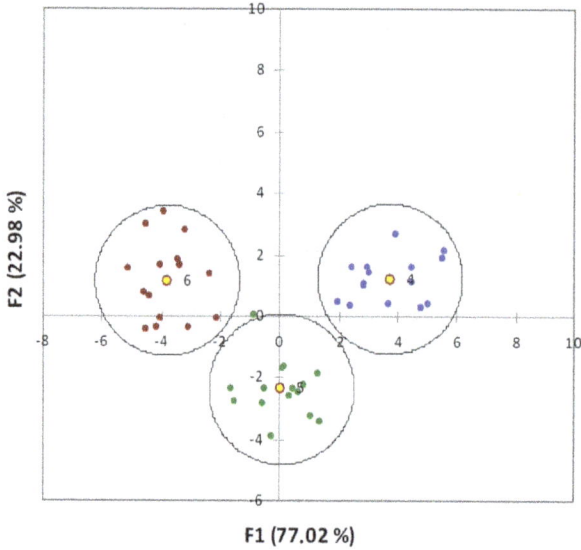
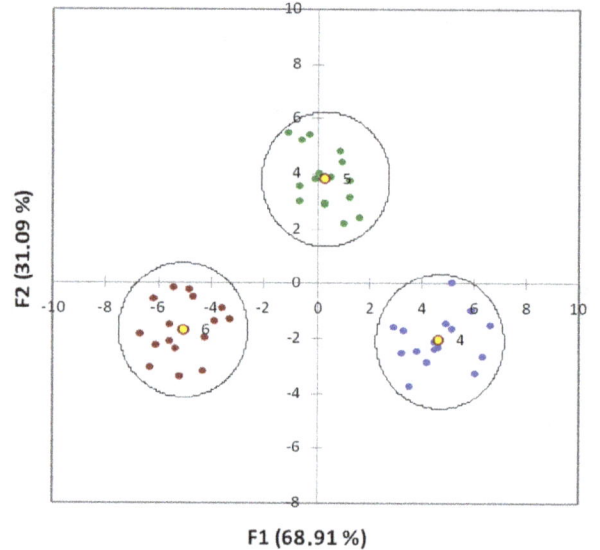

B   **lines CC, CCRI (progressors)**

non-immunized   **immunized**

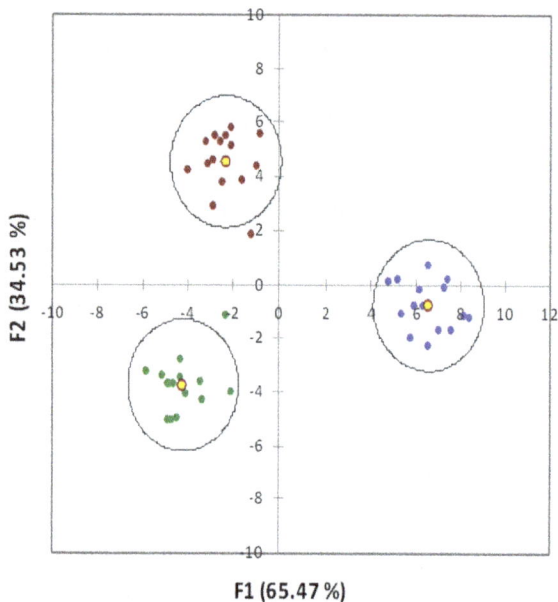
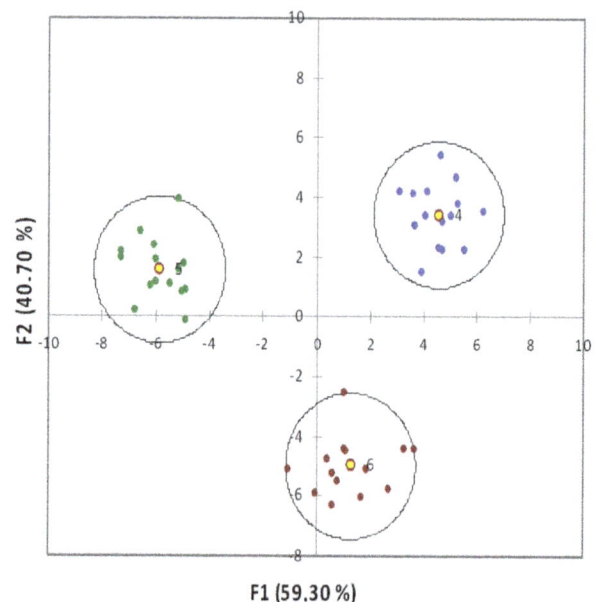

Figure 5 Comparison of the kinetics of cytokine pattern in RSV challenged chickens of different congenic lines. Classification of individual responses by PCA and discriminant analysis in immunized and non-immunized groups of regressors (**A**) and progressors (**B**). Samples were classified into three groups by using PCA (XLSTAT software). The first group (blue spots) includes samples taken on the time of challenge, the second group (green spots) includes samples obtained 14 days after challenge and the third group (brown spots) comprises samples obtained 28 days after challenge. F1 and F2 represent the two main components.

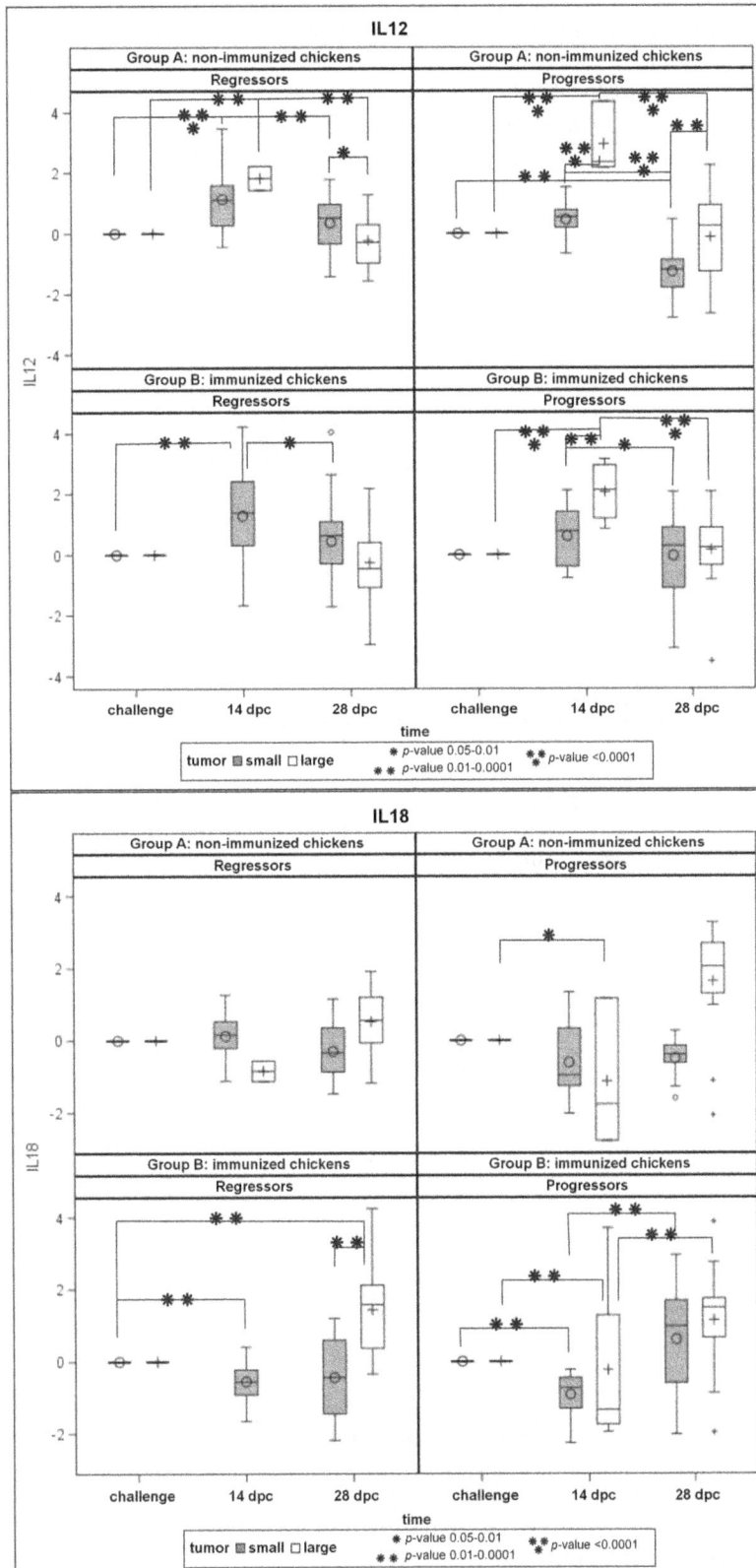

Figure 6 Single cytokine profiles of selected genes in progressor and regressor groups of immunized and non-immunized chickens.
The expression value after challenge was normalized to the basic value expression in the day of challenge. For more cytokines, see Additional file 5.

monoclonal antibody against chicken dendritic cell endocytic surface receptor CD205 (Ly75) and used it in the described antigen delivery system.

Using the newly prepared monoclonal anti chicken CD205 antibody, we observed chCD205 expression in different subsets of chicken leucocytes, mainly in antigen presenting cells as described by Vu Manh et al. [35]. Our observations were recently confirmed by Stainess et al. [4] who also found that CD205 expression was the highest in those chicken cells associated with antigen capture and presentation. We showed that the complex SA-RSV antigens-antibody was delivered specifically to the surface

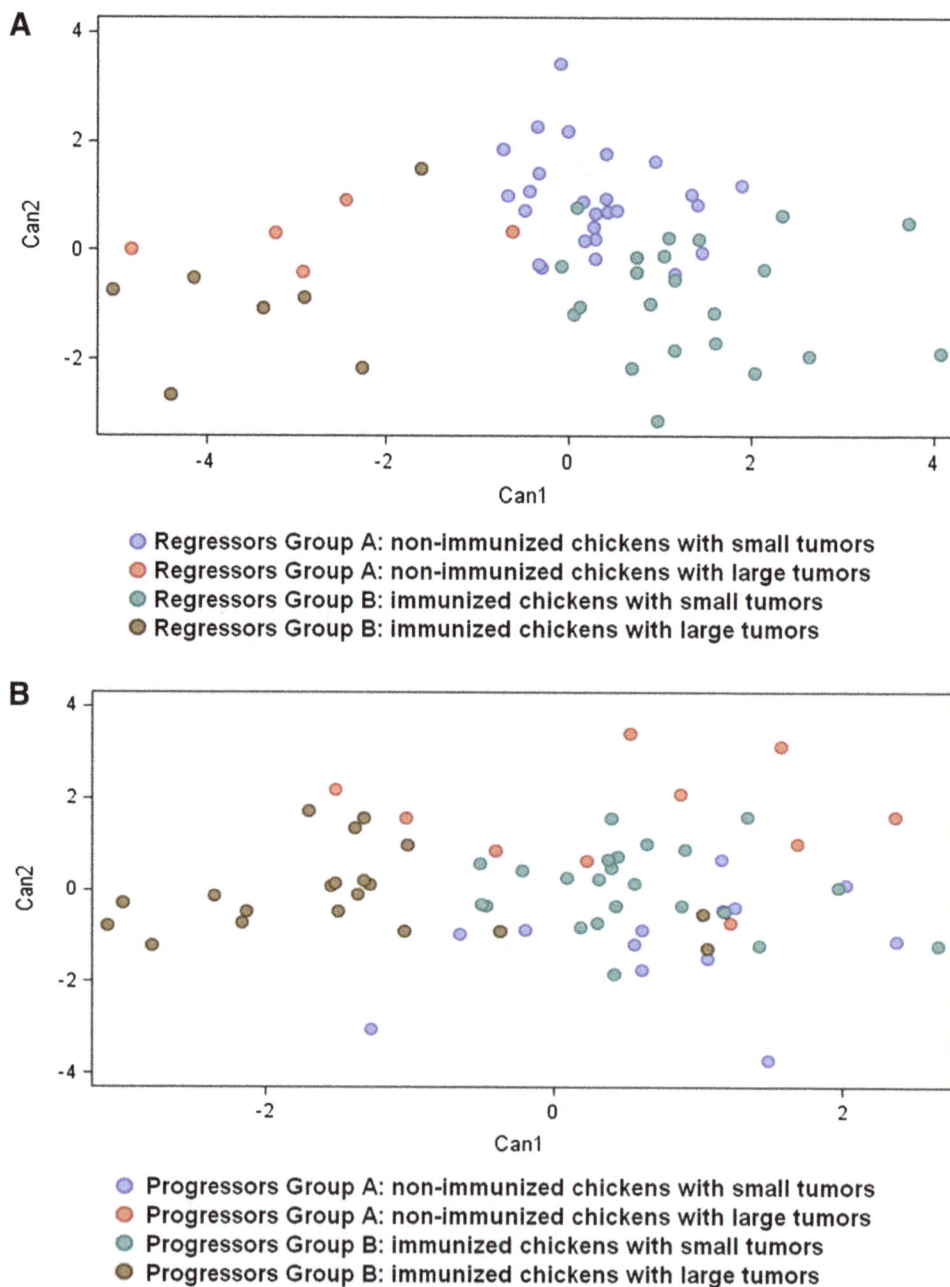

Figure 7 Analysis of correlation of cytokine pattern with RSV-induced tumor status by real-time PCR. Chickens were arbitrarily divided into two groups: small tumors—which stands for tumors up to 5 g (including completely regressed tumors) in the regressor lines CB and CB.R1 and for tumors up to 20 g in the progressor lines CC and CC.R1; large tumors—which stands for tumors above the weight 5 g in the CB and CB.R1 and above 20 g in the CC and CC.R1. **A** Classification of regressors individual responses by linear discriminant analysis. **B** Classification of progressors individual responses by linear discriminant analysis.

CD205 receptor and subsequently internalized. As pH in endosomes/lysosomes is between 4.5 and 5.5 [36], the FITC fluorescence signal was expected to decrease after receptor endocytosis and transfer of the complex into the cell endosome apparatus. This was confirmed by our internalization experiments where we showed decreased fluorescence signals after incubation of FITC-CD205-labeled chicken splenocytes at different temperatures.

In mammals, anti-CD205 antibodies are internalized via coated vesicles and are delivered to endosomal compartments [6]. The cytosolic domain of CD205 mediates efficient endocytosis and recycling through the late endosomes and MHCII-rich compartments [5]. In addition to its capacity to shuttle antigens from the extracellular space into specialized MHCII-rich lysosomal compartments, CD205 is also able to introduce antigens to the MHCI processing machinery.

We used poly I:C as an adjuvant, which acts as dsRNA recognized by TLR3 and thus mimics viral infection [37]. It is indicated that poly I:C can inhibit RSV

Table 1 Significant differences in cytokine expression profiles between groups with small or large tumors of immunized and non-immunized chickens at particular time points

	Imm.	Non-imm.		Imm.	Non-imm.
CB, CB.RI			CC, CC.RI		
14 dpc	+	Il-10*	14 dpc	–	IFNγ*
		Il-15**		Il-2**	–
		TLR*		Il-4**	Il-4*
28 dpc	Il-2**	–		Il-8**	–
	–	Il-4*		Il-12**	Il-12***
	Il-8**	–		–	Il-17*
	–	Il-12*		iNOS***	–
	Il-15***	Il-15**		XCL1*	XCL1*
	Il-18**	–		–	MIF***
	–	iNOS***		LITAF**	–
	–	XCL1**		TRAF5**	–
	–	MIF**	28 dpc	Il-1*	–
	TGF-β**	TGF-β *		Il-4*	Il-4*
	TLR7***	TLR7***		–	Il-12**
	TRAF5*	TRAF5**		–	Il-15***
				–	Il-17*
				–	XCL1***
				MIF**	–
				TGF-β*	–
				TLR7**	TLR7***
				LITAF**	–

For more detailed explanation, see Additional file 5.

+ At this time point, no large tumor was developed.

* p < 0.05; ** p < 0.01; *** p < 0.001.

transformation of chicken embryo fibroblasts in vitro [38], however, in our experiments we observed no such effect and, importantly, a rapid progression of tumors in susceptible lines CC and CC.R1 were not compromised at all. This distinction may be connected with e.g. in vivo use, different site of administration or a prolonged interval between immunization and challenge.

Antigen presentation by a subset of APC via MHCI molecules [39] provides a basis for protein vaccines when appropriately delivered. In this case, the genetic make-up of recipients, namely the ability of particular class I molecules to bind relevant peptides, is of great importance for successful protection. In our experiments, regressors, but not progressors, mount an effective CTL reaction against RSV tumor cell targets [13]. It turned out that this situation clearly corresponds to the presence of immunogenic peptide motifs within the RSV proteins that are stringently recognized by MHCI molecules (B-F12) of the regressor line, whereas only sparse relaxed motifs are available for MHCI molecules (B-F4) of the progressor line [17, 40]. A protective effect of vaccination with a single v-src-derived peptide identified to act against RSV challenge was demonstrated in the regressor chickens [41]. Many more peptides predicted to bind class I molecules from different disease-resistant chicken lines than from susceptible lines were found including Marek's disease virus (MDV), infectious bursal disease virus (IBDV) and avian influenza virus [42–45]. It has been shown that some peptides derived from IBDV can be used as effective vaccine in chickens harboring the dominantly expressed class I molecule of the B12 haplotype. However, only one predicted peptide used for vaccination provided effective protection against the IBDV challenge, whereas vaccination with another peptide failed. In fact, even more severe signs of disease were observed in this case [43]. Thus, the data presented both in our paper and in other experimental systems strongly suggest the decisive role of the genetic make-up of recipients on the efficiency and final outcome of vaccination.

After activation of different chicken DC populations by direct in vivo antigen targeting of their surface receptor, we assume, in the case of regressors, antigen-dependent activation of both CD8+ cytotoxic T lymphocytes and effector CD4+ T cells, as well as activation of innate immunity cells. Other cell types such as natural killer cells (NK) and macrophages may also play a role in the immune responses against RSV tumors. In the case of progressors we do not suppose activation of an effective CTL reaction against RSV.

In this experiment, the cytokine response analyses showed significant up-regulation of IL-12, IL-2, IL-15 and IL-18 in the progressors, which reflects an anti-tumor immunity in the rapidly growing tumors. In this context, we can assume that DC at later stages of differentiation may regulate the activity of NK cells through the release of IL-12, IL-15 and IL-18, as has been reported [46]. DC are known to induce the growth and function of NK cells and play a crucial role in naïve T-cell priming. NK cells can influence the capability of DC to promote Th1 polarization, and the prevalence of IL-12, IL-2, IL-18, or IL-4 at inflammatory sites may differentially modulate the NK-cell interaction with DC [47]. Interestingly, we detected significant up-regulation of IL-17 in the group of immunized progressors. This is in accordance with the hypothesis that Th17 cells facilitate chemoattraction of Th1 cells [48].

In mammals, Cooper et al. [49] showed that IL-12-, IL-15- and IL-18-induced NK cells were memory-like cells and exhibited responses upon restimulation with cytokines (IL-2 and IL-15). DC rapidly stimulate NK cells through production of cytokines, such as IL-2, IL-12, IL-15 and IL-18. It has been reported that DC vaccination generates long-term cell-based resistance against tumor cells in an antigen-independent manner [49]. In the process of oncogenesis, we observed intriguing down-regulation of LITAF mainly in the group of immunized progressors with large tumors. Simultaneously, we did not detect any significant increase in the expression of IFNγ mainly in the immunized groups of progressors, which would indicate involvement of NK cells in the tumor interactions.

In chickens, there are several C-type lectins that are similar to certain mammalian natural killer receptor genes located in the close vicinity of or even within the MHC-B [50–54]. Other novel families of potential chicken Ig-like receptors were also discovered [55]. B-NK was found on several T-cell subsets and also on CD3⁻CD8⁺ sorted splenocytes that were in vitro expanded by IL-2 and on embryonic splenocytes, both of which resemble chicken NK cells [56]. Our findings of specifically activated cytokines known to act in the NK-cell pathway point to their importance in our experimental system of MHC-B congenic lines of chickens, in addition to the previously described Th1 antitumor response. NK cell receptors could be considered as both activating and inhibitory and the balance of their effects determines the final character of the immune response. It is within the context of these subtle and diverse factors, that the data presented in this report must be considered. We performed in vitro restimulation of PBMC where we evaluated supernatant levels of three cytokines (IL-2, IL-12 and IFNγ). Unfortunately, the availability of specific antibodies against chicken cytokines is limited; other cytokines were not evaluated therefore. All cytokine levels were significantly increased in the immunized groups restimulated with v-src antigen. This suggests that the direct delivery of the antigens via CD205 receptor may also induce the classical Th1 immune profile.

Interestingly, both congenic lines sharing the B-G4 allele, CB.R1 (regressors) and CC (progressors), showed a rather adverse effect of vaccination (for the composition of the MHC-B haplotypes see the "Materials and methods"). The true function of the B-G genes—known as MHC-B class IV—is still elusive, namely with respect to their immunological functions [26]. The significant role of the B-G genes in the relative resistance to MDV-induced lymphoma has also been described in another experimental system of MHC-B recombinant chickens [28]. Our results suggest that the genotype in the B-G genes (MHC—class IV) correlates to some extent in the response to the vaccination despite the general status of regressors or progressors governed primarily by the B-F (MHCI) genes. So far, we can only speculate what putative suppressive signal of the B-G4 molecule might influence the significant aggravating of the vaccination response in our model system.

We report in this study the first description of a novel system of vaccination of chickens based on a novel tool for antigen delivery into chicken DC. A novel anti-chCD205 monoclonal antibody has been developed and the internalization of the antigen through this receptor has been confirmed. Cytokine expression profile differences in RSV-challenged progressor and regressor chicken lines have been described. Based on the increased expression of cytokines specific for activated DC (IL-12, IL-15 and IL-18) we have shown partial stimulation of specific cell types involved in cell-mediated immunity, although the only significant effect of immunization on the tumor size has been confirmed in IL-12. Further investigation is needed to elucidate the apparently complex mechanism of the response to vaccination and to optimize the system of antigen delivery to avoid unwanted suppressive effects.

Additional files

Additional file 1. Supplementary Materials and methods. Additional description of anti-chicken CD205 monoclonal antibody preparation, the construction, expression and purification of the recombinant SA-RSV fusion proteins and the description of amino acid sequence CD205 protein.

Additional file 2. List of primers used in the study. Sequences of primers used in anti-CD205 antigen cloning.

Additional file 3. List of primers used in the study. Sequences of primers used in anti-CD205 antigen cloning.

Additional file 4. List of primers used for RT-PCR in this study. Sequences of primers used in cytokine pattern analyses, primers length, amplicon size and amplified genes access PubMed database numbers.

Additional file 5. Cytokine profiles of selected genes in progressor and regressor groups of immunized and non-immunized chickens. These data show the expression profiles of all observed cytokines in progressor and regressor groups of immunized and non-immunized chickens. The expression value after challenge was normalized to the basic value of expression in the day of challenge.

Abbreviations

APC: antigen-presenting cells; DC: dendritic cells; dpc: days post challenge; FFU: focus-forming units; MHC: major histocompatibility complex; PBMC: peripheral blood mononuclear cells; NK: natural killer cells; PCA: principal component analysis; RSV: Rous sarcoma virus; RT-PCR: real-time polymerase chain reaction; SA: streptavidin; sc: subcutaneously.

Competing interests

The authors declare that they have no competing interests.

Authors' contributions

Conceived and designed the experiments: JM, JP, OS, PT. Performed the experiments: BB, JK, JM, JP, OS, PT. Analysed the data: JK, JM, JP. Interpreted the data: JM, JP. Prepared the manuscript: JH, JM, JP, OS. All authors read and approved the final manuscript.

Acknowledgements

This work was supported by Grant No. QJ1210041 funded by the Ministry of Agriculture of the Czech Republic. The authors would like to thank Professor Bernd Kaspers for kindly providing the putative anti-chicken CD11c monoclonal antibody, Dr Vlasta Korenková for help with Biomark analyses, Professor Miloslav Suchánek and Dr Vendula Novosadová for help with statistical analyses, and Lucie Parolová for her skilled assistance.

Author details

[1] BIOPHARM, Research Institute of Biopharmacy and Veterinary Drugs, Jílové U Prahy, Czech Republic. [2] Institute of Molecular Genetics, Academy of Sciences of the Czech Republic, Prague, Czech Republic. [3] Institute of Microbiology, Academy of Sciences of the Czech Republic, Prague, Czech Republic.

References

1. Gajewski TF, Schreiber H, Fu Y-X (2013) Innate and adaptive immune cells in the tumor microenvironment. Nat Immunol 14:1014–1022
2. Gabrilovich DI, Ostrand-Rosenberg S, Bronte V (2012) Coordinated regulation of myeloid cells by tumours. Nat Rev Immunol 12:253–268
3. Burkholder B, Huang R-Y, Burgess R, Luo S, Jones VS, Zhang W, Lv Z-Q, Gao C-Y, Wang B-L, Zhang Y-M, Huang R-P (2014) Tumor-induced perturbations of cytokines and immune cell networks. Biochim Biophys Acta 1845:182–201
4. Staines K, Young JR, Butter C (2013) Expression of chicken DEC205 reflects the unique structure and function of the avian immune system. PLoS One 8:e51799
5. Jiang W, Swiggard WJ, Heufler C, Peng M, Mirza A, Steinman RM, Nussenzweig MC (1995) The receptor DEC-205 expressed by dendritic cells and thymic epithelial cells is involved in antigen processing. Nature 375:151–155
6. Bonifaz L, Bonnyay D, Mahnke K, Rivera M, Nussenzweig MC, Steinman RM (2002) Efficient targeting of protein antigen to the dendritic cell receptor DEC-205 in the steady state leads to antigen presentation on major histocompatibility complex class I products and peripheral CD8 + T cell tolerance. J Exp Med 196:1627–1638
7. Trumpfheller C, Finke JS, López CB, Moran TM, Moltedo B, Soares H, Huang Y, Schlesinger SJ, Park CG, Nussenzweig MC, Granelli-Piperno A, Steinman RM (2006) Intensified and protective CD4 + T cell immunity in mice with anti-dendritic cell HIV gag fusion antibody vaccine. J Exp Med 203:607–617
8. Steinman RM (2008) Dendritic cells in vivo: a key target for a new vaccine science. Immunity 29:319–324
9. Stanek O, Linhartova I, Majlessi L, Leclerc C, Sebo P (2012) Complexes of streptavidin-fused antigens with biotinylated antibodies targeting

receptors on dendritic cell surface: a novel tool for induction of specific T-cell immune responses. Mol Biotechnol 51:221–232
10. Dong H, Stanek O, Salvador FR, Länger U, Morillon E, Ung C, Sebo P, Leclerc C, Majlessi L (2013) Induction of protective immunity against Mycobacterium tuberculosis by delivery of ESX antigens into airway dendritic cells. Mucosal Immunol 6:522–534
11. Brugge JS, Erikson RL (1977) Identification of a transformation-specific antigen induced by an avian sarcoma virus. Nature 269:346–348
12. Plachy J, Pink JR, Hála K (1992) Biology of the chicken MHC (B complex). Crit Rev Immunol 12:47–79
13. Plachy J, Hála K, Hejnar J, Geryk J, Svoboda J (1994) src-specific immunity in inbred chickens bearing v-src DNA- and RSV-induced tumors. Immunogenetics 40:257–265
14. Plachý JV, Hejnar JV, Trtková K, Trejbalová K, Svoboda J, Hála K (2001) DNA vaccination against v-src oncogene-induced tumours in congenic chickens. Vaccine 19:4526–4535
15. Taylor RL, Ewert DL, England JM, Halpern MS (1992) Major histocompatibility (B) complex control of the growth pattern of v-src DNA-induced primary tumors. Virology 191:477–479
16. Gelman IH, Hanafusa H (1993) src-specific immune regression of Rous sarcoma virus-induced tumors. Cancer Res 53:915–920
17. Kaufman J, Völk H, Wallny HJ (1995) A "minimal essential Mhc" and an "unrecognized Mhc": two extremes in selection for polymorphism. Immunol Rev 143:63–88
18. Kaufman J, Milne S, Göbel TW, Walker BA, Jacob JP, Auffray C, Zoorob R, Beck S (1999) The chicken B locus is a minimal essential major histocompatibility complex. Nature 401:923–925
19. Wallny H-J, Avila D, Hunt LG, Powell TJ, Riegert P, Salomonsen J, Skjødt K, Vainio O, Vilbois F, Wiles MV, Kaufman J (2006) Peptide motifs of the single dominantly expressed class I molecule explain the striking MHC-determined response to Rous sarcoma virus in chickens. Proc Natl Acad Sci U S A 103:1434–1439
20. Walker BA, Hunt LG, Sowa AK, Skjødt K, Göbel TW, Lehner PJ, Kaufman J (2011) The dominantly expressed class I molecule of the chicken MHC is explained by coevolution with the polymorphic peptide transporter (TAP) genes. Proc Natl Acad Sci U S A 108:8396–8401
21. Zhang L, Katselis GS, Moore RE, Lekpor K, Goto RM, Hunt HD, Lee TD, Miller MM (2012) MHC class I target recognition, immunophenotypes and proteomic profiles of natural killer cells within the spleens of day-14 chick embryos. Dev Comp Immunol 37:446–456
22. Hofmann M, Nussbaum AK, Emmerich NP, Stoltze L, Schild H (2001) Mechanisms of MHC class I-restricted antigen presentation. Expert Opin Ther Targets 5:379–393
23. Salomonsen J, Chattaway JA, Chan ACY, Parker A, Huguet S, Marston DA, Rogers SL, Wu Z, Smith AL, Staines K, Butter C, Riegert P, Vainio O, Nielsen L, Kaspers B, Griffin DK, Yang F, Zoorob R, Guillemot F, Auffray C, Beck S, Skjødt K, Kaufman J (2014) Sequence of a complete chicken BG haplotype shows dynamic expansion and contraction of two gene lineages with particular expression patterns. PLoS Genet 10:e1004417
24. Plachý J (1984) Hierarchy of the B (MHC) haplotypes controlling resistance to rous sarcomas in a model of inbred lines of chickens. Folia Biol (Praha) 30:412–425
25. Plachý J (1988) The B-G region genes of the chicken MHC are responsible for lethal graft-versus-host disease in newly hatched chickens. Folia Biol (Praha) 34:84–98
26. Kaufman J, Skjødt K, Salomonsen J (1991) The B-G multigene family of the chicken major histocompatibility complex. Crit Rev Immunol 11:113–143
27. Salomonsen J, Eriksson H, Skjødt K, Lundgren T, Simonsen M, Kaufman J (1991) The "adjuvant effect" of the polymorphic B-G antigens of the chicken major histocompatibility complex analyzed using purified molecules incorporated in liposomes. Eur J Immunol 21:649–658
28. Goto RM, Wang Y, Taylor RL, Wakenell PS, Hosomichi K, Shiina T, Blackmore CS, Briles WE, Miller MM (2009) BG1 has a major role in MHC-linked resistance to malignant lymphoma in the chicken. Proc Natl Acad Sci U S A 106:16740–16745
29. Plachý J, Vilhelmová M (1984) Syngeneic lines of chickens. VII. The lines derived from the recombinants at the B complex (MHC) of Rous sarcoma regressor and progressor inbred lines of chickens. Folia Biol (Praha) 30:189–201

30. Méric C, Spahr PF (1986) Rous sarcoma virus nucleic acid-binding protein p12 is necessary for viral 70S RNA dimer formation and packaging. J Virol 60:450–459

31. Hong YH, Lillehoj HS, Lillehoj EP, Lee SH (2006) Changes in immune-related gene expression and intestinal lymphocyte subpopulations following *Eimeria maxima* infection of chickens. Vet Immunol Immunopathol 114:259–272

32. Rothwell L, Young JR, Zoorob R, Whittaker CA, Hesketh P, Archer A, Smith AL, Kaiser P (2004) Cloning and characterization of chicken IL-10 and its role in the immune response to *Eimeria maxima*. J Immunol 173:2675–2682

33. Jolliffe IT (2002) Principal Component Analysis. Springer-Verlag, New York

34. Martin MM, Lindqvist L (1975) The pH dependence of fluorescein fluorescence. J Lumin 10:381–390

35. Vu Manh T-P, Marty H, Sibille P, Le Vern Y, Kaspers B, Dalod M, Schwartz-Cornil I, Quéré P (2014) Existence of conventional dendritic cells in *Gallus gallus* revealed by comparative gene expression profiling. J Immunol 192:4510–4517

36. Sorkin A, Von Zastrow M (2002) Signal transduction and endocytosis: close encounters of many kinds. Nat Rev Mol Cell Biol 3:600–614

37. Martins KAO, Bavari S, Salazar AM (2015) Vaccine adjuvant uses of poly-IC and derivatives. Expert Rev Vaccines 14:447–459

38. Dodge WH, Moscovici C (1972) Effect of poly I:C on transformation by Rous sarcoma virus. Proc Soc Exp Biol Med 139:1407–1412

39. Rock KL (1996) A new foreign policy: MHC class I molecules monitor the outside world. Immunol Today 17:131–137

40. Kaufman J, Wallny HJ (1996) Chicken MHC molecules, disease resistance and the evolutionary origin of birds. Curr Top Microbiol Immunol 212:129–141

41. Hofmann A, Plachy J, Hunt L, Kaufman J, Hala K (2003) v-src oncogene-specific carboxy-terminal peptide is immunoprotective against Rous sarcoma growth in chickens with MHC class I allele B-F12. Vaccine 21:4694–4699

42. Koch M, Camp S, Collen T, Avila D, Salomonsen J, Wallny HJ, van Hateren A, Hunt L, Jacob JP, Johnston F, Marston DA, Shaw I, Dunbar PR, Cerundolo V, Jones EY, Kaufman J (2007) Structures of an MHC class I molecule from B21 chickens illustrate promiscuous peptide binding. Immunity 27:885–899

43. Butter C, Staines K, van Hateren A, Davison TF, Kaufman J (2013) The peptide motif of the single dominantly expressed class I molecule of the chicken MHC can explain the response to a molecular defined vaccine of infectious bursal disease virus (IBDV). Immunogenetics 65:609–618

44. Hou Y, Guo Y, Wu C, Shen N, Jiang Y, Wang J (2012) Prediction and identification of T cell epitopes in the H5N1 influenza virus nucleoprotein in chicken. PLoS One 7:e39344

45. Reemers SS, van Haarlem DA, Sijts AJ, Vervelde L, Jansen CA (2012) Identification of novel avian influenza virus derived CD8 + T-cell epitopes. PLoS One 7:e31953

46. Andrews DM, Andoniou CE, Scalzo AA, van Dommelen SLH, Wallace ME, Smyth MJ, Degli-Esposti MA (2005) Cross-talk between dendritic cells and natural killer cells in viral infection. Mol Immunol 42:547–555

47. Agaugué S, Marcenaro E, Ferranti B, Moretta L, Moretta A (2008) Human natural killer cells exposed to IL-2, IL-12, IL-18, or IL-4 differently modulate priming of naive T cells by monocyte-derived dendritic cells. Blood 112:1776–1783

48. Khader SA, Bell GK, Pearl JE, Fountain JJ, Rangel-Moreno J, Cilley GE, Shen F, Eaton SM, Gaffen SL, Swain SL, Locksley RM, Haynes L, Randall TD, Cooper AM (2007) IL-23 and IL-17 in the establishment of protective pulmonary CD4 + T cell responses after vaccination and during *Mycobacterium tuberculosis* challenge. Nat Immunol 8:369–377

49. Cooper MA, Elliott JM, Keyel PA, Yang L, Carrero JA, Yokoyama WM (2009) Cytokine-induced memory-like natural killer cells. Proc Natl Acad Sci U S A 106:1915–1919

50. Kaufman J (1999) Co-evolving genes in MHC haplotypes: the "rule" for nonmammalian vertebrates? Immunogenetics 50:228–236

51. Rogers SL, Göbel TW, Viertlboeck BC, Milne S, Beck S, Kaufman J (2005) Characterization of the chicken C-type lectin-like receptors B-NK and B-lec suggests that the NK complex and the MHC share a common ancestral region. J Immunol 174:3475–3483

52. Rogers SL, Kaufman J (2008) High allelic polymorphism, moderate sequence diversity and diversifying selection for B-NK but not B-lec, the pair of lectin-like receptor genes in the chicken MHC. Immunogenetics 60:461–475

53. Shiina T, Briles WE, Goto RM, Hosomichi K, Yanagiya K, Shimizu S, Inoko H, Miller MM (2007) Extended gene map reveals tripartite motif, C-type lectin, and Ig superfamily type genes within a subregion of the chicken MHC-B affecting infectious disease. J Immunol 178:7162–7172

54. Rogers S, Shaw I, Ross N, Nair V, Rothwell L, Kaufman J, Kaiser P (2003) Analysis of part of the chicken Rfp-Y region reveals two novel lectin genes, the first complete genomic sequence of a class I alpha-chain gene, a truncated class II beta-chain gene, and a large CR1 repeat. Immunogenetics 55:100–108

55. Straub C, Neulen M-L, Sperling B, Windau K, Zechmann M, Jansen CA, Viertlboeck BC, Göbel TW (2013) Chicken NK cell receptors. Dev Comp Immunol 41:324–333

56. Viertlboeck BC, Wortmann A, Schmitt R, Plachý J, Göbel TW (2008) Chicken C-type lectin-like receptor B-NK, expressed on NK and T cell subsets, binds to a ligand on activated splenocytes. Mol Immunol 45:1398–1404

8

Innate immune responses induced by the saponin adjuvant Matrix-M in specific pathogen free pigs

Viktor Ahlberg[1], Bernt Hjertner[1], Per Wallgren[2], Stina Hellman[1], Karin Lövgren Bengtsson[3]
and Caroline Fossum[1]* ⓘ

Abstract

Saponin-based adjuvants have been widely used to enhance humoral and cellular immune responses in many species, but their mode of action is not fully understood. A characterization of the porcine transcriptional response to Matrix-M was performed in vitro using lymphocytes, monocytes or monocyte-derived dendritic cells (MoDCs) and in vivo. The effect of Matrix-M was also evaluated in specific pathogen free (SPF) pigs exposed to conventionally reared pigs. The pro-inflammatory cytokine genes *IL1B* and *CXCL8* were up-regulated in monocytes and lymphocytes after Matrix-M exposure. Matrix-M also induced *IL12B*, *IL17A* and *IFNG* in lymphocytes and IFN-α gene expression in MoDCs. Several genes were indicated as up-regulated by Matrix-M in blood 18 h after injection, of which the genes for IFN-α and TLR2 could be statistically confirmed. Respiratory disease developed in all SPF pigs mixed with conventional pigs within 1–3 days. Two out of four SPF pigs injected with saline prior to contact exposure displayed systemic symptoms that was not recorded for the four pigs administered Matrix-M. Granulocyte counts, serum amyloid A levels and transcription of *IL18* and *TLR2* coincided with disease progression in the pigs. These results support further evaluation of Matrix-M as a possible enhancer of innate immune responses during critical moments in pig management.

Introduction

Immunostimulatory effects of saponins from *Quillaja saponaria* Molina are known since nearly 100 years. These saponins have on numerous occasions been used in veterinary vaccines, but the mechanisms underlying the effects are not fully understood [1–4]. Purified fractions of *Quillaja* saponins combined with phospholipids and cholesterol can be formulated into nanoparticle ISCOM-Matrix adjuvants [5, 6], such as the Matrix-M™ (Novavax AB, Uppsala, Sweden). Immunization experiments using Matrix-M as adjuvant reveal an antigen specific immune response characterized by long-lasting antibody production, a balanced T_H1/T_H2 cytokine profile and induction of cytotoxic T cells [7–9]. These adjuvant properties of Matrix-M also seem to increase the otherwise poor immunogenicity of Ebola virus glycoproteins [10].

In the pig, experimental vaccines formulated with ISCOM-Matrix have provided protection against pseudorabies [11], rotavirus [12, 13], *Toxoplasma gondii* [14] and *Mycoplasma hyopneumoniae* [15]. Intramuscular injection of the adjuvant component Matrix-M alone in pigs resulted in cellular influx to the draining lymph node [16] as also seen for neutrophils, dendritic cells, monocytes and NK cells after subcutaneous injection of Matrix-M in mice [17, 18] and for monocytes in calves [19]. The innate immune reaction to intramuscular injection of Matrix-M in pigs was further characterized by a type I interferon-related transcriptional response both at the site of administration and in the draining lymph node [16, 20]. These indications that Matrix-M seems to activate the interferon system, amongst other innate immune parameters, raises the possibility for its strategic use in pigs that are extra vulnerable to infections.

*Correspondence: caroline.fossum@slu.se
[1] Department of Biomedical Sciences and Veterinary Public Health, Swedish University of Agricultural Sciences, SLU, Uppsala, Sweden
Full list of author information is available at the end of the article

In modern pig husbandry disease susceptibility has been associated with weaning, transport and mixing, especially of pigs with different health status [21]. Physiological stress and infectious agents co-operate and preventive treatments include administration of IFN-α [22, 23] and β-glucans [24, 25]. Immunomodulators as a tool to boost the immune system against possible infections can potentially also be used in emergency vaccines [26]. In recent years it has been proposed that vaccine induced short-term innate immune responses possess a type of memory manifesting itself in a prolonged activation of innate immune cells which also acts on heterologous targets [27]. These non-specific effects of vaccines are now often referred to as "trained innate immunity" implying that priming of monocyte-derived cells and NK-cells by vaccination affects their future response to non-related agents [28].

The aim of the present study was to expand our understanding of how the saponin adjuvant Matrix-M may affect the response to different stressors such as infection and/or transport, building on previously acquired results on effects of Matrix-M administration to the pig [16, 20]. Therefore, we further evaluated modulatory effects of Matrix-M on innate immune parameters in the pig. To accomplish this, the host response to Matrix-M was evaluated in a 6-day contact exposure model using specific pathogen free (SPF) pigs treated with Matrix-M or saline 1 day before transport and mixing with conventionally reared pigs. During this period leukocyte counts, serum amyloid A (SAA) and expression of immune related genes were monitored in blood. Furthermore, gene expression results from blood were complemented by those from in vitro exposure of porcine peripheral blood mononuclear cell (PBMC) subpopulations to Matrix-M.

Materials and methods
Animals
The SPF pigs (Yorkshire × Landrace) originated from a herd (Serogrisen, Ransta, Sweden) declared free from major swine pathogens. The conventionally reared pigs came from a farrow-to-finish herd with a high prevalence of respiratory lesions recorded at slaughter. Pigs in this herd were in general seronegative to *Actinobacillus pleuropneumoniae*, *Mycoplasma hyopneumoniae*, *Pasteurella multocida* and *Streptococcus suis* when transferred to fattening units at 11 weeks of age, but displayed high levels of serum antibodies to *A. pleuropneumoniae* and to *P. multocida* 8 weeks later. Porcine circovirus type 2 (PCV2) was known to be present in both herds but there were no clinical signs of PCV2-associated diseases. All pigs were aged 9–11 weeks when included in the contact exposure experiment.

In vitro exposure to Matrix-M
The transcriptional response to Matrix-M was studied in vitro using PBMCs collected from SPF pigs (Lövsta Research Station, Uppsala, Sweden). The PBMCs were isolated from heparinized blood by centrifugation for 45 min at 500g on FicollPaque PLUS (GE Healthcare Biosciences, Uppsala, Sweden), washed twice in PBS and resuspended in RPMI 1640 medium supplemented with 20 mM HEPES buffer, 2 mM L-glutamine, 200 IU penicillin/mL, 100 µg streptomycin/mL, 50 µM 2–mercaptoethanol and 5% FCS (Gibco, Life Technologies, Carlsbad, CA, USA). Cell viability was determined with Trypan blue exclusion test and $10–20 \times 10^6$ PBMCs were seeded into 6-well plates (Nunclon, Nunc, Roskilde, Denmark) for further enrichment into subpopulations.

Monocytes were enriched from PBMCs by plastic adherence for 2/3 h. Thereafter the non-adherent lymphocyte-enriched cells (referred to as "lymphocytes") were transferred to new 6-well plates. Monocyte-derived dendritic cells (MoDCs) were generated as previously described [29] by culturing monocytes for 5 days in the presence of rpIL-4 (40 ng/mL; R&D Systems, Minneapolis, MN, USA) and rpGM-CSF (20 ng/mL; R&D Systems), replacing one-third of the culture volume after 3 days. The cells were used after 5 days when they had acquired a dendritic morphology. The resulting cell cultures were exposed to Matrix-M (1 µg/mL; Isconova AB, Uppsala, Sweden) that is delivered as a solution in PBS and easily blended into the culture medium. Lymphocytes were cultured for 3 days, with Matrix-M present for the last 6 h or 3 days. Monocytes were cultured for 1 day, with Matrix-M present for the last 6 h. MoDCs were exposed to Matrix-M for 6 h after generation, or with Matrix-M present during the 5 days of generation. All cultures were grown in 2 mL of medium for indicated durations at 37 °C with 7% CO_2 in air.

Matrix-M administration and contact exposure of SPF pigs
All pigs in the contact exposure experiment were castrated males, aged 9–11 weeks. Two barrows from each of four SPF-litters received 150 µg Matrix-M ($n = 8$) suspended in 1 mL sterile endotoxin-free 0.9% NaCl solution (saline; Fresenius Kabi, Uppsala, Sweden), and two other barrows in these litters received saline only ($n = 8$). The intramuscular injection was made into the thigh at equal distance from the knee and the ischial tuberosity. After 16 h, all SPF pigs were transported during 2 h to the National Veterinary Institute. At arrival (18 h), the SPF pigs were allotted to four experimental groups and allocated to three rooms. Four hours later (22 h), four of the eight conventionally reared pigs from four litters were mixed with four pigs treated with Matrix-M (SPF^Matrix-M/Conv) and with four pigs treated with saline (SPF^Saline/Conv),

respectively, in different rooms according to a split-litter design. The remaining eight SPF pigs (SPF[Matrix-M/SPF] and SPF[Saline/SPF]) were housed in a third room. Thus, four experimental groups of four SPF pigs were established in three rooms with eight pigs in total per room (Figure 1). Each room of eight square metres, had individual ventilation and manure handling systems and an individual atrium for staff access. Pigs were fed 2% of their bodyweight with a commercial dry feed twice daily, and had free access to water and bedding material. The experiment was approved by the Uppsala Ethical Committee on Animal Experiments (Reg. No. C 105214/15).

The health status of the animals was recorded daily and graded as 0 = healthy; 1 = moderately affected; 2 = clearly affected; 3 = severely affected. Clinical signs of disease and respiratory signs were scored from 0 (none) to 3 (severe) as described [30]. Blood was collected by jugular venepuncture using vacuum tubes without additives or with EDTA (BD Vacutainer; BD Diagnostics, Franklin Lakes, NJ, USA), or PAXgene Blood RNA tubes (PreAnalytiX, Hombrechtikon, Switzerland), at time points indicated in Figure 1. Five days after mixing, all pigs were sacrificed by electrical stunning and subsequent exsanguination. Macroscopic alterations of the draining lymph node, bronchial lymph node, lung and joints were scored from 0 (none) to 3 (severe).

RNA extraction

RNA from the in vitro exposure experiment was extracted as described [31] using a combination of Trizol reagent (Invitrogen, Carlsbad, CA, USA) and RNA purification spin columns (E.Z.N.A. Total RNA Kit, Omega Biotek, Norcross, GA, USA). RNA from blood collected in PAXgene tubes during the in vivo experiment was extracted using the PAXgene Blood RNA Kit (PreAnalytiX) and samples with low RNA yield were concentrated with the E.Z.N.A. MicroElute RNA Clean Up Kit (Omega Biotek). RNA concentration (A_{260}) and purity ($A_{260/280}$ and $A_{260/230}$) was determined by spectrophotometry (NanoDrop 8000, NanoDrop Technologies, Montchamin, DE, USA). Integrity of RNA was determined by capillary gel electrophoresis (Experion, BioRad, Hercules, CA, USA).

Synthesis of cDNA

Total RNA (250–1000 ng) from the in vitro and in vivo experiments were treated with RQ1 RNase-Free DNase (Promega, Madison, WI, USA) and DNA-free DNA Removal Kit (Life Technologies), respectively, followed by synthesis of cDNA with the GoScript Reverse Transcription System (Promega). Each cDNA was diluted five times in nuclease free water and stored at −20 °C until analysis.

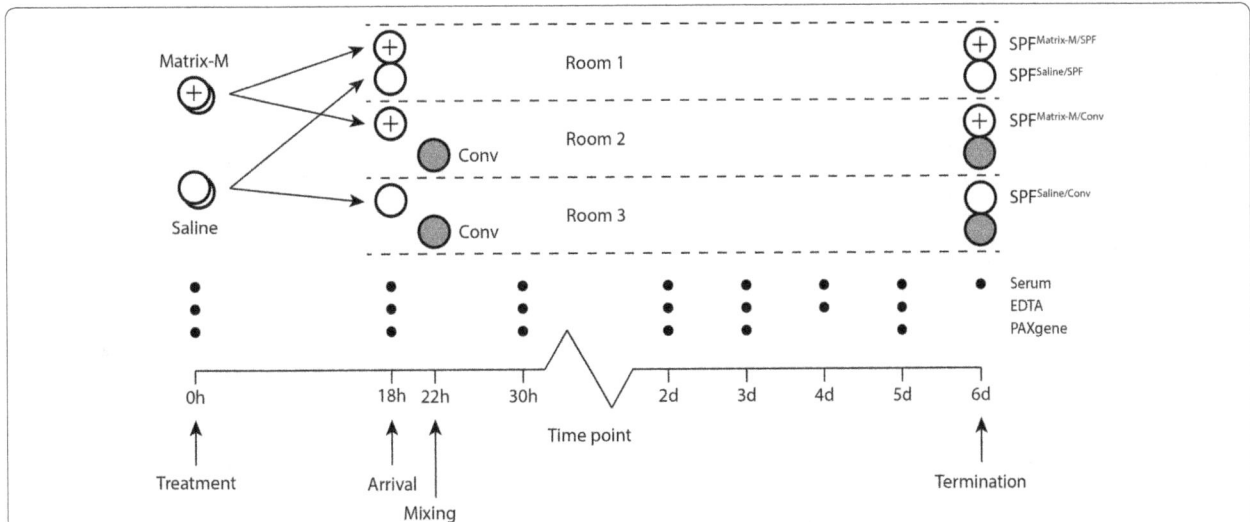

Figure 1 Experimental design. Sixteen SPF pigs were treated (0 h) with Matrix M (n = 8) or saline (n = 8) the evening before a 2-h transport to the animal facility. At arrival (18 h), the SPF pigs were allotted to three rooms. SPF pigs given Matrix-M or saline were mixed in the first room (SPF[Matrix-M/SPF] and SPF[Saline/SPF]; n = 4 + 4). Four hours later (22 h) eight conventionally reared pigs (Conv) arrived and were mixed with four of the SPF pigs given Matrix-M (SPF[Matrix-M/Conv]) or four of those given saline (SPF[Saline/Conv]; n = 4) in the other two rooms. Blood samples were collected from the SPF pigs in tubes without additives (serum), EDTA tubes and PAXgene Blood RNA tubes as indicated. Clinical examination was performed concurrently with blood sampling and at least once more each day. Post-mortem examination was performed on all pigs at termination of the experiment (6 days).

Real-time quantitative PCR (qPCR)

Transcripts specific for the genes CXCL8, IFITM3, IFNA, IFNB, IFNG, IL1B, IL6, IL10, IL12B, IL17A, SPP1, STING, TGFB1, TLR2, TLR4 and TNFA were quantified by qPCR using the QuantiTect SYBR Green PCR Kit (Qiagen) and an iQ5 Real Time PCR cycler (Bio-Rad). Each sample was amplified in duplicate 25 µL reactions with 2 µL cDNA (diluted × 5) and primers according to Table 1. The cycling conditions consisted of an initial cycle of 95 °C for 15 min followed by 40 cycles of 95 °C for 15 s, the gene-specific annealing temperature (Table 1) for 30 s and 72 °C for 30 s. A melt-curve analysis was done at the end of the program for product verification.

To evaluate the level of genomic DNA contamination in the samples, the IFNA assay was used either on aliquots run in the cDNA synthesis without reverse transcriptase

Table 1 Primer details and qPCR conditions

Gene	Primer sequence	Anneal temp (°C)	Primer conc (nM)	Eff (%)[a]	r^2	Melt point (°C)	References
CXCL8	F: AGCCAGGAAGAGACTAGAAAGAAA R: TTGGGGTGGAAAGGTGTG	56	500	97	0.998	81.5	New design
GAPDH[b]	F: ACACTCACTCTTCTACCTTTG R: CAAATTCATTGTCGTACCAG	56	500	94	0.998	80	[54]
HPRT[b]	F: GGTCAAGCAGCATAATCCAAAG R: CAAGGGCATAGCCTACCACAA	60	500	100	0.996	80	[55]
IFITM3	F: ATCAACATCCGAAGCGAGACC R: GGAAAATTACCAGGGAGCCAGTG	56	500	96	0.999	85.5	New design
IFN-α	F: AGCCTCCTGCACCAGTTCTG R: TCACAGCCAGGATGGAGTCC	60	500	100	0.997	84.5	[20]
IFN-β	F: TAGCACTGGCTGGAATGAAACC R: TCAGGTGAAGAATGGTCATGTCT	58	400	104	0.993	79.5	[20]
IFN-γ	F: TGGTAGCTCTGGGAAACTGAATG R: GGCTTTGCGCTGGATCTG	60	400	102	0.998	76.5	[31]
IL1B	F: GTGATGGCTAACTACGGTGACAA R: CTCCCATTTCTCAGAGAACCAAG	60	400	91	0.999	79.5	[56]
IL6	F: CTGGCAGAAAACAACCTGAACC R: TGATTCTCATCAAGCAGGTCTCC	60	400	98	0.994	77.5	[57]
IL10	F: CGGCGCTGTCATCAATTTCTG R: CCCCTCTCTTGGAGCTTGCTA	60	400	100	0.995	80.5	[57]
IL12B	F: TCTTGGGAGGGTCTGGTTTG R: AAGCTGTTCACAAGCTCAAGTATGA	61	400	96	0.999	76.5	[31]
IL17A	F: CAGACGGCCCTCAGATTACTCCA R: AGCCCACTGTCACCATCACTTTCT	61	400	91	0.993	84.5	New design
PPIA[b]	F: GCAGACAAAGTTCCAAAGACAG R: AGATGCCAGGACCCGTATG	60	400	92	0.999	80.5	[58]
RPL32[b]	F: CGGAAGTTTCTGGTACACAATGTAA R: TGGAAGAGACGTTGTGAGCAA	55	300	97	0.997	77	[20]
SPP1	F: TTGGACAGCCAAGAGAAGGACAGT R: GCTCATTGCTCCCATCATAGGTCTTG	56	300	93	0.997	82.5	[20]
STING	F: TTACATCGGGTACCTGCGGC R: CCGAGTACGTTCTTGTGGCG	56	500	101	0.992	82	[20]
TGFB1	F: TACGCCAAGGAGGTCACCC R: CAGCTCTGCCCGAGAGAGC	60	400	90	0.992	83	[59]
TLR2	F: GGCAAGTGGATTATTGACAACATC R: ACCACTCGCTCTTCACAAAGTTC	60	500	94	0.997	78.5	[60]
TLR4	F: CTTCACTACAGAGACTTCATTC R: ACACCACGACAATAACCT	54	500	89	0.999	79	[61]
TNFA	F: AGCCTCTTCTCCTTCCTCCTG R: GAGACGATGATCTGAGTCCTTGG	60	400	91	0.993	84	[31]
YWHAZ[b]	F: ATTGGGTCTGGCCCTTAACT R: GCGTGCTGTCTTTGTATGACTC	58	400	101	0.997	78.5	[20]

Conditions optimized or re-optimized for reagents and equipment described in "Materials and methods".

[a] PCR efficiency estimated on serial dilutions of reference cDNA.

[b] Reference gene used for normalization.

(in vitro samples) or on the DNased total RNA at a concentration taking into account the dilution factor generated at cDNA synthesis (in vivo samples).

For initial analyses, cDNA from four pigs each in two experimental groups (SPF$^{Matrix-M}$ and SPF^{Saline}) was pooled within each group and screened using a custom made (Additional file 1) dried-down qPCR plate array (PrimePCR, Bio-Rad). The expression of selected genes from the plate were further analysed in wet format (IL18, MYD88, NLRP3 and TLR9). All PrimePCR assays were run on the CFX96 Touch (Bio-Rad) using SsoAdvanced Universal SYBR® Green Supermix (Bio-Rad) according to the manufacturer's instructions. All reactions on the custom made plate were run as single reactions whereas assays in wet format were run in duplicates.

Reference genes and calculation of relative expression

Data acquired from the in vitro experiment was normalized to the reference genes RPL32 and YWHAZ [20]. For the in vivo experiment, a total of five reference genes were evaluated (GAPDH, HPRT, PPIA, RPL32, YWHAZ), of which GAPDH, RPL32 and YWHAZ were present on the qPCR plate array. Based on geNorm analysis within the program qBasePLUS (Biogazelle), PPIA and RPL32 were selected for normalization of data ($M = 0.345$). Relative gene expression (fold change, FC) in samples was calculated to a calibrator, either untreated controls (in vitro) or the 0 h time point (in vivo), and normalized [32] to the aforementioned reference genes

DNA extraction and screening for PCV2

Blood samples from SPF pigs (0, 18 h or 5 days after mixing) and conventionally reared pigs (22 h or 5 days after mixing) were screened for presence of PCV2. DNA from 200 μL blood collected with EDTA as additive was extracted using the QIAamp DNA mini kit (Qiagen, Hilden, Germany), eluted in 100 μL elution buffer and the concentration and purity was determined by spectrophotometry (Nanodrop 8000). The undiluted DNA was screened using a universal PCV2 assay (F: TAATTTTGC AGACCCGGAAAC; R: AGTAGATCATCCCACGGC AG) against the ORF1 reading frame [33] and the QuantiTect SYBR Green PCR Kit (Qiagen) as described above (56 °C annealing temperature; 96% efficiency). The presence of PCR inhibitors was evaluated by spiking selected negative samples with 2×10^5 copies of PCV2 DNA before analysis.

Blood and serum analyses

Total and differential white blood cell (WBC) counts were determined in blood collected with EDTA as additive using an automated cell counter (Exigo Veterinary Hematology System; Boule Diagnostics, Spånga,

Sweden). Blood samples without additives were centrifuged for 10 min at 800 g and serum was collected and stored at −20 °C until analysis. Serum amyloid A was determined using a commercial kit (Phase range Serum Amyloid A Assay; Tridelta Development, Maynooth, Ireland) according to the manufacturer's instructions. Serum antibodies to *M. hyopneumoniae* and *H. parasuis* were analysed by commercial kits according to the manufacturers' instructions (IDEXX *M. hyo.* Ab test, IDEXX, Westbrook, USA; Swinecheck HPS, Biovet, St Hyacinthe, Canada) and to *A. pleuropneumoniae* and *P. multocida* by indirect ELISA systems [30, 34].

Data and statistical analysis

Statistical analyses were performed in Excel (Microsoft) or Prism 5.0 (GraphPad Software). WBC counts are shown as mean ± SD and statistical differences analysed by Student's t test. Gene expression is reported as fold change (FC) and shown as median or geometrical mean with SD. Statistical differences in gene expression between experimental groups or treatments were determined using the Mann–Whitney U test or, where applicable, the Wilcoxon matched-pairs signed rank test. Spearman correlation was calculated between gene expression and WBC counts. For all tests, p values less than 0.05 were regarded as significant and a gene with a FC < 0.5 or > 2 was considered as differentially expressed.

Results

Transcriptional response to Matrix-M in vitro

The transcriptional response in lymphocytes, monocytes and MoDCs was measured after short-term (6 h) and long-term (3 or 5 days) stimulation with Matrix-M (Table 2). During these conditions, gene expression of the pro-inflammatory cytokines IL-1β and CXCL8, but not TNF-α or IL-6, was up-regulated by Matrix-M in both lymphocytes and monocytes. Increased transcription of IL-6 was only detected in MoDCs that had been generated for 5 days in the presence of Matrix-M.

Expression of the T$_H$-related cytokine genes IL-12p40, IL-17A and IFN-γ was increased in lymphocytes cultured for 3 days in the presence of Matrix-M. These long-term exposed lymphocytes displayed a decreased transcription of IL-10. IFN-α transcription was up-regulated in MoDCs but not in any other cell type. IFN-β, the interferon-regulated gene IFITM3 and the type I interferon-associated genes STING and SPP1 remained unaffected by Matrix-M. The expression of TLR2 was down-regulated in lymphocytes and in MoDCs exposed to Matrix-M.

In summary, in vitro exposure to Matrix-M affected the gene expression for immunomodulatory cytokines, including IFN-α in cultures of porcine blood mononuclear cells. These effects were most pronounced in

Table 2 Effects of Matrix-M on gene expression (relative gene expression versus untreated control) in cultures of porcine monocytes, lymphocytes and monocyte-derived dendritic cells (MoDC)

Target name	Lymphocytes 3 days[a]		Monocytes 1 day[a]	MoDC 5 days[a]	
	Matrix-M 6 h[b]	Matrix-M 3 days[b]	Matrix-M 6 h[b]	Matrix-M 6 h[b]	Matrix-M 5 days[b]
	$n = 8$[c]	$n = 8$[c]	$n = 10$[c]	$n = 6$[c]	$n = 6$[c]
IL-1β	2.0	9.6*	3.3*	–	–
IL-6	< >	3.9	2.1	< >	10.2*
TNF-α	2.5	< >	< >	–	–
CXCL8	2.4*	5.9**	3.2**	< >	< >
IL-12p40	2.6*	2.6*	nd	–	–
IL-17A	0.3	27.8*	nd	–	–
IFN-γ	< >	4.8*	nd	–	–
IL-10	0.2*	0.4*	< >	–	–
TGF-β	< >	< >	–	–	–
IFN-α	< >	< >	< >	< >	3.8*
IFN-β	nd	nd	nd	< >	2.8
IFITM3	< >[d]	< >[d]	< >	< >[d]	< >[d]
SPP1	< >[d]	< >[d]	< >[e]	< >[d]	0.2[d]
STING	< >[d]	< >[d]	–	< >[d]	< >[d]
TLR2	0.4**	0.2	< >	0.3*	0.2*

< >, gene not affected, i.e. $0.5 < FC < 2$.

nd not detected; too few samples showed any expression of the gene of interest to allow FC calculation, – not analysed.

* $p < 0.05$ and ** $p < 0.01$ for difference in expression between Matrix-M treated samples and medium control (i.e. $FC \neq 1$); Wilcoxon matched-pairs signed rank test.

[a] Total culture time.

[b] Matrix-M exposure time.

[c] Unless otherwise indicated.

[d] $n = 4$.

[e] $n = 6$.

long-term cultures, but were also indicated in cultures exposed to Matrix-M for 6 h.

Transcriptional response to Matrix-M in SPF pigs

The transcriptional response to Matrix-M was followed during 5 days in blood obtained from SPF pigs that were administered Matrix-M (SPF[Matrix-M/SPF]; $n = 4$) or saline (SPF[Saline/SPF]; $n = 4$) and subjected to a 2-h transport. Pooled samples from pigs administered Matrix-M ($n = 4$) were compared to pooled samples from pigs given saline ($n = 4$) using a qPCR plate array containing 92 genes representing innate immunity parameters. A transient increase in gene expression (FC > 2 compared to 0 h) was found for both groups after transport (Figure 2; Additional file 1). The increase appeared earlier in pigs administered Matrix-M (23 genes at 18 h, 19 genes at 30 h) than in those given saline (4 genes at 18 h, 24 genes at 30 h). Only a couple of genes were down-regulated (FC < 0.5) over this time period; CXCL10 and TLR7 in the Matrix-M group and TNFA and FOXP3 in the saline group. Comparing FC values between groups at 18 h confirmed

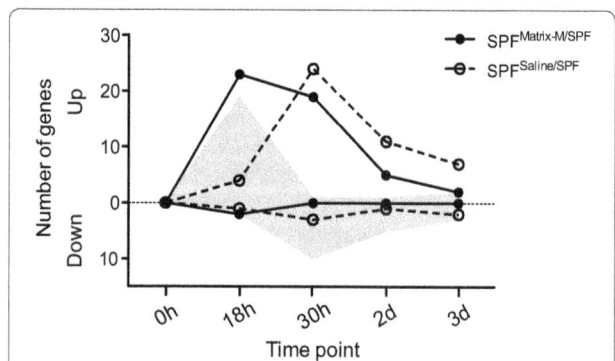

Figure 2 Gene regulation in pooled blood samples from pigs administered Matrix-M or saline. The number of up-regulated and down-regulated genes (fold change > 2 and < 0.5, respectively) in pooled blood from pigs administered Matrix-M ($n = 4$) or saline ($n = 4$), as analysed using a 92-gene qPCR plate array. The expression analysis is presented as the number of differentially expressed genes at each time point in relation to the 0 h time point (Matrix-M solid circles, saline open circles) or as the number of differentially expressed genes in Matrix-M pigs (up-regulated or down-regulated) in relation to the expression in saline pigs at each corresponding time point (depicted by the grey area).

a higher expression (> twofold) of 19 genes in the Matrix-M treated pigs (C3, CCR1, CD80, FOXP3, IFNGR1, IL18, IL1A, IRF7, JAK2, MYD88, NFKBIA, NLRP3, NOD1, NRAMP1, STAT3, TLR4, TLR8, TLR9 and TYK2).

Based on results from the pooled samples and the in vitro data, IFN-α, IFN-β, CXCL8, IL1B, IL6, IL18, MYD88, NLRP3, TLR2, TLR4 and TLR9 were selected for analysis of gene expression in individual samples. The gene expression of MYD88 and NLRP3 displayed a similar kinetic as depicted by the qPCR plate array, i.e., an earlier increase in pigs administered Matrix-M compared to those given saline (Figure 3A). In contrast, the expression of IL1B, TLR2 and TLR4 peaked at 18 h in both groups, whereas the expression of IL18 was highest at 30 h. Transcripts specific for CXCL8, IFN-β and IL-6 were hardly detected and the average FC values for IFN-α and TLR9 did not exceed 2 in blood from the SPF pigs, regardless of treatment. However, statistical analysis of the gene expression data including samples from all SPF pigs at 18 h, i.e. before contact exposure, revealed a significantly ($p < 0.05$) higher expression of IFN-α and TLR2 in pigs administered Matrix-M than in those given saline (Figure 3B). At autopsy, the draining lymph node was enlarged in four of the eight pigs injected with Matrix-M, indicating cell recruitment and/or cell proliferation (Table 3). No such reactions were recorded for any pig injected with saline.

Clinical effects of Matrix-M in SPF pigs at contact exposure

To evaluate if the indicated immune activation by Matrix-M had any clinical effect, SPF pigs where challenged by contact exposure to conventionally reared pigs 22 h after administration of Matrix-M (SPF$^{Matrix-M/Conv}$, Nos. 9–12) or saline (SPF$^{Saline/Conv}$, Nos. 13–16). The contact pigs were clinically healthy during the trial but lung lesions were recorded post-mortem in five of them (two out of four mixed with SPF$^{Matrix-M/Conv}$ and three out of four mixed with SPF$^{Saline/Conv}$ pigs). All conventionally reared pigs were seronegative to *H. parasuis*, whereas antibodies were detected in sera collected from eight SPF pigs originating from two litters. These antibody levels decreased significantly from day 0 to day 6 ($p < 0.05$; paired *t* test), indicating that they were of maternal origin. Both contact pigs and SPF pigs remained seronegative to *M. hyopneumoniae*, *A. pleuropneumoniae* and *P. multocida* throughout the study. The experimental conditions did not affect the PCV2 viral load as no PCV2 DNA was detected in blood from any of the SPF or contact pigs before or at the end of the experiment.

No signs of respiratory disease or lesions in the respiratory tract were recorded for SPF pigs that were mixed with other SPF pigs (SPF$^{Matrix-M/SPF}$ and SPF$^{Saline/SPF}$). None of the SPF pigs that were mixed with conventional pigs at 22 h showed any clinical signs of disease before the contact exposure. Thereafter all these SPF-pigs, irrespective of treatment, developed respiratory symptoms within 1–3 days that lasted throughout the study (Table 3). At necropsy, seven out of these eight SPF pigs displayed reactions in bronchial lymph nodes and/or lung. Lameness and decreased general condition were recorded in two out of the four SPF pigs administered saline (Nos. 14 and 16), with onset 2–4 days after mixing. These two pigs were the only ones displaying joint lesions at the post-mortem examination. In addition, ascetic fluid was found in the peritoneum of pig no. 14.

Thus, all challenged SPF pigs developed respiratory disease, but affected general health status and joint lesions were only recorded for pigs administered saline before the contact exposure. The draining lymph node was enlarged in four of the eight pigs receiving Matrix-M (Nos. 3, 10, 11, 12) but not in any pig administered saline. One SPF$^{Matrix-M/SPF}$ pig (No. 1) turned lame on day 5, which was associated to a superficial abscess in the fetlock joint.

Granulocyte counts, SAA levels and gene expression in Matrix-M treated SPF pigs during the contact exposure experiment

Granulocyte counts, SAA levels and gene expression were monitored for all SPF-pigs throughout the study. The granulocyte numbers increased after transport (18 h) in all SPF groups, from $5.5 \pm 1.4 \times 10^6$ to $10.6 \pm 3.3 \times 10^6$/mL blood in pigs treated with Matrix-M ($n = 8$) and from $5.6 \pm 2.2 \times 10^6$ to $8.9 \pm 3.3 \times 10^6$/mL blood in pigs given saline ($n = 8$). The granulocyte numbers then returned to baseline and remained so in SPF pigs mixed with other SPF pigs (Figure 4A), except in the pig with an abscess in the fetlock joint (pig no. 1), that had 10.5×10^6 granulocytes/mL blood at day 5. Increased levels of SAA were observed in all SPF groups at day 2, i.e. 1 day after allocation and mixing with other pigs. The SAA levels returned to baseline by day 4 in SPF pigs that were mixed with other SPF pigs (Figure 4B), but increased to 132 µg/mL in blood collected on day 6 from pig no. 1. This pig displayed increased gene expression of MyD88, IL18, NLRP3, TLR2 and TLR4 in blood collected day 5. No such alteration in gene expression was recorded for any of the other SPF pigs mixed with SPF-pigs, irrespective of treatment.

A second increase in granulocyte number was recorded following the contact exposure of SPF pigs to conventionally reared pigs (Figure 5). Among SPF pigs administered saline (SPF$^{Saline/Conv}$), the granulocyte counts remained elevated throughout the study and increased considerably for pig nos. 14 and 16 at days 4 and 5. In these two pigs the SAA levels increased above 500 µg/mL from

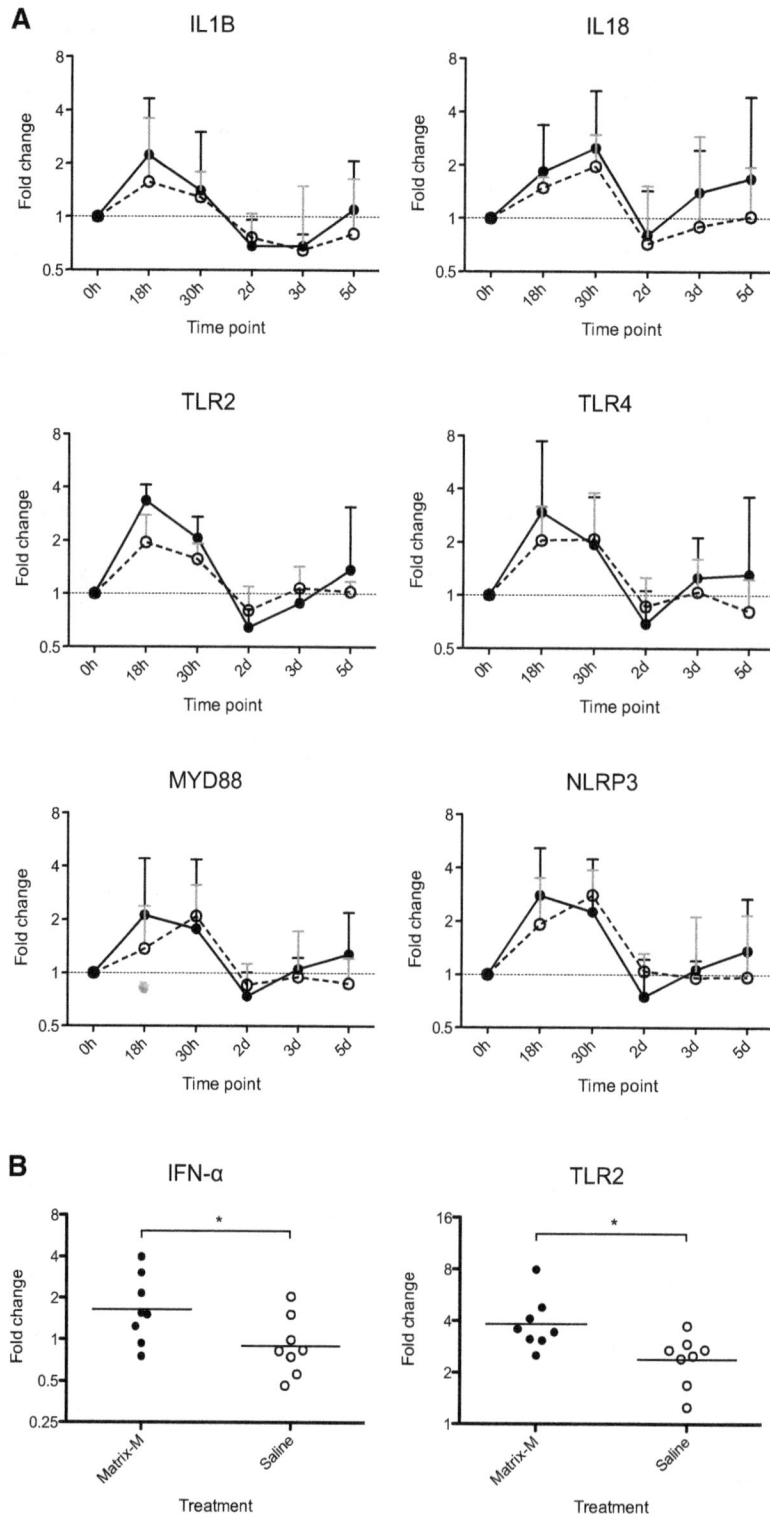

Figure 3 Gene expression in blood of SPF pigs administered Matrix-M (solid line) or saline (open line). A Alterations of the gene expression over a 5 day period following administration of Matrix-M or saline (0 h), transport and mixing with non-littermates (18 h). FC values at indicated times are calculated against the 0 h time point and given as geometric mean ± SD, $n = 4$. **B** Gene expression for all SPF pigs, measured 18 h after injection of Matrix-M ($n = 8$) or saline ($n = 8$). FC values are calculated against the 0 h time point and individual FC values and geometric mean are given for each treatment.

day 4 and onwards. An increased expression of IL18 and TLR2 was also obvious in blood samples collected from these pigs at the last occasions of sampling, i.e. when they displayed lameness and depressed general condition.

The granulocyte numbers in blood from pigs administered Matrix-M (SPF^Matrix-M/Conv) before the contact exposure remained at baseline until day 5 when it increased in three of the four pigs (Nos. 10, 11, 12). This increase coincided with an increase in both SAA levels and expression of IL18 and TLR2 (Figure 5) and IL1B, TLR4 and MYD88 (data not shown) in blood from these pigs. Pig no. 11 had the highest granulocyte count and SAA level on the last day recorded. Furthermore, it also had a higher expression of IL18 than the other pigs already at 18 h, which also was evident for MYD88 and NLRP3 (data not shown). In contrast, pig no. 9 had a

modest increase in granulocyte numbers and no increase in SAA levels on day 5 and 6, and generally showed the lowest variation in gene expression.

The expression of the IFN-α gene was not affected by contact exposure in either SPF^Matrix-M/Conv pigs or SPF^Saline/Conv pigs during the study (Figure 5). Similarly, IFN-β and IL-6 transcripts were only detected in a few of the SPF pigs, which were mixed with other SPF pigs (data not shown). The expression for IL1B, TLR4, MYD88 and NLRP3 generally increased in all pigs at 18 h but thereafter the individual variations were too large for conclusive results (data not shown).

Taken together, the expression pattern of several of the pro-inflammatory genes analysed correlated with changes in granulocyte counts and SAA levels. This relationship was further corroborated by a significant

Table 3　Clinical score and post-mortem findings recorded for the SPF pigs in the natural challenge experiment

Pig ID	Clinical findings					Post-mortem examination				
	General condition		Respiratory signs		Other	DLN	Lung	BLN	Joints	Other
	Score[a]	Onset[b] (day)	Score[a]	Onset[b] (day)						
SPF^Matrix-M/SPF										
#1	–	–	–	–	Lameness[c]	–	–	–	–	Abscess[d]
#2	–	–	–	–	–	–	–	–	–	–
#3	–	–	–	–	–	2	–	–	–	–
#4	–	–	–	–	–	–	–	–	–	–
SPF^Saline/SPF										
#5	–	–	–	–	–	–	–	–	–	–
#6	–	–	–	–	–	–	–	–	–	–
#7	–	–	–	–	–	–	–	–	–	–
#8	–	–	–	–	–	–	–	–	–	–
SPF^Matrix-M/Conv										
#9	–	–	0.5	1	–	–	0.5	1	–	–
#10	–	–	0.5	1	–	1	–	1	–	–
#11	–	–	0.5	2	–	1	0.5	–	–	–
#12	–	–	1	3	–	1	0.5	–	–	–
SPF^Saline/Conv										
#13	–	–	0.5	1	–	–	0.5	0.5	–	–
#14	2	3	1	1	Lameness[e]	–	3	1	3	Ascites[f]
#15	–	–	1	2	–	–	–	1	–	–
#16	1	2	1	1	Lameness[c]	–	–	–	2	–

Pigs were administered Matrix-M (Nos. 1–4 and 9–12) or saline (Nos. 5–8 and 13–16) and were challenged by contact exposure (Nos. 9–16) or mixed with non-littermate SPF pigs (Nos. 1–8).

DLN draining lymph node, *BLN* bronchial lymph node.

[a] Maximum score recorded.

[b] Days after mixing.

[c] Onset 4 days after mixing.

[d] Superficial abscess of 1 cm at fetlock joint.

[e] Onset 3 days after mixing.

[f] Ascetic fluid in the peritoneum.

A

B

Figure 4 Granulocyte counts and SAA levels in blood of SPF pigs administered Matrix-M or saline. A Alterations in granulocyte counts over a 5 day period following administration of Matrix-M or saline (0 h), transport and mixing with non-littermates at 18 h. Mean value ± SD, n = 4. **B** Alterations in SAA over a 5 day period following administration of Matrix-M or saline (0 h), transport and mixing with non-littermates at 18 h. Mean value ± SD, n = 4.

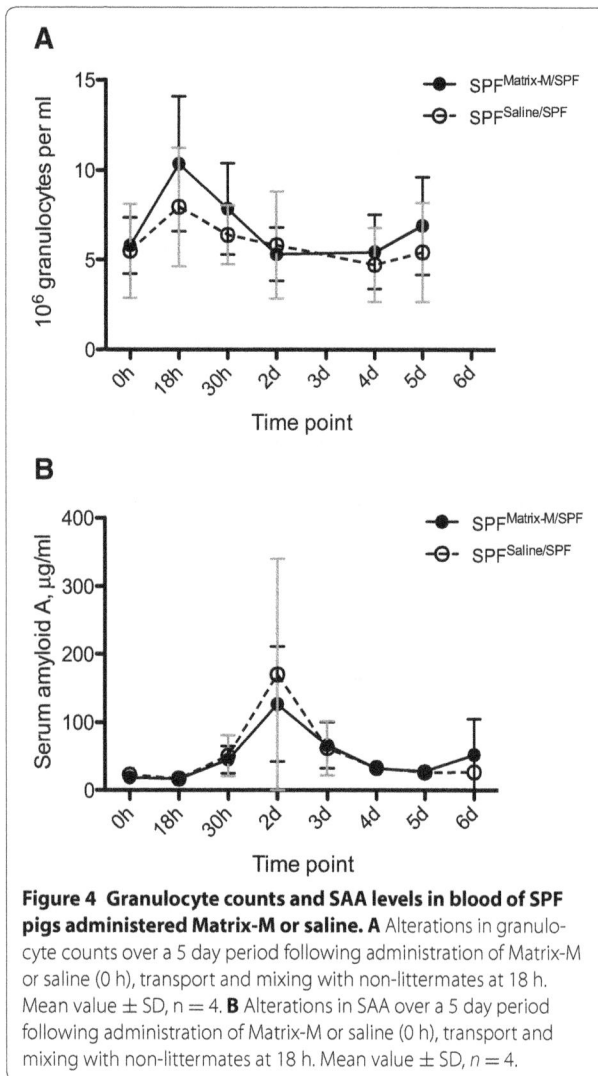

correlation between granulocyte counts and the expression of *TLR2* ($p < 0.001$; rho = 0.63; Spearman analysis for all pigs and time points).

Discussion

Immunomodulatory effects of Matrix-M were evaluated at contact exposure of SPF pigs to conventionally reared pigs. Although all contact SPF pigs in this model developed respiratory disease, only control pigs administered saline developed symptoms of systemic disease as evidenced by joint lesions. Granulocyte counts, levels of the acute-phase protein SAA and gene expression of IL-18 and TLR2 indicated a difference in kinetics of disease development between the two experimental groups. Pigs receiving intramuscular injection of Matrix-M, but not yet subjected to contact exposure, showed a statistically significant increase in expression of TLR2 and IFN-α in blood after 18 h.

Prior to the in vivo studies, in vitro effects of Matrix-M on partially enriched porcine mononuclear cell populations were evaluated. Clearly upregulated genes included proinflammatory cytokines (IL-1β, CXCL8), T_H cytokines (IFN-γ, IL-12p40, IL-17A) and IFN-α. This up-regulation was most pronounced in PBMCs devoid of adherent cells, i.e., lymphocytes, when cultured for 3 days in the presence of Matrix-M. Lymphocytes cultured for only 16 h and exposed to Matrix-M for 6 h did not change their expression of any of the genes analysed (data not shown), in agreement with previous results [20]. The lymphocyte preparations in the current study were only partially purified, with no attempts to phenotypic characterization of the cells. However, γδ T cells that can produce both IL-17 and IFN-γ reach high numbers in the porcine circulation [35, 36] that may have contributed to the relative increase in IL-17 and IFN-γ transcription in lymphocytes. IL-12 and IL-18 act synergistically on the IFN-γ production by porcine T cells [35] and IL-12p40 transcripts were detected in lymphocytes cultured in the presence of Matrix-M. Thus, both the period of exposure to Matrix-M and the total culture time as well as the cell composition appears important for the induction of cytokine gene expression by Matrix-M in vitro.

Most adjuvant effects are evaluated by in vivo or in vitro antigen re-stimulation. In such cases it is comparatively easy to profile the specific immunological response based on cytokine production, effector cell development and antibody isotypes. In the absence of antigen, adjuvant effects are solely monitored by innate immune parameters. However, innate immune reactions are influenced by mediators from several organs making them more problematic to assess in vitro. Using defined immunomodulators whole blood cultures have been used with some success to monitor cytokine profiles in man [37] and inflammatory biomarkers in pigs [38]. Still, the in vitro system does not always reflect the in vivo situation even in the case when defined immunomodulating molecules are used. PolyI:C and plasmid DNA both readily induced IFN-α in porcine tissue whereas these substances only induced low levels of IFN-α in porcine PBMC cultures, unless the inducers were pre-incubated with lipofectin [39, 40]. In accordance, previous in vivo characterization of the immunomodulatory capacity of ISCOM-Matrix formulations, such as production of cytokines and activation of dendritic cells, has not been successfully reproduced in vitro [41].

The transcriptional response to Matrix-M was further evaluated in vivo. For that purpose SPF pigs were administered Matrix-M or saline 16 h before a 2-h transport and subsequent mixing with contact pigs. In line with earlier observations [42, 43], the transport and mixing caused a transient increase in granulocyte counts

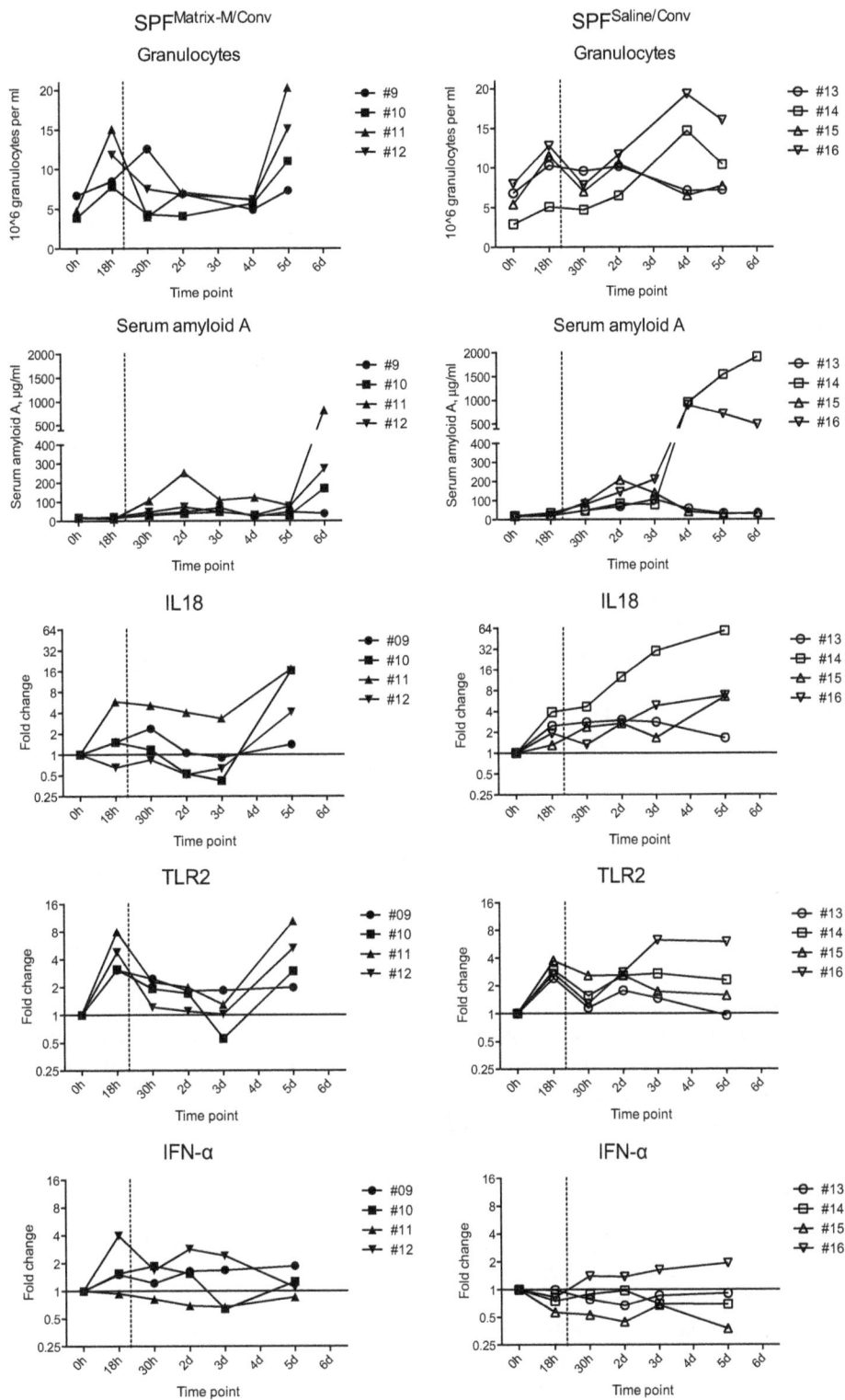

Figure 5 Granulocyte counts, SAA and gene expression in blood of SPF pigs administered Matrix-M or saline. The pigs were administered Matrix-M or saline (0 h), transport to the animal facility (arrival at 18 h) and exposed to conventional pigs (at 22 h, dashed vertical line). Individual FC values are presented for SPF$^{Matrix/Conv}$ pigs (closed symbols) and SPF$^{Saline/Conv}$ pigs (open symbols). FC is calculated against the 0 h time point for each individual.

(at 18 h) and SAA levels (at day 2) with no differences between pigs administered Matrix-M and those given saline. These effects were therefore attributed to the "stress" all pigs experienced. An increased transcription appeared for approximately 20% of the 92 innate immunity genes assessed in the pooled blood samples. This increase was evident in pooled samples collected both at 18 and 30 h from SPF$^{Matrix-M}$ pigs but only found at 30 h in pooled samples from SPF^{Saline} pigs. Of these genes only two (NFKBIA and S100A8) were identified as differentially expressed in a whole transcriptomic analysis of blood cells from pigs after ACTH administration [44]. However, SAA, IL-6, IgA and IL-18 are all suggested as biomarkers of "stress" in the pig [45]. Furthermore, studies in man indicate an intrinsic network between glucocorticosteroids, SAA, cytokines, chemokines, TLR2 and TLR4 [46]. Thus, it is likely that the physiological effect of transport masked effects on the transcription of innate immune genes caused by Matrix-M administration.

When individual samples at time point 18 h were analysed, only the expression of IFN-α and TLR2 was significantly increased in pigs administered Matrix-M compared to saline. This increased gene expression of IFN-α is in line with the induction of interferon-regulated genes in muscle and draining lymph node from pigs 24 h after administration of Matrix-M [16]. Subsequent analyses also demonstrated IFN-β transcripts as well as a low expression of SPP1 and STING in some of these lymph nodes [20]. When analysed in vitro, IFNB, STING and SPP1 showed no expression or were down-regulated whereas IFN-α was up-regulated in long-term cultures of MoDC. Similarly, the expression of TLR2 was down-regulated when analysed in vitro but significantly up-regulated in blood from the SPF-pigs administered Matrix-M. TLR2 was also highly up-regulated locally after intramuscular injection with Matrix-M in pigs [16] and analysis on archived material from that study revealed a tendency toward up-regulation of TLR2 in PBMCs isolated 17 h after the injection (data not shown). In blood, porcine TLR2 is mostly expressed on monocytes, with some expression on granulocytes and no expression on lymphocytes [47]. Thus, changes in the blood relative cellular composition for example caused by altered mononuclear cell migration and polymorphonuclear cell influxes need to be considered amongst other factors when evaluating gene expression in blood samples [48]. Differences between adjuvant effects recorded in vitro and in vivo may hinder the evaluation of mechanistic effects [49] and co-culture systems with endothelial cells can better reflect the in vivo situation when using PBMC for evaluation of immune activators [50].

Based on the results from in vitro data and previous reports on the immunostimulatory effect of Matrix-M [16] we hypothesized that Matrix-M could act prophylactic or therapeutic to affect the clinical outcome of a natural infection. Experience from porcine reproductive and respiratory syndrome virus [22] and PCV2 [51] demonstrate that infectious diseases in production animals are often multifactorial and may benefit from stressors such as weaning, transport and mixing of groups [21]. In an effort to imitate field conditions, SPF pigs were subjected to non-infectious stress from transport and mixing of groups and to infectious stress by contact exposure to conventionally reared pigs (Figure 1). Two of the SPF pigs that were administered saline before contact exposure developed signs of systemic disease that resembled Glässer's disease [52]. This syndrome is caused by *H. parasuis* infection and is commonly associated with transport and mixing of pigs of different health status. Post-mortem examination supported this diagnosis, but *H. parasuis* could not be recovered from affected organs by cultivation. However, the presence of *H. parasuis* was demonstrated by metagenomic sequencing of 16S rRNA genes (SciLifeLab, Uppsala, Sweden, data not shown) and the low level of serum antibodies to *H. parasuis* indicated that the pigs were at risk to develop disease. The affected pigs expressed high levels of SAA and granulocyte counts following the onset of clinical symptoms. Notably, the SAA levels correlated with severity of disease, as outlined in [53], as well as to the expression of IL18 and TLR2. The SAA levels and granulocyte counts returned to baseline after the initial peak in all other SPF pigs mixed with conventional pigs, irrespective of treatment. Thus, there appeared no systemic inflammation in these pigs, although all SPF pigs developed respiratory symptoms. However, in three out of four challenged SPF pigs receiving Matrix-M, both SAA levels, granulocytes counts and transcription of IL1B, IL18, MYD88, NLRP3, TLR2 and TLR4 increased on the last day recorded. All these parameters were also increased in the control pig (No. 1) suffering from an abscess, further supporting their use as indicators of inflammation. This suggests that Matrix-M did not fully protect against systemic disease, but affected the disease kinetics as innate immune responses appeared later after challenge in Matrix-M injected pigs (Figure 5).

Taken together, both the in vitro and in vivo results indicate an immunomodulatory effect of Matrix-M in the pig. In the contact exposure model, Matrix-M seemed to be able to reduce or delay systemic symptoms resembling Glässer's disease. There was no discernible effect on local respiratory symptoms but this might be overcome by employing a different route of administration. If these indications can be confirmed in the field, Matrix-M could be suitable to enhance innate immune responses during critical moments in pig management. Equally important, the capacity to a rapid activation of innate immune parameters is highly desirable in adjuvants used for emergency vaccination.

Additional file

Additional file 1. Gene expression in pooled blood samples from pigs administered Matrix-M or saline. The gene expression was analysed by a qPCR plate array in pooled blood samples collected at 0, 18, 30 h, 2 and 3 days after administration of Matrix-M (4 pigs) or saline (4 pigs). The relative gene expression is given as FC for each experimental group relative to 0 h (FC = 1). These values are then used to compare the gene expression after Matrix-M administration in relation to that after administration of saline.

Competing interests

KLB is employee of Novavax AB, manufacturer of saponin-based Matrix adjuvants. Employees may hold stock and/or stock options in the company. VA, BH, SH, PW and CF declare that they have no competing interests.

Authors' contributions

VA designed the study together with co-authors, performed the animal experiment together with PW and a majority of the laboratory experiments together with BH and SH. BH has made contributions to sample preparation and qPCR design, application and evaluation of data. PW was responsible for the animal experiment including clinical and post-mortem examinations and blood parameter analyses. KLB main contributions were related to adjuvant use and function. CF contributed to result evaluation and manuscript writing. All authors contributed to the manuscript draft. All authors read and approved the final manuscript.

Acknowledgements

This work was supported by grants from The Swedish Research Council for Environment, Agricultural Sciences and Spatial Planning. We thank Per Karlsson and Maria Persson for valuable technical assistance.

Author details

[1] Department of Biomedical Sciences and Veterinary Public Health, Swedish University of Agricultural Sciences, SLU, Uppsala, Sweden. [2] National Veterinary Institute, SVA, Uppsala, Sweden. [3] Novavax AB, Uppsala, Sweden.

References

1. de Paula Barbosa A (2014) Saponins as immunoadjuvant agent: a review. Afr J Pharm Pharmacol 8:1049–1057
2. McKee AS, MacLeod MK, Kappler JW, Marrack P (2010) Immune mechanisms of protection: can adjuvants rise to the challenge? BMC Biol 8:37
3. Sun HX, Xie Y, Ye YP (2009) Advances in saponin-based adjuvants. Vaccine 27:1787–1796
4. Rajput ZI, Hu SH, Xiao CW, Arijo AG (2007) Adjuvant effects of saponins on animal immune responses. J Zhejiang Univ Sci B 8:153–161
5. Morein B, Hu KF, Abusugra I (2004) Current status and potential application of ISCOMs in veterinary medicine. Adv Drug Deliv Rev 56:1367–1382
6. Lövgren K, Morein B (1988) The requirement of lipids for the formation of immunostimulating complexes (ISCOMS). Biotechnol Appl Biochem 10:161–172
7. Pedersen GK, Sjursen H, Nøstbakken JK, Jul-Larsen Å, Hoschler K, Cox RJ (2014) Matrix M(TM) adjuvanted virosomal H5N1 vaccine induces balanced Th1/Th2 CD4(+) T cell responses in man. Hum Vaccines Immunother 10:2408–2416
8. Quinn KM, Yamamoto A, Costa A, Darrah PA, Lindsay RW, Hegde ST et al (2013) Coadministration of polyinosinic: polycytidylic acid and immunostimulatory complexes modifies antigen processing in dendritic cell subsets and enhances HIV gag-specific T cell immunity. J Immunol 191:5085–5089
9. Madhun AS, Haaheim LR, Nilsen MV, Cox RJ (2009) Intramuscular Matrix-M-adjuvanted virosomal H5N1 vaccine induces high frequencies of multifunctional Th1 CD4+ cells and strong antibody responses in mice. Vaccine 27:7367–7376
10. Bengtsson KL, Song H, Stertman L, Liu Y, Flyer DC, Massare MJ et al (2016) Matrix-M adjuvant enhances antibody, cellular and protective immune responses of a Zaire Ebola/Makona virus glycoprotein (GP) nanoparticle vaccine in mice. Vaccine 34:1927–1935
11. Tsuda T, Sugimura T, Murakami Y (1991) Evaluation of glycoprotein gII ISCOMs subunit vaccine for pseudorabies in pig. Vaccine 9:648–652
12. González AM, Nguyen TV, Azevedo MS, Jeong K, Agarib F, Iosef C et al (2004) Antibody responses to human rotavirus (HRV) in gnotobiotic pigs following a new prime/boost vaccine strategy using oral attenuated HRV priming and intranasal VP2/6 rotavirus-like particle (VLP) boosting with ISCOM. Clin Exp Immunol 135:361–372
13. Iosef C, Van Nguyen T, Jeong K, Bengtsson KL, Morein B, Kim Y et al (2002) Systemic and intestinal antibody secreting cell responses and protection in gnotobiotic pigs immunized orally with attenuated Wa human rotavirus and Wa 2/6-rotavirus-like-particles associated with immunostimulating complexes. Vaccine 20:1741–1753
14. Garcia JL, Gennari SM, Navarro IT, Machado RZ, Sinhorini IL, Freire RL et al (2005) Partial protection against tissue cysts formation in pigs vaccinated with crude rhoptry proteins of *Toxoplasma gondii*. Vet Parasitol 129:209–217
15. Xiong Q, Wei Y, Feng Z, Gan Y, Liu Z, Liu M et al (2014) Protective efficacy of a live attenuated *Mycoplasma hyopneumoniae* vaccine with an ISCOM-matrix adjuvant in pigs. Vet J 199:268–274
16. Ahlberg V, Bengtsson KL, Wallgren P, Fossum C (2012) Global transcriptional response to ISCOM-Matrix adjuvant at the site of administration and in the draining lymph node early after intramuscular injection in pigs. Dev Comp Immunol 38:17–26
17. Magnusson SE, Reimer JM, Karlsson KH, Lilja L, Bengtsson KL, Stertman L (2012) Immune enhancing properties of the novel Matrix-M adjuvant leads to potentiated immune responses to an influenza vaccine in mice. Vaccine 31:1725–1733
18. Reimer JM, Karlsson KH, Bengtsson KL, Magnusson SE, Fuentes A, Stertman L (2012) Matrix-M adjuvant induces local recruitment, activation and maturation of central immune cells in absence of antigen. PLoS One 7:e41451
19. Lund H, Boysen P, Åkesson CP, Lewandowska-Sabat AM, Storset AK (2016) Transient migration of large numbers of CD14(++) CD16(+) monocytes to the draining lymph node after onset of inflammation. Front Immunol 7:322
20. Fossum C, Hjertner B, Ahlberg V, Charerntantanakul W, McIntosh K, Fuxler L et al (2014) Early inflammatory response to the saponin adjuvant Matrix-M in the pig. Vet Immunol Immunopathol 158:53–61
21. Amadori M, Zanotti C (2016) Immunoprophylaxis in intensive farming systems: the way forward. Vet Immunol Immunopathol 181:2–9
22. Amadori M, Razzuoli E (2014) Immune control of PRRS: lessons to be learned and possible ways forward. Front Vet Sci 1:2
23. Dec M, Puchalski A (2008) Use of oromucosally administered interferon-alpha in the prevention and treatment of animal diseases. Pol J Vet Sci 11:175–186
24. Stuyven E, Cox E, Vancaeneghem S, Arnouts S, Deprez P, Goddeeris BM (2009) Effect of beta-glucans on an ETEC infection in piglets. Vet Immunol Immunopathol 128:60–66
25. Volman JJ, Ramakers JD, Plat J (2008) Dietary modulation of immune function by beta-glucans. Physiol Behav 94:276–284
26. Foster N, Berndt A, Lalmanach AC, Methner U, Pasquali P, Rychlik I et al (2012) Emergency and therapeutic vaccination—is stimulating innate immunity an option? Res Vet Sci 93:7–12
27. Netea MG, Joosten LAB, Latz E, Mills KH, Natoli G, Stunnenberg HG et al (2016) Trained immunity: a program of innate immune memory in health and disease. Science 352:aaf1098
28. Jensen KJ, Benn CS, van Crevel R (2016) Unravelling the nature of non-specific effects of vaccines—a challenge for innate immunologists. Semin Immunol 28:377–383
29. Johansson E, Domeika K, Berg M, Alm GV, Fossum C (2003) Characterisation of porcine monocyte-derived dendritic cells according to their cytokine profile. Vet Immunol Immunopathol 91:183–197

30. Sjölund M, Fossum C, Martín de la Fuente AJ, Alava M, Juul-Madsen HR, Lampreave F et al (2011) Effects of different antimicrobial treatments on serum acute phase responses and leucocyte counts in pigs after a primary and a secondary challenge infection with *Actinobacillus pleuropneumoniae*. Vet Rec 169:70

31. Wikström FH, Fossum C, Fuxler L, Kruse R, Lövgren T (2011) Cytokine induction by immunostimulatory DNA in porcine PBMC is impaired by a hairpin forming sequence motif from the genome of Porcine circovirus type 2 (PCV2). Vet Immunol Immunopathol 139:156–166

32. Vandesompele J, De Preter K, Pattyn F, Poppe B, Van Roy N, De Paepe A et al (2002) Accurate normalization of real-time quantitative RT-PCR data by geometric averaging of multiple internal control genes. Genome Biol 3:RESEARCH0034

33. Bálint A, Tenk M, Deim Z, Rasmussen TB, Uttenthal A, Csagola A et al (2009) Development of primer-probe energy transfer real-time PCR for the detection and quantification of Porcine circovirus type 2. Acta Vet Hung 57:441–452

34. Wallgren P, Persson M (2000) Relationship between the amounts of antibodies to *Actinobacillus pleuropneumoniae* serotype 2 detected in blood serum and in fluids collected from muscles of pigs. J Vet Med B Infect Vet Public Health 47:727–737

35. Sedlak C, Patzl M, Saalmüller A, Gerner W (2014) IL-12 and IL-18 induce interferon-γ production and de novo CD2 expression in porcine γδ T cells. Dev Comp Immunol 47:115–122

36. Stepanova H, Mensikova M, Chlebova K, Faldyna M (2012) CD4+ and γδTCR+ T lymphocytes are sources of interleukin-17 in swine. Cytokine 58:152–157

37. May L, van Bodegom D, Kuningas M, Meij JJ, de Craen AJM, Frölich M et al (2009) Performance of the whole-blood stimulation assay for assessing innate immune activation under field conditions. Cytokine 45:184–189

38. Peters SM, Yancy H, Bremer E, Monroe J, Paul D, Stubbs JT 3rd et al (2011) In vitro identification and verification of inflammatory biomarkers in swine. Vet Immunol Immunopathol 139:67–72

39. Magnusson M, Johansson E, Berg M, Eloranta ML, Fuxler L, Fossum C (2001) The plasmid pcDNA3 differentially induces production of interferon-alpha and interleukin-6 in cultures of porcine leukocytes. Vet Immunol Immunopathol 78:45–56

40. Wattrang E, Wallgren P, Fuxler L, Lindersson M, Fossum C (1997) Tissue chambers—a useful model for in vivo studies of cytokine production in the pig. Vet Immunol Immunopathol 56:133–150

41. Wilson NS, Yang B, Morelli AB, Koernig S, Yang A, Loeser S et al (2012) ISCOMATRIX vaccines mediate CD8+ T-cell cross-priming by a MyD88-dependent signaling pathway. Immunol Cell Biol 90:540–552

42. Salamano G, Mellia E, Candiani D, Ingravalle F, Bruno R, Ru G et al (2008) Changes in haptoglobin, C-reactive protein and pig-MAP during a housing period following long distance transport in swine. Vet J 177:110–115

43. Piñeiro M, Piñeiro C, Carpintero R, Morales J, Campbell FM, Eckersall PD et al (2007) Characterisation of the pig acute phase protein response to road transport. Vet J 173:669–674

44. Sautron V, Terenina E, Gress L, Lippi Y, Billon Y, Larzul C et al (2015) Time course of the response to ACTH in pig: biological and transcriptomic study. BMC Genomics 16:961

45. Martínez-Miró S, Tecles F, Ramón M, Escribano D, Hernández F, Madrid J et al (2016) Causes, consequences and biomarkers of stress in swine: an update. BMC Vet Res 12:171

46. De Buck M, Gouwy M, Wang JM, Van Snick J, Proost P, Struyf S et al (2016) The cytokine-serum amyloid A-chemokine network. Cytokine Growth Factor Rev 30:55–69

47. Alvarez B, Revilla C, Domenech N, Pérez C, Martínez P, Alonso F et al (2008) Expression of toll-like receptor 2 (TLR2) in porcine leukocyte subsets and tissues. Vet Res 39:13

48. Chaussabel D, Pascual V, Banchereau J (2010) Assessing the human immune system through blood transcriptomics. BMC Biol 8:84

49. Ghimire TR (2015) The mechanisms of action of vaccines containing aluminum adjuvants: an in vitro vs in vivo paradigm. Springerplus 4:181

50. Findlay L, Sharp G, Fox B, Ball C, Robinson CJ, Bird C et al (2011) Endothelial cells co-stimulate peripheral blood mononuclear cell responses to monoclonal antibody TGN1412 in culture. Cytokine 55:141–151

51. Darwich L, Mateu E (2012) Immunology of Porcine circovirus type 2 (PCV2). Virus Res 164:61–67

52. Oliveira S, Pijoan C (2004) Haemophilus parasuis: new trends on diagnosis, epidemiology and control. Vet Microbiol 99:1–12

53. Cray C, Zaias J, Altman NH (2009) Acute phase response in animals: a review. Comp Med 59:517–526

54. Nygard AB, Jørgensen CB, Cirera S, Fredholm M (2007) Selection of reference genes for gene expression studies in pig tissues using SYBR green qPCR. BMC Mol Biol 8:67

55. Feng X, Xiong Y, Qian H, Lei M, Xu D, Ren Z (2010) Selection of reference genes for gene expression studies in porcine skeletal muscle using SYBR green qPCR. J Biotechnol 150:288–293

56. Shirkey TW, Siggers RH, Goldade BG, Marshall JK, Drew MD, Laarveld B et al (2006) Effects of commensal bacteria on intestinal morphology and expression of proinflammatory cytokines in the gnotobiotic pig. Exp Biol Med 231:1333–1345

57. Duvigneau JC, Hartl RT, Groiss S, Gemeiner M (2005) Quantitative simultaneous multiplex real-time PCR for the detection of porcine cytokines. J Immunol Methods 306:16–27

58. McCulloch RS, Ashwell MS, O'Nan AT, Mente PL (2012) Identification of stable normalization genes for quantitative real-time PCR in porcine articular cartilage. J Anim Sci Biotechnol 3:36

59. von der Hardt K, Kandler MA, Fink L, Schoof E, Dötsch J, Brandenstein O et al (2004) High frequency oscillatory ventilation suppresses inflammatory response in lung tissue and microdissected alveolar macrophages in surfactant depleted piglets. Pediatr Res 55:339–346

60. Borca MV, Gudmundsdottir I, Fernandez-Sainz IJ, Holinka LG, Risatti GR (2008) Patterns of cellular gene expression in swine macrophages infected with highly virulent classical swine fever virus strain Brescia. Virus Res 138:89–96

61. Tang ZX, Chen GX, Liang MY, Rong J, Yao JP, Yang X et al (2014) Selective antegrade cerebral perfusion attenuating the TLR4/NF-kappaB pathway during deep hypothermia circulatory arrest in a pig model. Cardiology 128:243–250

9

Differential protein expression in chicken macrophages and heterophils in vivo following infection with *Salmonella* Enteritidis

Zuzana Sekelova[1], Hana Stepanova[1], Ondrej Polansky[1], Karolina Varmuzova[1], Marcela Faldynova[1], Radek Fedr[2,3], Ivan Rychlik[1*] and Lenka Vlasatikova[1]

Abstract

In this study we compared the proteomes of macrophages and heterophils isolated from the spleen 4 days after intravenous infection of chickens with *Salmonella* Enteritidis. Heterophils were characterized by expression of MMP9, MRP126, LECT2, CATHL1, CATHL2, CATHL3, LYG2, LYZ and RSFR. Macrophages specifically expressed receptor proteins, e.g. MRC1L, LRP1, LGALS1, LRPAP1 and a DMBT1L. Following infection, heterophils decreased ALB and FN1, and released MMP9 to enable their translocation to the site of infection. In addition, the endoplasmic reticulum proteins increased in heterophils which resulted in the release of granular proteins. Since transcription of genes encoding granular proteins did not decrease, these genes remained continuously transcribed and translated even after initial degranulation. Macrophages increased amounts of fatty acid elongation pathway proteins, lysosomal and phagosomal proteins. Macrophages were less responsive to acute infection than heterophils and an increase in proteins like CATHL1, CATHL2, RSFR, LECT2 and GAL1 in the absence of any change in their expression at RNA level could even be explained by capturing these proteins from the external environment into which these could have been released by heterophils.

Introduction

Macrophages and heterophils represent professional phagocytes acting as effectors and modulators of innate immunity as well as orchestrators of adaptive immunity [1]. Heterophils, the avian counterparts of mammalian neutrophils, belong among the first responders to bacterial infections and sensing of pathogen associated molecular patterns (PAMPs) stimulates heterophils for phagocytosis as well as release of bactericidal proteins stored in heterophil granules into the extracellular environment [2]. In agreement with their general function in host protection against pathogens, heterophils play a crucial role in the protection of chickens against *Salmonella* infection and chickens with heterophil depletion are not protected against colonization of systemic sites [3–5]. However, although there are several reports on

specific heterophil functions during infection of chickens with *Salmonella enterica*, their genome-wide response to infection has not been characterized so far.

Macrophages are professional phagocytes responsible for the destruction and clearance of pathogens. When activated, macrophages increase their antibacterial activity by the expression of antimicrobial peptides like cathepsins B, C, D and S, avidin, ferritin or ovotransferrin [6], and production of NO radicals from arginine by inducible NO synthase. The antimicrobial proteins expressed by macrophages are commonly produced also by heterophils though it is not known to what extent these may differ in their immediate availability and total amount produced by both cell types. Macrophages can also regulate the immune response by the expression of cytokines e.g. IL1β, IL6, IL8, IL18 or LITAF [7] and are capable of antigen presentation [8–10]. However, similar to heterophils, an unbiased report on total proteome expressed by chicken macrophages is absent.

*Correspondence: rychlik@vri.cz
[1] Veterinary Research Institute, Hudcova 70, 621 00 Brno, Czech Republic
Full list of author information is available at the end of the article

In our previous study we showed that heterophils and macrophages increase in the spleen of chickens when intravenously infected with *Salmonella* Enteritidis (*S.* Enteritidis) [7]. Next we characterized the gene expression at the tissue level in the whole spleen and expression of selected transcripts was tested in sorted leukocyte subpopulations [6]. However, none of this provided general data on the protein expression in chicken heterophils and macrophages. Although intravenous infection of chickens only partially represents specific *Salmonella*—chicken interactions which are mixed up with a general response to bacteremia caused by Gram negative bacterium, this way of infection represents a model for the understanding heterophil and macrophage functions during early response to infection. In the current study we therefore isolated heterophils and macrophages from chicken spleens by fluorescence-activated cell sorting (FACS), purified proteins from these cells and identified them by mass spectrometry. This allowed us to (1) characterize the total proteome of heterophils and macrophages, (2) define proteins which exhibited differential abundance in chicken heterophils compared to macrophages and (3) identify proteins that changed in abundance following the intravenous infection with *S.* Enteritidis in either of these populations. Since we also included a group of chickens which was vaccinated prior to challenge, we also addressed whether there are any proteins specifically expressed by the macrophages or heterophils from the vaccinated chickens. Using this approach we identified over one hundred proteins characteristic of either chicken heterophils or macrophages which allowed us to further refine their function in chickens.

Materials and methods
Ethics statement
The handling of animals in this study was performed in accordance with current Czech legislation (Animal protection and welfare Act No. 246/1992 Coll. of the Government of the Czech Republic). The specific experiments were approved by the Ethics Committee of the Veterinary Research Institute (permit number 5/2013) followed by the Committee for Animal Welfare of the Ministry of Agriculture of the Czech Republic (permit number MZe 1480).

Bacterial strains and chicken line
Newly hatched ISA Brown chickens from an egg laying line (Hendrix Genetics, Netherlands) were used in this study. Chickens were reared in perforated plastic boxes with free access to water and feed and each experimental or control group was kept in a separate room. The chickens were vaccinated with *S.* Enteritidis mutant completely lacking *Salmonella* pathogenicity island 1 (SPI-1)

constructed as described earlier [11] and infected with isogenic wild type *S.* Enteritidis 147 spontaneously resistant to nalidixic acid. The strains were grown in LB broth at 37 °C for 18 h followed by pelleting bacteria at $10\,000 \times g$ for 1 min and re-suspending the pellet in the same volume of PBS as was the original volume of LB broth.

Experimental infection
There were 3 groups of chickens. Six chickens from the control group were sacrificed on day 48 of life. An additional 6 chickens (group 2) were infected intravenously with 10^7 CFU of wild type *S.* Enteritidis in 0.1 mL PBS on day 44 of life. The last 6 chickens (group 3) were orally vaccinated on day 1, revaccinated on day 21 of life with 10^7 CFU of *S.* Enteritidis SPI-1 mutant in 0.1 mL of inoculum and challenged intravenously with 10^7 CFU of wild type *S.* Enteritidis on day 44 of life. Intravenous mode of infection was used mainly to stimulate macrophage and heterophil response rather than to model natural infection of chickens with *S.* Enteritidis. All chickens in groups 2 and 3 were sacrificed 4 days post infection, i.e. when aged 48 days. The spleens from the chickens from all three groups were collected into PBS during necropsy. To confirm *S.* Enteritidis infection, approximately 0.5 g of liver tissue was homogenised in 5 mL of peptone water, tenfold serially diluted and plated in XLD agar, as described previously [11].

Collecting heterophil and macrophage subpopulations by flow cytometry
The cell suspensions were prepared by pressing the spleen tissue through a fine nylon mesh followed by 2 washes with 30 mL of cold PBS. After the last washing step, the splenic leukocytes were re-suspended in 1 mL of PBS and used for surface marker staining.

In total 10^8 of cells were incubated for 20 min with anti-monocyte/macrophage:FITC (clone KUL01 from Southern Biotech) and CD45:APC (clone LT40 from Southern Biotech), followed by wash with PBS. Monocytes/macrophages (CD45+KUL01+) and heterophils (identified based on FSC/SSC characteristics within CD45+ cells) were sorted using a FACSFusion flow cytometer operated by FACSDiva software (BD Biosciences). Only for simplicity, the monocytes/macrophages population will be called as "macrophage (Ma)" in the rest of this paper. Sorted cells were collected in PBS and immediately processed as described below. A small aliquot from each sample was subjected to immediate purity analysis. The purity of macrophages was $88.6 \pm 5.3\%$ and of heterophils $88.1 \pm 4.2\%$ when counting cell of expected staining, and FSC and SSC parameters out of all particles. When we gated at the area with live cells, the purity of macrophages and heterophils was between 97 and 98%.

Majority of contaminants therefore represented cellular debris and only around 2.5% of contaminants were formed by non-target cells.

Protein and RNA isolation from sorted cells, reverse transcription of mRNA and quantitative real time PCR (qPCR)

Sorted leukocyte subpopulations were lysed in 500 μL of Tri Reagent (MRC) for parallel isolation of RNA and proteins. Upon addition of 4-bromoanisole and 15 min centrifugation at 14 000 × g, proteins were precipitated with acetone from the lower organic phase. RNA present in upper aqueous phase was further purified using RNeasy purification columns according to the instructions of the manufacturer (Qiagen). The concentration of RNA was determined spectrophotometrically (Nanodrop, Thermo Scientific) and 1 μg of RNA was immediately reverse transcribed into cDNA using MuMLV reverse transcriptase (Invitrogen) and oligo dT primers. After reverse transcription, the cDNA was diluted 10 times with sterile water and stored at −20 °C prior qPCR. qPCR was performed in 3 μL volumes in 384-well microplates using QuantiTect SYBR Green PCR Master Mix (Qiagen) and a Nanodrop pipetting station from Innovadyne for PCR mix dispensing following MIQE recommendations [12]. Amplification of PCR products and signal detection were performed using a LightCycler II (Roche) with an initial denaturation at 95 °C for 15 min followed by 40 cycles of 95 °C for 20 s, 60 °C for 30 s and 72 °C for 30 s, followed by the determination of melting temperature of resulting PCR products to exclude false positive amplification. Each sample was subjected to qPCR in duplicate and the mean values of the Cq values of genes of interest were normalized (ΔCt) to an average Cq value of three reference genes (GAPDH, TBP and UB). The relative expression of each gene of interest was finally calculated as $2^{-\Delta Cq}$. Statistical analysis using a two sample t test for means equality was performed when comparing levels of mRNA expression between chicken groups and results with p value ≤ 0.05 were considered as significantly different in expression. Sequence of reference genes GAPDH, TBP and UB have been published elsewhere [13, 14]. Sequences of all newly designed primers used in this study including their location within different exons and sizes of PCR products are listed in Additional file 1.

Sample preparation for LC–MS/MS analysis

Precipitated proteins were washed with acetone and dried. The pellets were dissolved in 300 μL of 8 M urea and processed by the filter aided sample preparation method [15] using Vivacon 10 kDa MWCO filter (Sartorius Stedim Biotech). Proteins were washed twice with 100 μL of 8 M urea and reduced by 100 μL of 10 mM DTT. After reduction, proteins were incubated with 100 μL of 50 mM IAA and washed twice with 100 μL of 25 mM TEAB. Trypsin (Promega) was used at 1:50 ratio (w/w) and the digestion proceeded for 16 h at 30 °C.

For comparative analysis, peptide concentration was determined spectrophotometrically (Nanodrop, Thermo Scientific) and samples from the same group of chickens were pooled. Pooled samples were then labelled using the stable isotope dimethyl labelling protocol as described previously [16]. Labeled samples were mixed and 3 subfractions were prepared using Oasis MCX Extraction Cartridges (Waters). The samples were desalted on SPE C18 Extraction Cartridges (Empore) and concentrated in a SpeedVac (Thermo Scientific) prior to LC–MS/MS.

LC–MS/MS analysis

Protein samples were analysed on LC–MS/MS system using an UltiMate 3000 RSLCnano liquid chromatograph (Dionex) connected to LTQ-Orbitrap Velos Pro mass spectrometer (Thermo Scientific). Chromatographic separation was performed on EASY-Spray C18 separation column (25 cm × 75 μm, 3 μm particles, Thermo Scientific) with 2 h long (label free) or 3 h long (label based) 3–36% acetonitrile gradient.

High resolution (30 000 FWHM at 400 m/z) MS spectra were acquired for the 390–1700 m/z interval in an Orbitrap analyser with an AGC target value of 1×10^6 ions and maximal injection time of 100 ms. Low resolution MS/MS spectra were acquired in Linear Ion Trap in a data-dependent manner and the top 10 precursors exceeding a threshold of 10 000 counts and having a charge state of +2 or +3 were isolated within a 2 Da window and fragmented using CID.

Data processing, protein identification and quantification

Raw data were analysed using the Proteome Discoverer (v.1.4). MS/MS spectra identification was performed by SEQUEST using the *Gallus gallus* protein sequences obtained from Uniprot database. Precursor and fragment mass tolerance were 10 ppm and 0.6 Da, respectively. Carbamidomethylation (C) and oxidation (M) were set as static and dynamic modifications, respectively. Dimethylation (N-term and K) was set as static modification in the label-based analysis. Only peptides with a false discovery rate FDR $\leq 5\%$ were used for protein identification.

Spectral counting, the protocol in which abundance of a protein is expressed as the total number of tandem mass spectra matching its peptides (peptide spectrum matches, PSM), was used for comparative label-free analysis of heterophil and macrophage proteomes [17]. For a general comparison of protein abundance between heterophils and macrophages, PSMs belonging to a particular protein from all three groups of chickens, i.e. 18

samples, were summed up. The identification of at least two distinct peptides belonging to the particular protein and the threshold of at least 5 PSMs in at least one sample was required for its reliable identification [18, 19]. All data were normalized to the total number of PSMs in individual samples. Statistical analysis using a t test was performed and the proteins with p value ≤ 0.05 and with at least four fold differences in its amounts were considered as significantly different in their abundance between the subpopulations.

In the label-based quantification, only unique peptide sequences with at least 20 PSMs were considered for peptide ratio calculations. Subsequent analysis of label-based data was performed in R (https://www.R-project.org). For each protein, its individual peptide ratios were $\log_2$ transformed, mean values were calculated and tested with a one sample t test. Benjamini-Hochberg correction for multiple testing was then applied to the obtained p values. Only proteins having $\geq$ twofold change and adjusted p value ≤ 0.05 were considered as being significantly different in abundance.

Bioinformatic analysis
Protein interaction networks were built using the online database resource Search Tool for the Retrieval of Interacting Genes (STRING). Proteins were further analyzed using Gene Ontology (GO) database and the Kyoto Encyclopedia of Genes and Genomes (KEGG) for their classification into specific pathways. PCA plots were calculated and created in R (https://www.R-project.org).

Results
S. Enteritidis infection
Intravenous *S.* Enteritidis infection resulted in a high colonization of systemic sites. Average $\log_{10}$ *S.* Enteritidis counts were 5.03 ± 0.54 and 3.06 ± 0.99 CFU/g of liver in the infected chickens and the vaccinated and infected chickens, respectively. Despite this, no fatalities were observed among infected chickens. No *S.* Enteritidis was detected in any of the control non-infected chickens.

Identification of heterophil and macrophage specific proteins
Proteins specific for chicken heterophils or macrophages were determined irrespective whether these were obtained from the infected or non-infected chickens.

Altogether, 858 proteins from heterophils and 1032 proteins from macrophages were detected. Out of these, 654 proteins were expressed both in heterophils and macrophages. Two-hundred and eight proteins were detected in macrophages only and an additional 126 proteins were 4 times or more abundant in macrophages than in heterophils. On the other hand, 34 proteins were

detected in heterophils only and an additional 44 proteins were 4 times or more abundant in heterophils than in macrophages (Additional file 2).

Proteins characteristic for heterophils
Out of 78 proteins characteristic for heterophils (Additional file 2), 20 with the highest PSM difference between heterophils and macrophages are listed in Table 1. These included MRP126, LECT2, CATHL1, CATHL2, CATHL3, LYG2, LYZ and RSFR proteins, all with antibacterial functions. STOM and RAB27A proteins controlling storage and release of granular proteins in neutrophils also belonged among the characteristic and highly expressed proteins in heterophils. Two serine protease inhibitors, SERPINB10 and SERPINB1, were also found among the 20 most characteristic heterophil proteins (Table 1). Only a single KEGG pathway was specifically enriched in heterophils and this was the starch and sucrose metabolism pathway comprising PYGL, PGM1 and PGM2 proteins ($p = 1.7E-4$). Despite the KEGG pathway designation, all these proteins represent enzymes involved in glycogen metabolism [20].

Proteins characteristic for macrophages
Out of 334 proteins specific for macrophages (Additional file 2), 20 with the highest PSM difference between macrophages and heterophils are listed in Table 2. Five of these represented receptor proteins MRC1L, LRP1, LGALS1, LRPAP1 and DMBT1L, the last one containing the scavenger receptor cysteine-rich (SRCR) domain. CTSB, CKB, MECR, PHB2, H9KZK0 and p41/Li are involved in phagocytosis and antigen presentation. An additional 4 proteins UQCR, UQCRC1, ACO2 and HADHB are localized to the mitochondria. Only 3 proteins, MRC1L, HSP70 and p41/Li, were already recorded in chicken macrophages [21–23] although except for NAT3, PLB and SSB, the expression of the remaining proteins (out of the most abundant listed in Table 2) has been already recorded in murine or human macrophages. Proteins enriched in macrophages belonged to oxidative phosphorylation ($p = 4.7E-8$), fatty acid metabolism ($p = 1.73E-6$), citrate cycle ($p = 4.2E-6$), arginine and proline metabolism ($p = 8.5E-8$) and proteasome ($p = 4.5E-4$).

Heterophil proteins responding to in vivo infection with *S.* Enteritidis
Altogether, 153 proteins were present in different abundance in the heterophils before and after *S.* Enteritidis infection. Of these, 109 proteins increased and 44 proteins decreased in abundance (Additional files 3 and 4 for all quantified heterophil proteins). Proteins belonging to 2 KEGG categories were enriched in heterophils

Table 1　Twenty most characteristic proteins of heterophils (Het) compared to macrophages (Ma)

Acc. no.	Protein name	Gene ID	ΔPSM[a]	Fold ratio Het:Ma	Response to the infection	Function
P28318	MRP126, calprotectin	MRP126	7170	9.07	No	Calcium and zinc binding
P08940	Myeloid protein 1	LECT2	5532	6.32	Decrease	Chemotactic factor for Het
P02789	Ovotransferrin	OTFB	2351	4.87	Decrease	Iron binding, immune response
O73790	Heterochromatin-associated protein MENT	SERPINB10	1760	6.00	No	DNA condensation, cysteine protease inhibitor
E1C0K1	Extracellular fatty acid-binding protein	ExFABP	1742	4.94	No	Fatty acid and bacterial sidero-phores binding
F1NG13	Transglutaminase 3	TGM3	1572	19.94	No	Transglutaminase
Q2IAL7	Cathelicidin 2	CATHL2	1402	7.49	Decrease	Antimicrobial peptide
P27042	Lysozyme G	LYG2	989	4.57	Decrease	Antimicrobial peptide
Q2IAL6	Cathelicidin 3	CATHL3	936	5.37	No	Antimicrobial peptide
P00698	Lysozyme C	LYZ	839	5.17	Decrease	Antimicrobial peptide
Q6QLQ5	Cathelicidin 1	CATHL1	833	4.62	Decrease	Antimicrobial peptide
E1BTH1	Leukocyte elastase inhibitor	SERPINB1	627	Only Het	Decrease	Protection against own proteases
F1P284	Leukotriene A(4) hydrolase	LTA4H	603	5.78	Decrease	Epoxide hydrolase and amin-opeptidase
F1NGT3	Matrix metallopeptidase 9	MMP9	600	Only Het	Decrease	Degradation of the extracellular matrix
F2Z4L6	Serum albumin	ALB	557	4.79	Decrease	Plasma carrier
P30374	Ribonuclease homolog	RSFR	548	6.89	Decrease	Lysosomal cysteine protease
R9PXN7	Hematopoietic prostaglandin D synthase	HPGDS	504	17.79	No	Cytosolic glutathione S-trans-ferases
E1BTV1	Stomatin	STOM	502	23.82	No	Integral membrane protein
D2D3P4	Rab27a	Rab27a	435	88.08	No	Small GTPase, exocytosis
R4GI24	Integrin alpha-D	ITGAD	379	7.73	No	Adhesion of leukocytes

[a] The difference in PSM counts of particular protein in Het and Ma.

following *S.* Enteritidis infection. These included the category translation with 39 proteins ($p = 2.58E-62$) and protein processing in endoplasmic reticulum (12 proteins, $p = 1.74E-11$). Twenty proteins with the highest increase in abundance, except for those belonging to the category translation, are listed in Table 3. Among others, these included AVD, F13A, ANXA2, ANXA7 or CTSC.

Forty-four proteins decreased in abundance in heterophils following *S.* Enteritidis infection and 20 of these with the highest decrease are listed in Table 4. Proteins with decreased abundance were those found in heterophil granules such as MPO, LYZ, LYG2, CTSG, CTSL1, CATHL1, CATHL2, RSFR, MMP9 and LECT2. Another set of proteins which decreased in heterophils following *S.* Enteritidis infection included ALB, FN1 and OTFB (Table 4).

Macrophage proteins responding to in vivo infection with *S. Enteritidis*

Four KEGG pathways were specifically enriched when testing proteins of increased abundance in macrophages following *S.* Enteritidis infection. These included fatty acid elongation pathway (MECR and HADHB proteins,

$p = 2.49E-4$), lysosomal proteins CTSB and CTSC ($p = 6.98E-3$), phagosomal proteins RAB7A and STX7 ($p = 9.23E-3$) and LDHA and HADHB from the microbial metabolism in diverse environments pathway ($p = 9.4E-3$). Other proteins with increased abundance in macrophages following *S.* Enteritidis infection were MRP126, CATHL1, CATHL2, GAL1, CTSB, CTSC, RSFR, SOD1, LECT2, LY86 and FTH, all with antibacterial functions (Table 5). Proteins which decreased in abundance in macrophages following *S.* Enteritidis infection included RBMX, NDUFA4, FNBP1, FAM107, STMN1, GLOD4 and OLA1 (Table 5; Additional files 5, 6 for all quantified macrophage proteins).

RNA expression

Finally we verified the expression of 37 genes coding for selected proteins listed in Tables 1, 2, 3, 4 and 5. Expression of 4 genes, LRP1, MPO, PPIB and TUBA3A was too low and these genes were excluded from further consideration (Additional file 7).

Six genes (LGALS1, MRC1L, GDA, MECR, DMBT1, LRPAP1) out of 7 proteins selected as specific for macrophages were transcribed in macrophages at a higher

Table 2 Twenty most characteristic proteins for macrophages (Ma) compared to heterophils (Het)

Acc. no.	Protein name	Gene ID	ΔPSM[a]	Fold ratio Ma:Het	Response to the infection	Function
M1XGZ4	Macrophage mannose receptor 1 like	MRC1L	993	Only Ma	No	C-Type lectin
P98157	Low-density lipoprotein receptor-related protein 1	LRP1	810	Only Ma	No	Endocytic receptor
P07583	Galectin 1	LGALS1	607	Only Ma	No	Beta-galactoside-binding lectin
P43233	Cathepsin B	CTSB	538	8.42	Increase	Cysteine protease
F1NZ86	Heat shock 70 protein, mortalin	HSP70	508	5.30	No	Chaperon
P05122	Creatine kinase B-type	CKB	467	34.77	No	Energy transduction
F1NDD6	LDL receptor related protein associated protein 1	LRPAP1	374	Only Ma	No	LDL receptors trafficking
F1NIX4	Trans-2-enoyl-CoA reductase	MECR	356	33.16	Increase	Fatty acid elongation
F1P180	Aspartate aminotransferase	GOT2	350	7.27	No	Transaminase
P13914	Arylamine *N*-acetyltransferase	NAT3	350	23.92	No	Conjugating enzyme
H9KZK0	Protein containing the scavenger receptor cysteine-rich (SRCR) domain	DMBT1L	318	Only Ma	No	Scavenger receptor
E1BZF7	Putative phospholipase B	PLB	317	6.23	No	Removing fatty acids from phospholipids
Q6J613	Invariant chain isoform p41	Li	312	6.87	No	Chaperone
F1P582	Mitochondrial ubiquinol-cytochrome-c reductase complex core protein 2	UQCR	309	4.36	No	Oxidative phosphorylation
Q5ZMW1	Aconitate hydratase, mitochondrial	ACO2	306	6.17	No	TCA cycle
F1NAC6	Cytochrome b-c1 complex subunit 1	UQCRC1	289	6.42	No	Oxidative phosphorylation
F6R1X6	Lupus la protein	SSB	288	6.90	No	Protecting of 3′ poly(U) terminus of transcribed RNA
E1BTT4	Trifunctional enzyme subunit beta, mitochondrial	HADHB	287	30.61	Increase	β-Oxidation of fatty acids
Q5ZMN3	Prohibitin-2	PHB2	282	10.52	No	Not clear
F1NJD6	Guanine deaminase, cypin	GDA	275	Only Ma	No	Oxidizes hypoxanthine to xanthine

[a] The difference in PSM counts of particular protein in Ma and Het.

level than in heterophils. Only HSP70 was transcribed in macrophages and heterophils at the same level though it was present in higher abundance at the protein level in macrophages. Nine genes (MRP126, OTFB, LYG2, LYZ, SERPINB1, CATHL1, CATHL2, MMP9, LECT2) out of 14 heterophil specific proteins were transcribed in heterophils at a higher level than in macrophages. Two genes of this group (GPX, CTSG) were transcribed in heterophils and macrophages at the same level and the remaining 2 genes (RSFR, LTA4H) were transcribed at a higher level in macrophages though protein mass spectrometry indicated their higher abundance in heterophils.

Expression of 11 proteins which increased in abundance in macrophages following infection of chickens with *S.* Enteritidis was also tested at the RNA level. Except for MRP126, 10 of these (MECR, CTSC, ERAP1, RSFR, SOD1, CALR, CATHL1, CATHL2, LECT2, GAL1) did not exhibit any difference at the transcriptional level.

6 of 7 proteins (ANXA2, F13A, CTSC, ERAP1, AVD, HSP90B1) exhibiting an increased abundance in heterophils following infection of chickens with *S.* Enteritidis, also increased their expression at the level of transcription. Only IFITM did not change its expression at the RNA level. Finally we verified the expression of 11 proteins which decreased in abundance in heterophils following infection of chickens with *S.* Enteritidis. Eight of them (FN1, ALB, CTSL1, OTFB, LYZ, CATHL1, MMP9, LECT2) did not change their expression at the level of transcription and transcripts of 3 of them (RSFR, LYG2, CSTC) even increased following infection.

Similar to the results of protein mass spectrometry, RNA levels of the tested genes in the heterophils or macrophages from the vaccinated chickens were in between the expression in non-infected chickens and chickens infected without previous vaccination. Only 3 genes in heterophils did not follow this scheme and CATHL1,

Table 3 Proteins which increased in abundance in heterophils in response to *S.* Enteritidis infection

Acc. no.	Protein name	Gene ID	Fold ratio Inf: noninf	Fold ratio vac: noninf	Function
P02701	Avidin	AVD	55.57*	32.06*	Biotin binding
F1P4F4	Translocon-associated protein	SSR1	9.22*	6.36	Protein translocase
P17785	Annexin A2	ANXA2	6.44*	2.11	Activates macrophages for cytokine production
E1BWG1	Coagulation factor XIIIA	F13A	5.63*	2.60*	Crosslinking of fibrin chains, entrapment of bacteria
R4GJX3	Interferon-induced transmembrane protein	IFITM	4.99*	1.73	Acidification of the endosomal compartments, mediator of the host antiviral response
F1NK96	Protein disulfide-isomerase A6	PDIA6	4.33*	2.66*	Protein foldase
F1NVA4	Nucleophosmin	NPM1	3.68*	1.87	Alarmin, nuclear chaperon
F1NT28	Inorganic pyrophosphatase	PPA1	3.52*	1.67	Hydrolysis of inorganic pyrophosphate (PPi)
Q90593	78 kDa glucose-regulated protein	BiP	3.44*	1.94	Chaperon
F1NWB7	Endoplasmin	HSP90B1	3.33*	1.99	Chaperon
E1C1D1	Annexin 7	ANXA7	3.27*	2.68*	Granular membranes fusion and degranulation
P24367	Peptidyl-prolyl cis–trans isomerase B	PPIB	3.26*	2.23*	Regulation of protein folding and maturation
E1C2S1	Talin-1	TLN1	3.12*	2.56*	Activation of neutrophils
Q49B65	EF hand-containing protein 1	EFHD1	3.12*	1.72	Calcium binding
F1NWG2	Cathepsin C	CTSC	3.10*	1.99	Activates serine proteases (elastase, cathepsin G and granzymes)
F1NDY9	Protein disulfide-isomerase A4	PDIA4	2.93*	1.86	Protein foldase
E1C8M9	Calnexin	CANX	2.88*	1.75	Integral protein of the endoplasmic reticulum
E1BQN9	Calcyclin-binding protein	CACYBP	2.88*	2.38*	Calcium-dependent ubiquitination
H9L340	ATP synthase subunit beta	ATP5B	2.82*	1.56	Energy metabolism
F1NB92	Endoplasmic reticulum aminopeptidase 1	ERAP1	2.78*	0.89	Antigen processing and presentation of endogenous peptide via MHC class I

* Significantly different from the expression in heterophils from the non-infected chickens.

CATHL2 and LECT2 were expressed in heterophils from the vaccinated chickens at significantly higher level than in the heterophils from infected chickens.

Discussion

Until now, chicken heterophils and macrophages have been characterized only by their specific characteristics like cytokine signaling or production of antimicrobial peptides [2, 6, 7, 24, 25] and an unbiased report characterizing their total proteome, before and after infection, has been missing. In the current study we therefore isolated proteins from heterophils and macrophages and quantified their abundance before and after infection with *S.* Enteritidis by mass spectrometry. We have to remind that mass spectrometry provides reliable data for approximately 800 the most abundant proteins. The lowly represented proteins, despite their potential specificity or responsiveness to infection, could not be therefore detected.

Chicken macrophages differed from heterophils in 3 specific features. First, macrophages specifically expressed receptors such as MRC1L, LRP1, LGALS1, LRPAP1 and DMBT1L. Second, macrophages exhibited higher mitochondrial activity including fatty acid degradation, TCA cycle and oxidative phosphorylation. And third, macrophages specifically expressed enzymes involved in arginine and proline metabolism (Figure 1). Receptors specifically expressed by macrophages indicate their potential to sense signals from the external environment which allows them to modulate immune response [6, 7] including their own polarization [26, 27]. The dependency of macrophages on oxidative phosphorylation and mitochondria functions was already described for human macrophages and neutrophils [28]. Macrophages were also enriched in arginine and proline metabolism since one of their bactericidal activities is the production of NO radicals by iNOS and arginine [29]. Following infection with *S.* Enteritidis, macrophages

Table 4 **List of proteins which decreased in abundance in heterophils in response to *S.* Enteritidis infection**

Acc. no.	Protein name	Gene ID	Fold ratio inf: noninf	Fold ratio vac: noninf	Function
F1P1U6	Myeloperoxidase	MPO	0.013*	0.071*	Oxidative burst
E1C677	Natural killer cell activator	Gga.18306	0.026*	0.21*	GO prediction: regulation of cytokine biosynthetic process
F1NJT3	Fibronectin	FN1	0.11*	0.56	Binds components of extracellular matrix
F1NFQ7	Serine protease 57	PRSSL1	0.15*	0.37*	Serine-type endopeptidase activity
P00698	Lysozyme C	LYZ	0.16*	0.37*	Antimicrobial peptide
H9L027	Cathepsin G	CTSG	0.19*	0.30*	Lysosomal cysteine protease
Q6QLQ5	Cathelicidin-1	CATHL1	0.20*	0.51	Bactericidal, fungicidal and immu-nomodulatory activity
F1NZ37	Cathepsin L1	CTSL1	0.22*	0.48*	Controlling element of neutrophil elastase activity
P30374	Ribonuclease homolog	RSFR	0.23*	0.51	Lysosomal cysteine protease
P27042	Lysozyme G	LYG2	0.24*	0.60	Antimicrobial peptide
F2Z4L6	Serum albumin	ALB	0.24*	0.67	Plasma carrier
P02789	Ovotransferrin	OTFB	0.26*	0.55	Iron binding, immune response
F1NGT3	Matrix metallopeptidase 9	MMP9	0.26*	0.77	Degradation of the extracellular matrix
F1NVM1	G-protein coupled receptor 97	GPR97	0.27*	0.66	Regulates migration
Q2IAL7	Cathelicidin-2	CATHL2	0.31*	0.78	Antimicrobial peptide
Q2UZR2	Phosphoglucomutase 1	PGM1	0.35*	0.43*	Glucose metabolic process
E1BZS2	Nucleosome assembly protein 1-like	NAP1L1	0.36*	0.22*	Chaperone for the linker histone
P08940	Myeloid protein 1	LECT2	0.37*	0.62	Chemotactic factor
R4GH86	Glutathione peroxidase	GPX	0.41*	0.57	Protects organism from oxidative damage
F1NYH8	Ena/VASP-like protein	EVL	0.42*	0.70	Regulators of the actin cytoskeleton and cell migration

* Significantly different from the expression in heterophils from the non-infected chickens.

increased the expression of lysosomal and phagosomal proteins what could be associated not only with *S.* Enteritidis inactivation but also with macrophage ability of antigen presentation.

Heterophils specifically expressed granular proteins MPO, LYZ, LYG2, RSFR, LECT2, CATHL1, CATHL2, CTSL1, CTSG, OTFB, SERPINB1 and MMP9, and endoplasmic reticulum proteins SSR1, PDIA4, PDIA6, PPIB, BiP, HSP90B1 and CANX. The latter group of proteins is activated when lumenal conditions in endoplasmic reticulum are altered or chaperone capacity is overwhelmed by unfolded or misfolded proteins [30]. Induction of an unfolded protein response leads to neutrophil degranulation in mice [31] and based on our results, a similar response can be predicted also in chicken heterophils.

Granular proteins decreased in heterophils in response to infection. Since transcription of genes encoding these proteins did not change and the number of ribosomal proteins increased, these genes must have remained continuously transcribed and translated even after initial

degranulation [24, 32–35]. However, not all proteins that decreased in heterophils following *S.* Enteritidis infection were assigned to pathogen inactivation. Matrix metalloproteinase MMP9 is used for degradation of the extracellular matrix to enable leukocyte infiltration to the site of inflammation [36], and ALB and FN1, are found at the surface of granulocytes and inhibit their migration [37, 38]. The decrease of ALB and FN1 together with the degradation of extracellular matrix by MMP9 leads to heterophil translocation from the blood circulation to the site of inflammation.

Comparing expression at the protein and RNA levels provided several unexpected results. Changes in expression at the RNA level in response to infection were more pronounced in heterophils than in macrophages. We can exclude any technical issues in macrophage gene expression analysis since there were at least 3 genes inducible at the RNA level also in macrophages (AVD, MRP126 and F13A). Unlike macrophages, there were also greater differences in the expression profiles of heterophils

Table 5 Proteins of increased or decreased abundance in macrophages in response to *S.* Enteritidis infection

Acc. no.	Protein name	Gene ID	Fold ratio inf:noninf	Fold ratio vac:noninf	Function
P28318	MRP126, calprotectin	MRP126	15.67*	5.01*	Calcium and zinc binding
Q6QLQ5	Cathelicidin-1	CATHL1	7.32*	2.95*	Antimicrobial peptide
P30374	Ribonuclease homolog	RSFR	5.84*	1.66	Lysosomal cysteine protease
F1NIX4	Trans-2-enoyl-CoA reductase	MECR	5.47*	3.99*	Fatty acid elongation
P46156	Gallinacin 1	GAL1	4.15*	1.12	Antimicrobial protein
F1N8Q1	Superoxide dismutase	SOD1	4.01*	2.58	Oxygen scavenger
P08940	Myeloid protein 1	LECT2	3.87*	1.35	Chemotactic factor for Het
F1P4F3	Lymphocyte antigen 86, MD-1	LY86	3.53*	3.03	Inhibits LPS response of immune cells
F1NS91	60S ribosomal protein L9	RPL9	3.51*	3.82	Structural part of ribosome
E1BTT4	Trifunctional enzyme subunit beta, mitochondrial	HADHB	3.38*	3.54*	β-Oxidation of fatty acids
P43233	Cathepsin B	CTSB	2.88*	2.57*	Lysosomal cysteine protease
B4X9P4	Microsomal glutathione S-transferase 1	MGST1	2.87*	1.46	Membrane protection from oxidative stress
Q5ZMP2	Syntaxin 7	STX7	2.72*	2.94*	Late endosome–lysosome fusion
E1C0F3	Ras-related protein Rab-7a	RAB7A	2.69*	2.38*	Involved in endocytosis, phagosome–lysosome fusion
F1N9J7	Tubulin alpha-3 chain	Tuba3a	2.63*	1.96	Major constituent of microtubules
P08267	Ferritin heavy chain	FTH	2.62*	2.33*	Storage of iron in a soluble, nontoxic state
P02263	Histone H2A-IV	H2A4	2.61*	3.64*	Formation of nucleosome
F1NWG2	Cathepsin C	CTSC	2.48*	2.46*	Activates serine proteases
Q2IAL7	Cathelicidin-2	CATHL2	2.45*	1.01	Antimicrobial peptide
Q6EE32	Calreticulin	CALR	2.33*	2.21*	Molecular chaperon
Q9I9D1	Voltage-dependent anion-selective channel protein 2	VDAC2	2.27*	2.07*	Inhibits mitochondrial way of apoptosis
P02607	Myosin light polypeptide 6	MYL6	2.7*	1.66	Found in phagosome
F1NB92	Endoplasmic reticulum aminopeptidase 1	ERAP1	2.21*	2.04	Antigen processing and presentation of endogenous peptide via MHC class I
E1BTT8	Lactate dehydrogenase A	LDHA	2.07*	1.71	Glycolysis
R4GM10	Fructose-bisphosphate aldolase C	ALDOC	2.07*	2.33	Glycolysis
P24367	Peptidyl-prolyl cis–trans isomerase B	PPIB	2.00*	0.97	Regulation of protein folding and maturation
Q5ZKQ9	RNA binding motif protein, X-linked	RBMX	0.49*	0.59	Regulation of pre- and post-transcriptional processes
R4GGZ2	NADH dehydrogenase [ubiquinone] 1 alpha subcomplex subunit 4	NDUFA4	0.38*	0.65	Oxidative phosphorylation
E1BYF8	Formin-binding protein 1	FNBP1	0.33*	0.47*	Role in late stage of clathrin-mediated endocytosis
R4GJP1	Family with sequence similarity 107, member B	FAM107	0.32*	0.30*	Candidate tumor suppressor gene
P31395	Stathmin 1	STMN1	0.27*	0.51	Promotes disassembly of microtubules
E1BQI4	Glyoxalase domain-containing protein 4	GLOD4	0.21*	0.18*	Unknown
Q5ZM25	Obg-like ATPase 1	OLA1	0.12*	0.11	Negative role in cell adhesion and spreading

* Significantly different from the expression in macrophages from the non-infected chickens.

obtained from vaccinated chickens in comparison to those obtained from naive but infected animals and an increase in CATHL2 and LECT2 in the heterophils from the vaccinated chickens following *S.* Enteritidis challenge appeared as a specific positive marker of vaccination. Despite this, expression in heterophils and macrophages in naive but infected chickens tended to approach a similar expression profile (Figure 2).

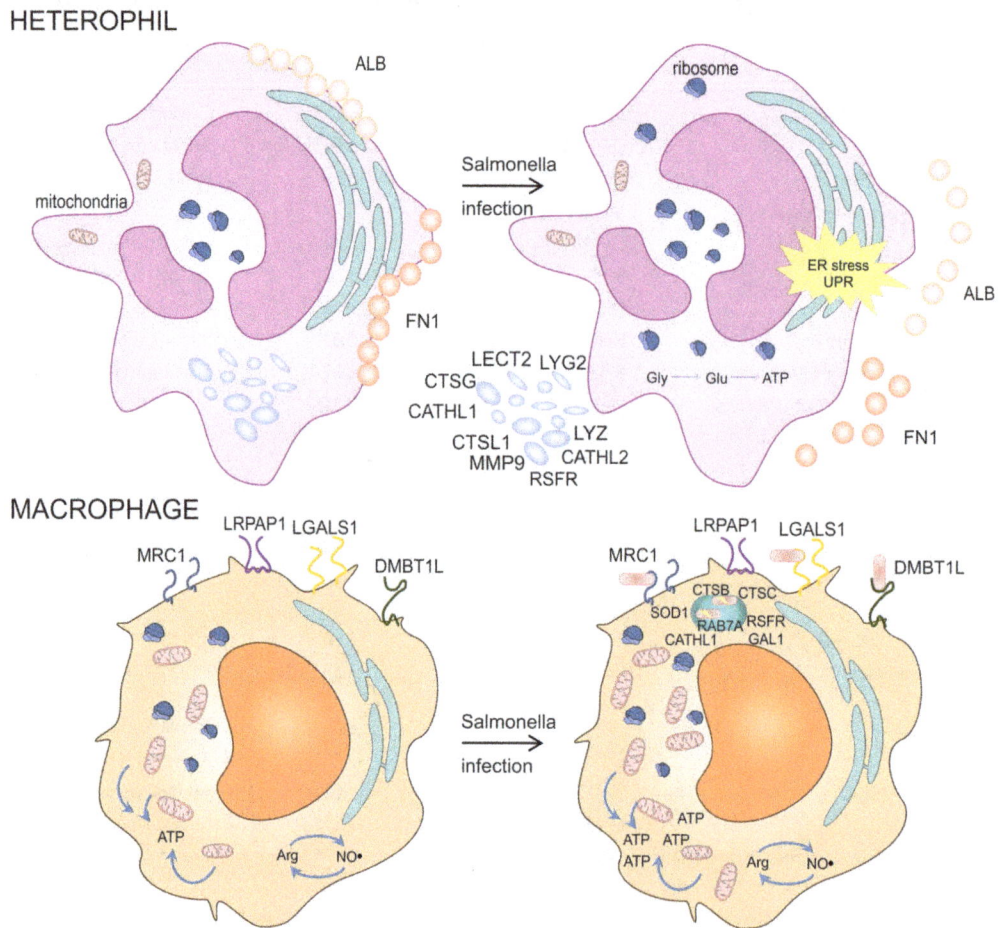

Figure 1 The most characteristic proteins and their functions in chicken heterophils and macrophages. Heterophils express MMP9, MRP126, LECT2, CATHL1, CATHL2, CATHL3, LYG2, LYZ and RSFR proteins. Following *S.* Enteritidis infection, heterophils decreased fibrinogen FN1 and albumin ALB, and increased ribosomal proteins. In addition, endoplasmic reticulum proteins are activated which results in the release of granular proteins. Heterophils expressed glycogen (Gly) metabolism pathway which allows for rapid glucose (Glu) availability and anaerobic ATP generation via glycolysis while macrophages increased mitochondrial activity. Macrophages expressed receptor proteins MRC1, LGALS1, LRPAP1 and DMBT1L, mitochondria-localized proteins and arginine metabolism proteins. Following infection with *S.* Enteritidis, macrophages increased the expression of lysosomal and phagosomal proteins (CTSB, CTSC, RAB7A, CATHL1, RSFR, GAL1, SOD1).

In this study we characterized protein expression in chicken heterophils and macrophages in response to intravenous infection with *S.* Enteritidis. Heterophils decreased ALB and FN1, and released MMP9 to enable their translocation to the site of infection. Secondly the endoplasmic reticulum proteins increased in heterophils which resulted in the release of granular proteins. On the other hand, macrophages were less responsive to acute infection and an increase in proteins like CATHL1, CATHL2, RSFR, LECT2 and GAL1 in the absence of any

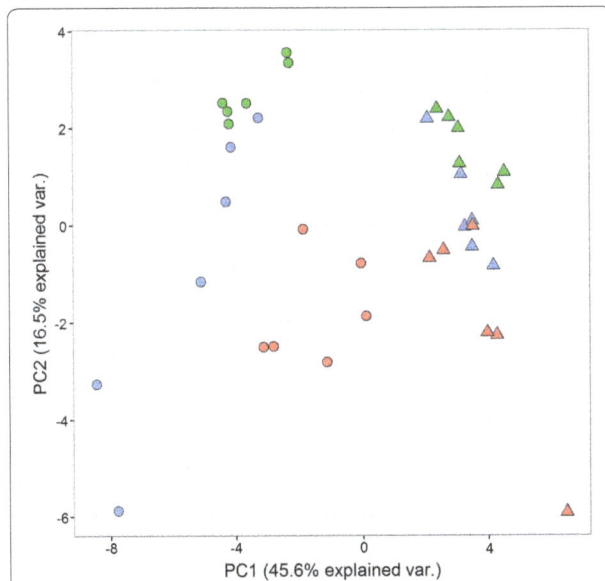

Figure 2 PCA cluster analysis of chicken heterophils and macrophages using expression data from qPCR. Each spot represents heterophils (circles) or macrophages (triangles) isolated from non-infected (green color), infected (red color), and vaccinated and infected chickens (blue color), 6 chickens per group. Heterophils from vaccinated chickens responded to infection more than macrophages from the same chicken. Transcription of heterophils and macrophages from naive but infected chickens approached the same profile.

change in their expression at RNA level could even be explained by capturing these proteins from the external environment into which these could have been released by heterophils.

Additional files

Additional file 1. List of primers used in quantitative RT PCR in the study.

Additional file 2. Identification of heterophil and macrophage specific proteins using label-free LC MS/MS and PSM quantification.

Additional file 3. Heterophil proteins responding to in vivo infection with S. Enteritidis.

Additional file 4. All heterophil proteins quantified in this study.

Additional file 5. Macrophage proteins responding to in vivo infection with S. Enteritidis.

Additional file 6. All macrophage proteins quantified in this study.

Additional file 7. Expression of selected genes at RNA level determined by quantitative RT PCR.

Competing interests
The authors declare that they have no competing interests.

Authors' contributions
ZS and OP purified proteins and performed protein mass spectrometry. HS and RF sorted splenic leukocytes by flow cytometry. KV and MF were

responsible for RNA purification and qPCR. IR and LV designed the study, analysed data and wrote the manuscript. All authors read and approved the final manuscript.

Acknowledgements
Authors would like to thank Peter Eggenhuizen for language corrections and acknowledge the excellent technical assistance of Andrea Durisova.

Author details
[1] Veterinary Research Institute, Hudcova 70, 621 00 Brno, Czech Republic. [2] Department of Cytokinetics, Institute of Biophysics of the CAS, Kralovopolska 135, 612 65 Brno, Czech Republic. [3] Center of Biomolecular and Cellular Engineering, International, Clinical Research Center, St. Anne's University Hospital Brno, Pekarska 53, 656 91 Brno, Czech Republic.

Funding
This work has been supported by project from P502-13-31474P of the Czech Science Foundation, AdmireVet project CZ.1.005/2.1.00/01.0006–ED0006/01/01 from the Czech Ministry of Education and RO0516 project of the Czech Ministry of Agriculture. RF was supported by the project LQ1605 from the National Program of Sustainability II (MEYS CR). The funders had no role in the study design, data collection and analysis, decision to publish, or preparation of the manuscript.

References
1. Silva MT (2010) When two is better than one: macrophages and neutrophils work in concert in innate immunity as complementary and cooperative partners of a myeloid phagocyte system. J Leukoc Biol 87:93–106
2. Genovese KJ, He H, Swaggerty CL, Kogut MH (2013) The avian heterophil. Dev Comp Immunol 41:334–340
3. Kogut MH, McGruder ED, Hargis BM, Corrier DE, DeLoach JR (1995) In vivo activation of heterophil function in chickens following injection with Salmonella Enteritidis-immune lymphokines. J Leukoc Biol 57:56–62
4. Kogut MH, Tellez G, Hargis BM, Corrier DE, DeLoach JR (1993) The effect of 5-fluorouracil treatment of chicks: a cell depletion model for the study of avian polymorphonuclear leukocytes and natural host defenses. Poult Sci 72:1873–1880
5. Barrow PA (2007) Salmonella infections: immune and non-immune protection with vaccines. Avian Pathol 36:1–13
6. Matulova M, Rajova J, Vlasatikova L, Volf J, Stepanova H, Havlickova H, Sisak F, Rychlik I (2012) Characterization of chicken spleen transcriptome after infection with Salmonella enterica serovar Enteritidis. PLoS One 7:e48101
7. Matulova M, Stepanova H, Sisak F, Havlickova H, Faldynova M, Kyrova K, Volf J, Rychlik I (2012) Cytokine signaling in splenic leukocytes from vaccinated and non-vaccinated chickens after intravenous infection with Salmonella Enteritidis. PLoS One 7:e32346
8. Qureshi MA (2003) Avian macrophage and immune response: an overview. Poult Sci 82:691–698
9. Swaggerty CL, Pevzner IY, Kaiser P, Kogut MH (2008) Profiling pro-inflammatory cytokine and chemokine mRNA expression levels as a novel method for selection of increased innate immune responsiveness. Vet Immunol Immunopathol 126:35–42
10. Singh R, Jain P, Pandey NK, Saxena VK, Saxena M, Singh KB, Ahmed KA, Singh RP (2012) Cytokines expression and nitric oxide production under induced infection to Salmonella Typhimurium in chicken lines divergently selected for cutaneous hypersensitivity. Asian-Australas J Anim Sci 25:1038–1044
11. Rychlik I, Karasova D, Sebkova A, Volf J, Sisak F, Havlickova H, Kummer V, Imre A, Szmolka A, Nagy B (2009) Virulence potential of five major pathogenicity islands (SPI-1 to SPI-5) of Salmonella enterica serovar Enteritidis for chickens. BMC Microbiol 9:268
12. Bustin SA, Benes V, Garson JA, Hellemans J, Huggett J, Kubista M, Mueller R, Nolan T, Pfaffl MW, Shipley GL, Vandesompele J, Wittwer CT (2009) The MIQE guidelines: minimum information for publication of quantitative real-time PCR experiments. Clin Chem 55:611–622

13. De Boever S, Vangestel C, De Backer P, Croubels S, Sys SU (2008) Identification and validation of housekeeping genes as internal control for gene expression in an intravenous LPS inflammation model in chickens. Vet Immunol Immunopathol 122:312–317

14. Li YP, Bang DD, Handberg KJ, Jorgensen PH, Zhang MF (2005) Evaluation of the suitability of six host genes as internal control in real-time RT-PCR assays in chicken embryo cell cultures infected with infectious bursal disease virus. Vet Microbiol 110:155–165

15. Wiśniewski JR, Zougman A, Nagaraj N, Mann M (2009) Universal sample preparation method for proteome analysis. Nat Methods 6:359–362

16. Boersema PJ, Raijmakers R, Lemeer S, Mohammed S, Heck AJ (2009) Multiplex peptide stable isotope dimethyl labeling for quantitative proteomics. Nat Protoc 4:484–494

17. Lundgren DH, Hwang SI, Wu L, Han DK (2010) Role of spectral counting in quantitative proteomics. Expert Rev Proteomics 7:39–53

18. Old WM, Meyer-Arendt K, Aveline-Wolf L, Pierce KG, Mendoza A, Sevinsky JR, Resing KA, Ahn NG (2005) Comparison of label-free methods for quantifying human proteins by shotgun proteomics. Mol Cell Proteomics 4:1487–1502

19. Wong JW, Sullivan MJ, Cagney G (2008) Computational methods for the comparative quantification of proteins in label-free LCn-MS experiments. Brief Bioinform 9:156–165

20. Adeva-Andany MM, González-Lucán M, Donapetry-García C, Fernández-Fernández C, Ameneiros-Rodríguez E (2016) Glycogen metabolism in humans. BBA Clin 5:85–100

21. Staines K, Hunt LG, Young JR, Butter C (2014) Evolution of an expanded mannose receptor gene family. PLoS One 9:e110330

22. Li YZ, Cheng CS, Chen CJ, Li ZL, Lin YT, Chen SE, Huang SY (2014) Functional annotation of proteomic data from chicken heterophils and macrophages induced by carbon nanotube exposure. Int J Mol Sci 15:8372–8392

23. Ye H, Xu FZ, Yu WY (2009) The intracellular localization and oligomerization of chicken invariant chain with major histocompatibility complex class II subunits. Poult Sci 88:1594–1600

24. van Dijk A, Molhoek EM, Veldhuizen EJ, Bokhoven JL, Wagendorp E, Bikker F, Haagsman HP (2009) Identification of chicken cathelicidin-2 core elements involved in antibacterial and immunomodulatory activities. Mol Immunol 46:2465–2473

25. van Dijk A, Tersteeg-Zijderveld MH, Tjeerdsma-van Bokhoven JL, Jansman AJ, Veldhuizen EJ, Haagsman HP (2009) Chicken heterophils are recruited to the site of *Salmonella* infection and release antibacterial mature Cathelicidin-2 upon stimulation with LPS. Mol Immunol 46:1517–1526

26. Novak R, Dabelic S, Dumic J (2012) Galectin-1 and galectin-3 expression profiles in classically and alternatively activated human macrophages. Biochim Biophys Acta 1820:1383–1390

27. May P, Bock HH, Nofer JR (2013) Low density receptor-related protein 1 (LRP1) promotes anti-inflammatory phenotype in murine macrophages. Cell Tissue Res 354:887–889

28. Kramer PA, Ravi S, Chacko B, Johnson MS, Darley-Usmar VM (2014) A review of the mitochondrial and glycolytic metabolism in human platelets and leukocytes: implications for their use as bioenergetic biomarkers. Redox Biol 2:206–210

29. Hussain I, Qureshi MA (1997) Nitric oxide synthase activity and mRNA expression in chicken macrophages. Poult Sci 76:1524–1530

30. Lai E, Teodoro T, Volchuk A (2007) Endoplasmic reticulum stress: signaling the unfolded protein response. Physiology (Bethesda) 22:193–201

31. Hu R, Chen ZF, Yan J, Li QF, Huang Y, Xu H, Zhang XP, Jiang H (2015) Endoplasmic reticulum stress of neutrophils is required for ischemia/reperfusion-induced acute lung injury. J Immunol 195:4802–4809

32. Rosenberg HF (2008) RNase A ribonucleases and host defense: an evolving story. J Leukoc Biol 83:1079–1087

33. Veldhuizen EJ, Brouwer EC, Schneider VA, Fluit AC (2013) Chicken cathelicidins display antimicrobial activity against multiresistant bacteria without inducing strong resistance. PLoS One 8:e61964

34. Johnson DA, Barrett AJ, Mason RW (1986) Cathepsin L inactivates alpha 1-proteinase inhibitor by cleavage in the reactive site region. J Biol Chem 261:14748–14751

35. Baumann M, Pham CT, Benarafa C (2013) SerpinB1 is critical for neutrophil survival through cell-autonomous inhibition of cathepsin G. Blood 121:3900–3907

36. Bradley LM, Douglass MF, Chatterjee D, Akira S, Baaten BJ (2012) Matrix metalloprotease 9 mediates neutrophil migration into the airways in response to influenza virus-induced toll-like receptor signaling. PLoS Pathog 8:e1002641

37. Nathan C, Xie QW, Halbwachs-Mecarelli L, Jin WW (1993) Albumin inhibits neutrophil spreading and hydrogen peroxide release by blocking the shedding of CD43 (sialophorin, leukosialin). J Cell Biol 122:243–256

38. Everitt EA, Malik AB, Hendey B (1996) Fibronectin enhances the migration rate of human neutrophils in vitro. J Leukoc Biol 60:199–206

10

Variation in susceptibility of different breeds of sheep to *Mycobacterium avium* subspecies *paratuberculosis* following experimental inoculation

D. J. Begg, A. C. Purdie, K. de Silva, N. K. Dhand, K. M. Plain and R. J. Whittington[*]

Abstract

Exposure to *Mycobacterium avium* subspecies *paratuberculosis* (MAP) does not always lead to Johne's disease. Understanding differences in disease susceptibility of individual animals is a key aspect to controlling mycobacterial diseases. This study was designed to examine the susceptibility or resistance of various breeds of sheep to MAP infection. Merino, Suffolk first cross Merino, Border Leicester, and Poll Dorset sheep were orally inoculated with MAP and monitored for 14 months. Clinical disease occurred more frequently in the Merino (42%) and Suffolk first cross Merino (36%) compared to the Border Leicester (12%) and Poll Dorset (11%) breeds. Infection risk, as determined by culture of gut and associated lymphoid tissues, ranged from 75% for the Suffolk first cross Merino to 47% for the Poll Dorset sheep. Significant differences were identified in the site in the intestines of the most severe histopathological lesions and the immune responses to infection between the breeds. However, there was no difference in faecal MAP shedding by clinical cases between breeds. All breeds tested were susceptible to MAP infection, as determined by infection and clinical disease development, although there were differences in the proportions of diseased animals between the breeds. Poll Dorset and Border Leicester sheep were more resilient to MAP infection but there was evidence that more animals could have developed disease if given more time. These findings provide evidence of potential differential disease susceptibility between breeds, further our understanding of disease pathogenesis and risks of disease spread, and may have an influence on control programs for *paratuberculosis*.

Introduction

Mycobacterium avium subspecies *paratuberculosis* (MAP) causes Johne's disease in ruminant hosts globally and is a source of economic loss. For this reason, and because of a potential zoonotic link [1] control programs for MAP have been implemented in many developed countries. These are based on hygiene measures and the removal of cases from affected herds and flocks. Increasing the level of resistance at population level through vaccination is also possible [2, 3]. However, increasing the level of genetic resistance or resilience to MAP infection

is relatively unstudied. Rather than being a slowly progressive and eventually fatal infection in all cases, it is now known that not all animals exposed to MAP develop Johne's disease (JD) and some appear to clear the infection spontaneously [4]. Furthermore, it is suspected that some breeds of ruminants are more resistant to MAP infection than others, but objective information is limited as no controlled experimental infection trials have been conducted to directly compare different breeds. Some breeds may be more susceptible than others, based on anecdotal evidence and one cross sectional survey of farmers, which suggested that fine wool Merino sheep were more likely to develop clinical JD [5]. It is known that many different breeds of sheep can develop clinical JD including Merino, Churra, Blackface, Texel, Bleu du

*Correspondence: richard.whittington@sydney.edu.au
Farm Animal and Veterinary Public Health, Sydney School of Veterinary
Science and School of Life and Environmental Sciences, Faculty
of Science, The University of Sydney, 425 Werombi Rd, Camden, NSW
2570, Australia

Maine, East Friesian, Romney, Highland cross and Rocky Mountain bighorn sheep [6–9].

Other studies have shown that genetics may play a role in the susceptibility to JD in ruminants [10, 11] and there is evidence that different breeds can vary in the amount of serum antibody produced in response to MAP exposure [12, 13]. It is difficult to determine in these studies whether the differences were due to differential antibody production, different stages of disease, and differences in the response to infection or were due to different trading patterns, which could result in differing levels of MAP exposure.

The aim of this study was to examine the susceptibility to MAP infection of four breeds of sheep. Relevant sheep breeds were identified following consultation with industry experts in Australia. The representatives of the Sheepmeat Council of Australia and WoolProducers Australia provided advice on which breeds to examine, those most commonly used in Australia. Lambs of each breed from MAP-free flocks were inoculated and the animals were monitored for disease development with the severity of disease confirmed. The findings indicate that all of the breeds tested can develop JD, but differences in susceptibility may exist between breeds.

Materials and methods
Animals
The use of animals in this study was approved by the University of Sydney Animal Ethics committee protocol number N00/10-2010/3/5372.

One hundred and sixty-nine sheep comprising more than 40 sheep of each of four different breeds were purchased from farms participating in the Australian Market Assurance Program for *paratuberculosis*. All farms were in the Armidale region of New South Wales, Australia, and had a program score of Monitored Negative 3. This is the highest assurance that a farm is free of MAP infected sheep [14]. The farms were also chosen as they had a similar lambing time so that all lambs were approximately 5 months of age at inoculation.

Forty-six Merino, 41 Poll Dorset, 41 Border Leicester and 41 Suffolk first cross Merino lambs were used in the experiment. The Merino breed was used as a control group, as previous experimental inoculation trials have been run in this breed with the same methodology [15]. The old British breeds of Poll Dorset, Border Leicester and Suffolk were chosen as they are the most commonly farmed sheep in Australia after the Merino. Due to an unexpected operational issue, pure breed Suffolk lambs could not be supplied, and only Suffolk first cross Merino lambs were available. All suppliers were asked to provide castrated males, but when the sheep arrived it

was discovered that the Poll Dorset and Border Leicester lambs were predominantly females.

The animals for each breed were allocated by systematic sampling into two groups by drafting off every fourth Merino or every tenth animal of the other breeds. The first group consisted of 10 Merino, 5 Poll Dorset, 5 Border Leicester and 5 Suffolk first cross Merino lambs. This group was used as an un-inoculated control group. The second group consisted of 36 lambs of each breed, and these were inoculated with MAP. The control animals were held on separate pasture adjacent to the inoculated animals; the pastures housing the controls had not held MAP-infected sheep in the past. The animals were managed under conventional Australian sheep farming conditions by grazing in open paddocks on unimproved pasture with reticulated water in elevated troughs; supplementary feeding with grain/lucerne chaff was provided as necessary. The lambs from different breeds were grazed together based on their status as controls or MAP-inoculated.

Experimental inoculation of the lambs
The oral inoculations of the sheep were as described by Begg et al. [15] using a pure culture S strain of MAP (Telford 9.2). Three doses were delivered over a one month period giving a total dose of 2.74×10^9 viable MAP. The same batches of prepared inoculum were used for all breeds.

Ante-mortem sampling and examinations
Blood and faecal samples were collected at regular intervals (2–4 months) from each lamb. All animals were monitored by visual inspection at least three times weekly. From eight and a half months post inoculation, bodyweights visual inspections were initially carried out on a monthly basis and the frequency was increased to weekly inspections to aid identification of individuals with clinical disease.

Necropsy and tissue collection
Sheep were culled from the experiment if they lost ≥10% of their body weight in 1 month. Any animal culled for weight loss also had a visual assessment to determine weight loss. All animals remaining at 14 months post inoculation were culled. Four inoculated animals died or were euthanised for reasons other than JD. These were Border Leicester ($n = 2$) and Merino ($n = 2$) sheep and the reasons for culling were misadventure, congenital disorder, liver disorder and one case of caseous lymphadenitis. Tissue culture data from two of these animals, both Merino, were included in the analysis, as their necropsy was conducted greater than 8 months post inoculation, a

period considered to be sufficient for the infection to be detected.

Euthanasia of the animals and tissues sampled were as described by Begg et al. [15] with minor modifications. The tissues collected from each animal for culture and histology were terminal ileum, middle jejunum, posterior and middle jejunal lymph nodes and a section of the liver. Sections were either frozen at −80 °C for MAP detection or placed in 10% neutral buffered formalin.

Histopathology

Formalin fixed tissues were embedded in paraffin, sectioned at 5 μm and stained with haematoxylin and eosin and Ziehl–Neelsen methods. Intestinal sections were graded as a score 0, 1, 2, 3a (paucibacillary) 3b (multibacillary), or 3c (severe paucibacillary) using established criteria [16]. Granulomatous lesions observed in the lymph nodes were graded as 1 (mild focal), 2 (mild multifocal) or 3 (severe multifocal to diffuse). Each animal was classified based on the highest grade of lesion observed.

MAP detection

Culture of MAP from faeces and tissues including intestine, associated lymph nodes and liver was performed using liquid culture media M7H9C as described previously [17, 18].

qPCR detection of MAP in faeces

Faecal samples were stored at −80 °C to ensure the integrity of the sample. Detection of MAP DNA from the samples was performed as described previously [19]. Briefly, a suspension of 1.2 g (dry) or 1.5 g (moist) faeces was prepared in 10 mL 0.85% w/v sterile saline. After vigorous shaking, this was allowed to settle for 30 min and 3–5 mL of supernatant was centrifuged at $1231 \times g$ for 30 min. To the pellet, 600 μL Lysis/binding solution (597.2 μL Buffer RLT and 2.8 μL Carrier RNA; Biosprint® 96 One-For-All Vet kit, Qiagen) was added, then transferred to a 2 mL screw capped tube containing 0.3 g of Zirconia/Silica beads (BioSpec Products Inc, Daintree Scientific) and disrupted using a mechanical cell disruptor/bead beater. The supernatant (400 μL) was transferred to a deep 96 well plate, with 40 μL Proteinase K and 300 μL Magnetic Bead mix (Biosprint® 96 One-For-All Vet kit, Qiagen). The DNA was eluted following the "BS96 Vet 100″ instrument protocol run on an automated magnetic particle processor (BioSprint 96, Qiagen). Positive and negative faecal controls, a process control (all buffers), and an extraction plate control were included in every experiment.

MAP DNA was detected by qPCR for the IS900 gene on an Mx3000P real-time PCR instrument (Stratagene, Agilent), using SensiMix SYBR Low-ROX qPCR master mix (Bioline) with forward and reverse primers at 250 nM (MP10-1 forward 5′-ATGCGCCACGACTT-GCAGCCT-3′; MP11-1 reverse 5′-GGCACGGCTCTT-GTTGTAGTCG-3′). The cycling parameters were: 95 °C for 8.5 min, 40 cycles at 95 °C for 30 s, 68 °C for 60 s, and melt curve analysis from 65 to 95 °C. A standard curve of MAP genomic DNA was included in every qPCR experiment (10–0.001 pg/reaction). The criteria for positive results (≥0.001 pg MAP genomic DNA) was determined by prior validation.

MAP specific antibody

The level of MAP specific antibodies was measured using a commercially available kit (Institut Porquier from IDEXX) following the manufacturer's instructions. The data are presented as S/P%, which was calculated as: (OD sample − OD negative control)/(OD positive control − OD negative control) × 100.

MAP specific IFNγ detection

The IFNγ stimulation was carried out using whole blood stimulated with MAP-specific antigen, a French pressed whole cell 316v strain of MAP(316v) or media for 48 h and the ELISA was performed as previously described [20]. On each ELISA plate sheep specific IFNγ positive and negative controls were used to calculate the SP ratio. The same batch of each control was used on all test plates. The raw data were transformed into S/P%, which was calculated as: (OD sample − OD negative control)/(OD positive control − OD negative control) × 100. The SP% of the media stimulated response was subtracted from the MAP antigen response to obtain the MAP-specific response.

Case definitions

An animal was classified as having clinical disease if the following criteria were met: it lost ≥ 10% of its body weight over 1 month, MAP was cultured from tissues after necropsy, and histopathological lesions consistent with JD were observed.

Statistical analysis

Contingency tables of breed with each of the binary outcome variables were created using FREQ procedure in SAS (© 2002–2012 by SAS Institute Inc., Cary, NC, USA) and cumulative incidence calculated. Log-linked binomial models were then fitted for each binary outcome variable with breed as an explanatory variable using Genmod procedure in SAS. Relative risk and its 95% confidence limits were calculated by exponentiation of the parameter estimate and their confidence limits.

Summary statistics and graphical summaries of serum antibody and IFN-γ responses were prepared to evaluate their distributions. General linear models were fitted with log transformed MAP-specific serum antibody or IFN-γ response as outcome variables and breed, months post infection and their interaction as fixed effects. Predicted means for log MAP-specific serum antibody and log IFN-γ responses for four breeds at various time points after infection were estimated and exponentiated to obtain geometric means. Standard errors of geometric means were approximated using the Delta method [21]. Assumptions of general linear models were evaluated using residual diagnostics.

All p-values reported in the manuscript are two sided. A 5% level of significance was considered for all analyses. Analyses were conducted using SAS Statistical program unless indicated otherwise.

Results

Clinical Johne's disease

Clinical cases of JD were identified in all breeds (Figure 1). It was not possible to identify individuals developing clinical disease by visual assessment of the Poll Dorset breed, although several met the definition of a clinical case (≥ 10% loss of body weight in a month, confirmed by histopathology and culture) (Figure 1D). Clinical disease

was seen more often in the Merino (42%) and Suffolk first cross Merino (36%) than in the Border Leicester (12%) and Poll Dorset (11%) sheep in the time frame examined, up to 14 months post inoculation, when the trial was terminated (Table 1). There was a significant difference in the frequency of development of clinical disease between the breeds (Table 1). The MAP inoculated Merino sheep were used as the positive control as the experimental infection model was previously validated in this breed [15]. In comparison to Merino, the Border Leicester and Poll Dorset breeds had significantly less risk of animals developing clinical disease ($p = 0.01$), but no significant difference was observed between the Merino and White Suffolk × Merino breeds (Table 1). The peak time of clinical case detection for the Merino and Suffolk first cross Merino sheep was at approximately 12 months post inoculation. The Border Leicester and Poll Dorset breeds had an increasing number of clinical cases in the final weeks of the trial, i.e. approaching 14 months post inoculation (data not shown).

Rates of infection and dissemination

At least 45% of sheep from each breed were infected at the time of necropsy; the Merino (69%) and Suffolk first

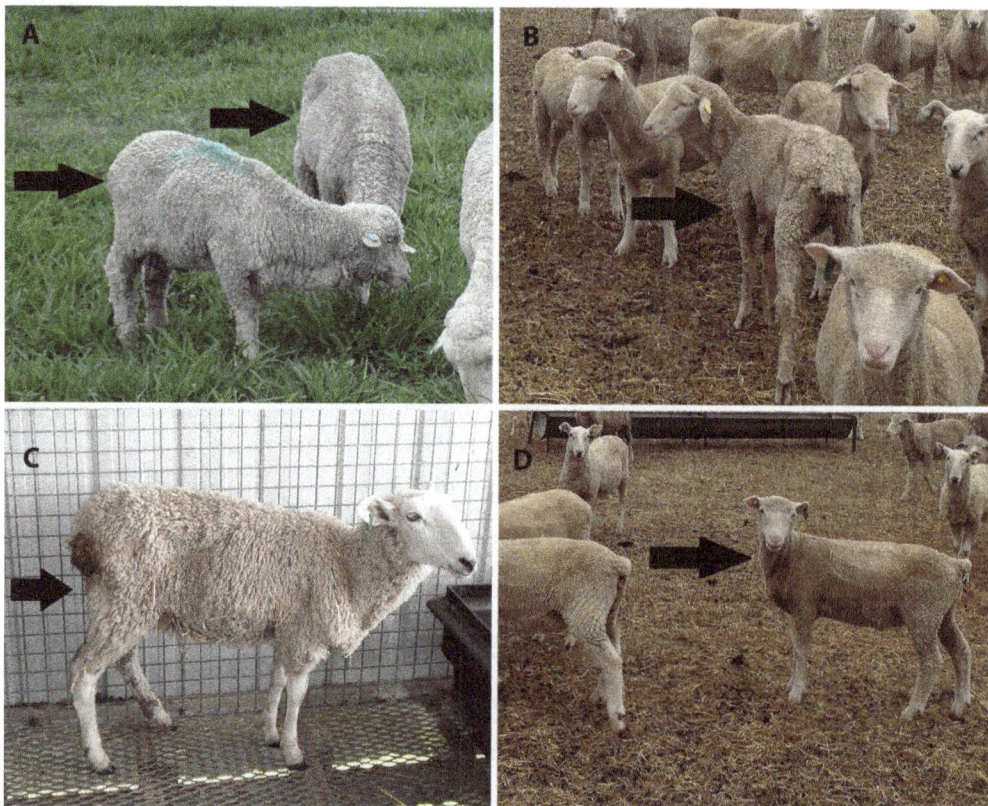

Figure 1 Clinical cases of JD in different sheep breeds. Arrows point to the clinical cases. **A** Merino, **B** Suffolk first cross Merino, **C** Border Leicester and **D** Poll Dorset; the clinical case determined by weight loss is difficult to observe by visual assessment alone in the Poll Dorset breed.

Table 1 Occurrence of clinical disease in four breeds of sheep 14 months after MAP inoculation based on a trial conducted in Australia in 2012

Breed	Total number of animals	Number of sheep developing clinical disease	Occurrence (%)	Relative risk	(95% CI)	p value
Merino	36	15	42	1.00[a]		
White Suffolk × Merino	36	13	36	0.87	(0.48–1.55)	0.63
Border Leicester	34	4	12	0.28	(0.10–0.77)	0.01
Poll Dorset	36	4	11	0.27	(0.10–0.73)	0.01

[a] Reference group.

cross Merino (75%) breeds had a greater proportion of animals with viable MAP in their tissues (i.e. were infected) (Table 2), compared to Border Leicester (53%) and Poll Dorset (47%) sheep.

Dissemination of MAP to tissues outside of the gut was examined by culture of a section of liver. Dissemination rates varied from 9 to 39% among the different breeds (Table 3). Both the Poll Dorset and Border Leicester breeds had significantly fewer sheep with MAP cultured from the liver ($p = 0.03$ and $p = 0.01$) compared to the Merinos (Table 3). In most cases these were the animals that developed clinical disease, although not all of the clinical cases had disseminated infection and one of the Poll Dorset animals that had disseminated infection did not have clinical disease.

Slightly fewer animals had histopathological lesions consistent with JD in their intestines than had MAP detected in their tissues. There was no significant difference in the occurrence of histopathological lesions greater than grade 1 [16] between breeds (Table 4). The

Merino and Suffolk first cross Merino breeds were more likely to have multibacillary lesions or to have no lesions (lesion score 0) (Figure 2). All the breeds had a similar proportion of animals that did not develop any histopathological lesions (33–47%). The Border Leicester breed was most likely to have paucibacillary lesions but had a range of lesions from multibacillary to the least severe grade 1 lesions. The Poll Dorset breed tended to have lower grades of lesion (lesion score 0, 1 and 2).

Of the two matching intestinal and lymph node sections used for histopathological analysis (terminal ileum/posterior jejunal lymph node and middle jejunum/middle jejunal lymph node), there was a significant difference ($p = 0.04$) in the location of the most severe histological lesion between the breeds (Table 5). Data from animals with histological lesions greater than 1 were included for analysis. The Merino, Suffolk first cross Merino and Border Leicester breeds were more likely to have the most severe lesions observed in the terminal ileum or posterior jejunal lymph node. The Poll Dorset breed animals

Table 2 Occurrence of infection in four breeds of sheep at necropsy (up to 14 months after MAP inoculation) as determined by culture from gut associated tissues

Breed	Total number of animals	Number of sheep with MAP infection	Occurrence (%)	Relative risk	(95% CI)	p value
Merino	36	25	69	1.00[a]		
White Suffolk × Merino	36	27	75	1.08	(0.81–1.44)	0.60
Border Leicester	34	18	53	0.76	(0.52–1.12)	0.17
Poll Dorset	36	17	47	0.68	(0.45–1.02)	0.06

[a] Reference group.

Table 3 Analysis of disseminated infection after MAP inoculation as determined by culture of the liver

Breed	Total[a]	Number of sheep with disseminated MAP infection	Occurrence (%)	Relative risk	(95% CI)	p value
Merino	33	13	39	1.00[b]		
White Suffolk × Merino	34	13	38	0.97	(0.53–1.77)	0.92
Border Leicester	33	3	9	0.23	(0.07–0.74)	0.01
Poll Dorset	36	5	14	0.35	(0.14–0.88)	0.03

[a] Total number of animals which had liver samples cultured.

[b] Reference breed.

Table 4 Analysis of histopathological lesions after MAP inoculation

Breed	Total[a]	Number of sheep with MAP histological lesions[b]	Occurrence (%)	Relative risk	(95% CI)	p value
Merino	35	20	57	1.00[c]		
White Suffolk × Merino	34	16	47	0.82	(0.52–1.30)	0.41
Border Leicester	34	16	47	0.82	(0.52–1.30)	0.41
Poll Dorset	36	15	42	0.73	(0.45–1.18)	0.20

[a] Total number of animals that had sections examined for histology.

[b] Animals were considered to have MAP associated histopathology if the lesion score [16] was greater than 1.

[c] Reference group.

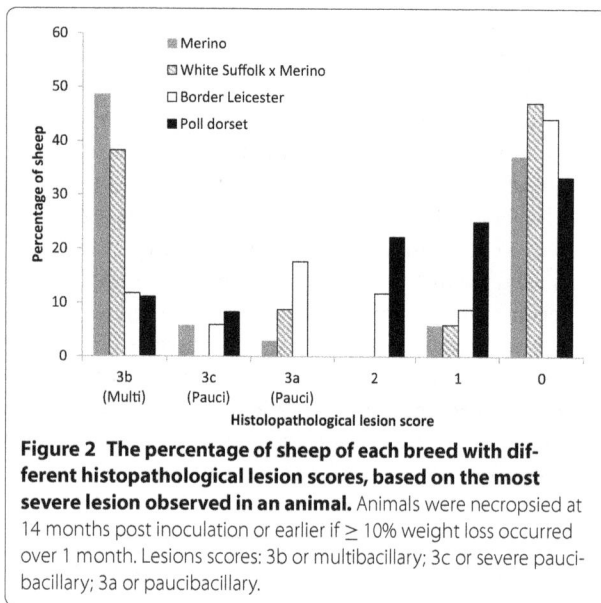

Figure 2 The percentage of sheep of each breed with different histopathological lesion scores, based on the most severe lesion observed in an animal. Animals were necropsied at 14 months post inoculation or earlier if ≥ 10% weight loss occurred over 1 month. Lesions scores: 3b or multibacillary; 3c or severe paucibacillary; 3a or paucibacillary.

were significantly ($p = 0.04$) more likely to have the most severe lesion in the middle jejunum and/or lymph node, with a prevalence of 67%.

Faecal shedding of MAP

Faecal samples were pooled from 6 animals of the same breed, creating 6 pools per breed. The animals were always allocated into the same pool at all sampling points. The Merino and Suffolk first cross Merino were the only breeds to shed MAP at 3 months post inoculation (Figure 3A). As the trial progressed, the Border Leicester and Poll Dorset breeds had increasing numbers of pools with MAP detected, indicating increasing faecal shedding. At 12 months post inoculation, the number of pooled faecal cultures of the Suffolk × Merino breed decreased from 6 to 5; this was primarily due to removal of some sheep of this breed due to clinical disease.

MAP shedding by the clinically diseased sheep was examined from faecal samples collected at necropsy or at the last sampling point from each animal. The amount of MAP shed in the faeces of sheep with clinical disease was estimated using qPCR and was not significantly different between the breeds (Figure 3B).

Host immune response to MAP

MAP-specific serum antibody responses were measured throughout the experiment. There were significant time and breed interactions observed ($p < 0.0001$). At the sampling prior to inoculation, the Suffolk first cross Merino animals had a lower mean MAP-specific antibody response compared to the Merino and Border Leicester breeds ($p < 0.05$) (Figure 4A). The MAP specific antibody responses from the un-inoculated sheep remained at baseline levels with average SP% less than 5 for all breeds (data not shown). At 12 and 14 months post inoculation, mean responses from the Suffolk first cross Merino animals were significantly lower compared to the other breeds ($p < 0.05$) (Figure 4A). By 14 months

Table 5 Analysis of the site of the most severe intestinal histopathological lesion after MAP inoculation

Breed	Total[a]	Number of sheep with the most severe lesion in the mid JJ or LN[c]	Occurence (%)	Relative risk	(95% CI)	p value
Merino	20	6	30	1.00[b]		
White Suffolk × Merino	16	4	25	0.83	(0.28–2.46)	0.74
Border Leicester	16	4	25	0.83	(0.28–2.46)	0.74
Poll Dorset	15	10	67	2.22	(1.04–4.75)	0.04

[a] Any animal with a histopathological lesion greater than 1 was used for analysis [16].

[b] Reference group.

[c] Mid JJ and LN: middle jejunum/middle jejunal lymph node sections.

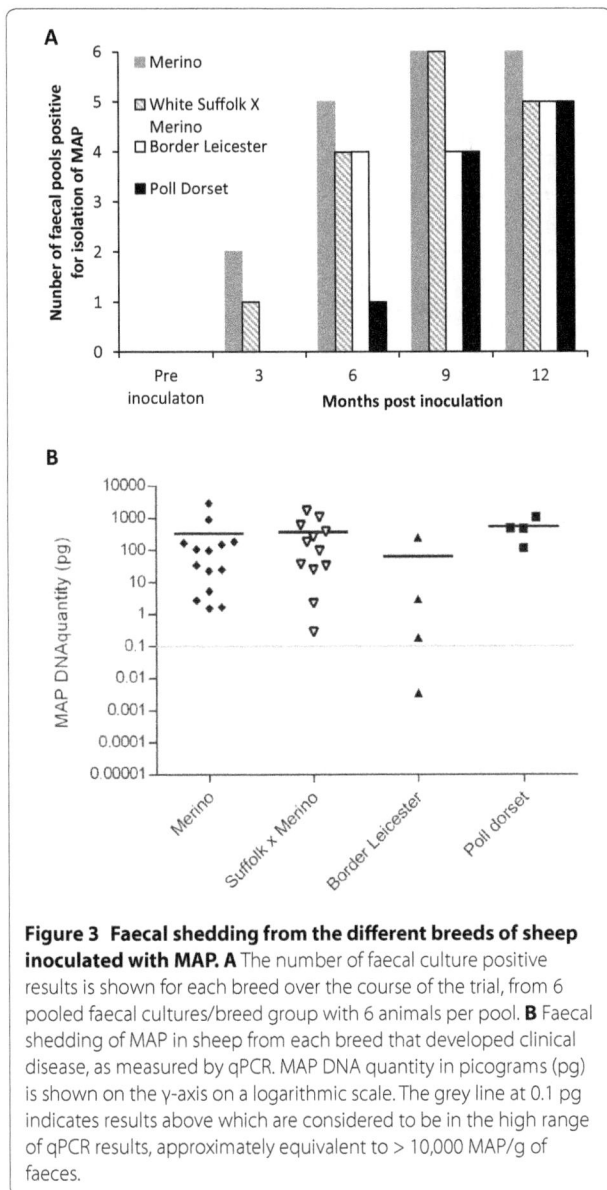

Figure 3 Faecal shedding from the different breeds of sheep inoculated with MAP. A The number of faecal culture positive results is shown for each breed over the course of the trial, from 6 pooled faecal cultures/breed group with 6 animals per pool. **B** Faecal shedding of MAP in sheep from each breed that developed clinical disease, as measured by qPCR. MAP DNA quantity in picograms (pg) is shown on the y-axis on a logarithmic scale. The grey line at 0.1 pg indicates results above which are considered to be in the high range of qPCR results, approximately equivalent to > 10,000 MAP/g of faeces.

cross Merino sheep had the lowest mean MAP specific IFN-γ response (Figure 4C). The Poll Dorset sheep had strong early responses, which were significantly different from all the other breeds at 3 months post inoculation ($p < 0.0001$) (Figure 4C). The responses from all breeds had decreased at 12 months post inoculation, with the White Suffolk first cross Merino animals having a significantly lower response ($p < 0.05$) compared to the other breeds.

Discussion

The outcomes of this trial indicated that all of the breeds examined were susceptible to development of JD in this experimental model, and that the Merino and Suffolk first cross Merino breeds developed the disease earlier than did the other breeds. When the trial was terminated at 14 months post inoculation, 47–75% of sheep from all breeds were infected with MAP and animals of every breed had developed clinical signs and were infectious. High quantities of MAP DNA were detected in the faeces of clinical cases independent of breed. As the experimental infection model is repeatable in Merino sheep, and representative of natural infection in terms of prevalence and spectrum of final disease states [15, 22], it is likely that the results for other breeds have external validity and would apply in natural infections of similar S strains of MAP.

In this experiment the sheep were assessed until 14 months post MAP exposure and by then 25% had developed clinical disease; had the trial continued it is possible that more sheep would have developed clinical disease. In a prior trial of 2.5 years duration in ($n = 20$) Merino sheep, 7 of 8 affected sheep succumbed to clinical disease during a 4 month period commencing 14 months post inoculation, and the total proportion of clinical cases was 35% [23]. Consistent with these findings, the Merino and Suffolk first cross Merino breeds had 42 and 36% clinical cases, respectively, with disease manifesting over a period of approximately 4 months commencing 10–14 months post inoculation, while the other breeds had a lower incidence of clinical cases. It is possible that more sheep from the Poll Dorset and Border Leicester breeds may have progressed to a more severe stage or to clinical disease if the trial had continued beyond 14 months. This view is supported by the increasing number of clinical cases in the final weeks of the trial for these two breeds, the increasing number of positive faecal pools detected by faecal culture as the trial progressed, and the fact that similar numbers of sheep from these two breeds had histological lesions consistent with JD at the end of the trial compared to the Merino breed, but the lesion grades were less severe indicative of an earlier stage of disease pathogenesis.

Detection of MAP from the tissues of the different breeds of sheep indicated that there were no significant

post inoculation both the Suffolk first cross Merino and Merino breeds had had animals culled due to clinical JD, and it would be expected that the mean antibody level would wane as these sheep were removed from the study.

Examination of the antibody responses of the clinical cases from the last sampling timepoint, taken before necropsy or at the time of necropsy, indicated a wide range of responses between individual animals (Figure 4B). Half of the total combined clinically affected animals from all breeds were classified as test positive, with the remainder falling below the threshold for a positive antibody response.

The IFN-γ response showed significant breed and time interactions ($p < 0.0001$). Overall, the White Suffolk first

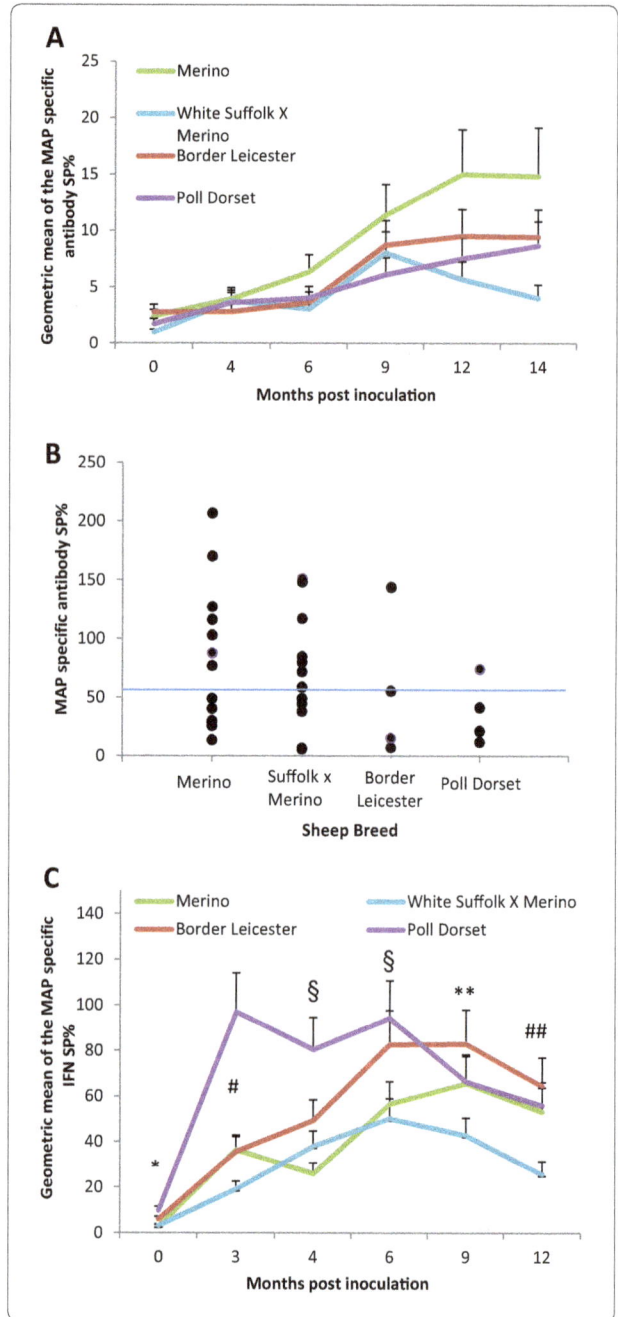

Figure 4 Specific immune responses from the different breeds of sheep inoculated with MAP. A MAP specific antibody responses. Data shown are Geometric means of the MAP specific SP% from the assay for each breed over the trial. Error bars indicate the standard error. ×, Significant difference between the White Suffolk × Merino animals and the Border Leicester and Merino breeds ($p < 0.05$). *, significant differences between the White Suffolk × Merino and Merino breeds ($p < 0.05$). **, significant differences between the White Suffolk × Merino and the other breeds ($p < 0.05$). **B** MAP specific antibody responses from animals with clinical disease, quantified at the last sampling taken before or at necropsy. MAP specific antibody responses were measured by a commercial ELISA (Institut Porquier from IDEXX); the blue horizontal line at SP% 55 represents the positive–negative cut point for the assay. **C** MAP specific interferon gamma responses from the different breeds of experimentally inoculated sheep. Data shown are geometric means of the MAP specific SP% from the assay. Error bars indicate the standard error. Poll Dorset and Border Leicester animals had a significantly ($p > 0.01$) greater than the Merino and White Suffolk × Merino. #Poll Dorset animals had a significantly greater mean response to the other breeds ($p > 0.0001$), the White Suffolk had a significantly lower response that the Merino and Border Leicester ($p > 0.05$). §Poll Dorset animal's response significantly greater response than the Merino and White Suffolk × Merino breeds ($p > 0.005$). **The Border Leicester breed had a significantly greater response than White Suffolk × Merino ($p > 0.01$). ##At 12 months post inoculation the White Suffolk × Merino breed had a significantly lower response than the other breeds ($p > 0.05$).

differences in infection rates between the Merino and other breeds examined. Similarly, all of the breeds had comparable numbers of animals positive for JD histopathological lesions. As has been found in previous studies, disseminated infection is normally limited to sheep with clinical disease and/or severe histopathological lesion grades [24]. In this experiment there was only one exception: a Poll Dorset animal that had no gross lesions, minor histopathological lesions in the gut and mesenteric lymph nodes but which had viable MAP in its liver.

It is accepted that the predilection site for MAP infections in ruminants is the ileum [25] and that gross and histopathological lesions are most prominent in the terminal ileum, but may extend from the caecum to duodenum [26]. This study is the first to show that the breed of animal may have a significant impact on the site where the most severe lesions were observed; in the Poll Dorset sheep histopathological lesions were more likely to be observed in the middle jejunum and/or lymph node rather than terminal ileum and posterior jejunal lymph node. Therefore, detection of JD in different breeds of sheep by histopathological examination may be improved by examining multiple sites along the ileum and jejunum.

As MAP infection in ruminants progresses, the level of faecal shedding of MAP also increases. One of the questions we aimed to answer was: do different breeds infected

with the same strain and amount of MAP at the same age become equally infectious? All of the clinically affected animals, irrespective of breed, were highly infectious, although the faecal shedding of MAP in the Poll Dorset and Border Leicester breeds was slower to develop than in Merino sheep. If left unmanaged on farm, the number of clinically affected sheep will increase. For some breeds the mortalities may take longer to become apparent, possibly creating a trading risk for farmers if not diagnosed.

Variation in susceptibility of different breeds of sheep to Mycobacterium avium subspecies...

131

The early cell-mediated immune response patterns amongst the breeds support previous results demonstrating that an early low IFNγ response is associated with susceptibility to disease and faecal shedding in Merinos [27]. The breed that had the lowest number of clinically diseased and infected animals, the Poll Dorset, also had sheep with the strongest early IFNγ responses. The responses in the other breeds also support our hypothesis that the magnitude of the early IFNγ response is associated with protection. Other studies by our group have also indicated that this early cell-mediated immune response is important in the divergence of disease outcomes [28, 29].

The MAP specific serum antibody level was significantly different between breeds at later time points (> 6 months post inoculation). Breed differences in anti-MAP antibody production in cattle have been previously reported [30]. In that study, 1–2 blood samples per animal were examined in naturally infected Brahman, Angus or cross bred cows. A pure bred Brahman cow was more likely than the others to have a high antibody level or ELISA score.

Unlike the IFNγ response, the magnitude of the antibody response did not match the severity of disease outcome. The Merino and Suffolk first cross Merino sheep had similar disease outcomes but the latter had significantly lower serum anti-MAP antibody levels as the disease progressed. Interestingly, the majority of clinically diseased Border Leicester and Poll Dorset sheep would not have been diagnosed by serum ELISA tests using current recommendations for the positive–negative cutpoint. This was exacerbated by the inability to detect some Poll Dorset animals with weight loss using a visual inspection. These findings have fundamental implications for disease diagnosis. Breed-specific cut points for serum antibody ELISA may need to be developed.

The sensitivity of the ELISA for detection of clinical cases was approximately 50%. As JD progresses the amount of MAP specific antibody increases especially in those animals with multibacillary lesions [31, 32], with sensitivities of ELISAs for affected sheep ranging from 36 to 85% [33]. Most of the clinical cases in this trial had multibacillary lesions, irrespective of the breed, indicating that the ELISA used in this study had a sensitivity at the lower end of the range.

One of the operational issues that occurred in this study was that the suppliers of the Border Leicester and Poll Dorset lambs provided mostly female animals. However, there are no reports of a difference in the susceptibility to develop clinical JD in relation to the sex of an animal. In humans, tuberculosis is typically observed more often in males than in females (1.9:1) although regional differences in these proportions do occur [34, 35]. In tuberculoid leprosy, the disease ratio is reversed, 0.82:1 [36]. Consequently, it is possible that there was gender bias in the results of this trial, but it is not possible to confirm this without further specific studies in sheep.

It is known that in deer of the same breed there are differences in susceptibility or resistance to MAP infection attributable to sire effects [37]. Within-breed MAP susceptibility differences are likely to occur in other ruminant species but have not been examined in detail. In this study, although the sheep of each breed were sourced from a single farm, they may have been derived from different sires. A study to examined intra and inter-breed differences would be complex and require large numbers of animals; it was beyond the scope of this trial.

In conclusion, a susceptibility to MAP infection was observed in all breeds that were examined in this study, as determined by infection and clinical disease development. However, there were differences in the disease outcomes observed: Merino and Suffolk cross Merino had more clinically affected animals in the timeframe examined; Poll Dorset and Border Leicester sheep had a slower disease progression. Importantly, all clinical cases, regardless of breed, were equally infectious, shedding large numbers of MAP. Thus for design of control programs it should be assumed that sheep of all breeds can become infectious following MAP exposure. The slower development of disease in Poll Dorset and Border Leicester sheep may provide an opportunity for farmers, as a move to these breeds may reduce environmental contamination of MAP by reduced faecal shedding, and they may have a longer economic life. On the other hand, infection could be harder to detect in these breeds due to delayed seroconversion and/or difficulty of assessing weight loss by visual means. These findings have important implications for decision making related to control and management strategies for MAP at farm and regional levels.

Competing interests

The authors declare that they have no competing interests.

Authors' contributions

DJB involved in the study conception, design, acquisition of data, analysis/interpretation of data, and manuscript preparation. ACP involved in the study conception, design, acquisition of data and manuscript preparation. KdS involved in the study conception, design, acquisition of data, and manuscript preparation. NKD involved in the study design, analysis/interpretation of data, and manuscript preparation. KMP involved in the study conception, design, acquisition of data, analysis/interpretation of data, and manuscript preparation. RJW involved in the study conception, design, analysis/interpretation of data, and manuscript preparation. All authors read and approved the final manuscript.

Acknowledgements

The authors would like to thank Nicole Carter, Ann Michele Whittington, Rebecca Maurer, Gina Attard and Anna Waldron for providing laboratory assistance. Craig Kristo, Nobel Toribio, Lee white and James Dalton assisted with the field work. Dr Graeme Eamens, Department of Primary Industry, Elizabeth Macarthur Agricultural Institute who supplied the MAP 316v antigen. This work was supported by Meat and Livestock Australia and by Cattle Council of Australia, Sheepmeat Council of Australia and WoolProducers Australia through Animal Health Australia.

Funding

This work was supported by Meat and Livestock Australia and by Cattle Council of Australia, Sheepmeat Council of Australia and WoolProducers Australia through Animal Health Australia. The funding bodies had no role in the design of the study and the collection, analysis, and interpretation of data or in writing the manuscript. The advice of the funding bodies and their members was only used in the selection of the breeds of sheep used in the study.

References

1. Waddell LA, Rajic A, Sargeant J, Harris J, Amezcua R, Downey L, Read S, McEwen SA (2008) The zoonotic potential of *Mycobacterium avium* spp. *paratuberculosis*: a systematic review. Can J Public Health 99:145–155
2. Reddacliff L, Eppleston J, Windsor P, Whittington R, Jones S (2006) Efficacy of a killed vaccine for the control of *paratuberculosis* in Australian sheep flocks. Vet Microbiol 115:77–90
3. Report of the Committee on Tuberculosis (1964) Proc Annu Meet US Anim Health Assoc. 68:356–359
4. Dennis MM, Reddacliff LA, Whittington RJ (2011) Longitudinal study of clinicopathological features of Johne's disease in sheep naturally exposed to *Mycobacterium avium* subspecies *Paratuberculosis*. Vet Pathol 48:565–575
5. Lugton IW (2004) Cross-sectional study of risk factors for the clinical expression of ovine Johne's disease on New South Wales farms. Aust Vet J 82:355–365
6. Smeed JA, Watkins CA, Rhind SM, Hopkins J (2007) Differential cytokine gene expression profiles in the three pathological forms of sheep *paratuberculosis*. BMC Vet Res 3:18
7. Delgado L, Marin JF, Muñoz M, Benavides J, Juste RA, García-Pariente C, Fuertes M, González J, Ferreras MC, Pérez V (2013) Pathological findings in young and adult sheep following experimental infection with 2 different doses of *Mycobacterium avium* subspecies *paratuberculosis*. Vet Pathol 50:857–866
8. Forde T, Kutz S, De Buck J, Warren A, Ruckstuhl K, Pybus M, Orsel K (2012) Occurrence, diagnosis, and strain typing of *Mycobacterium avium* subspecies *paratuberculosis* infection in Rocky Mountain bighorn sheep (*Ovis canadensis canadensis*) in southwestern Alberta. J Wildl Dis 48:1–11
9. Smith SI, West DM, Wilson PR, de Lisle GW, Collett MG, Heuer C, Chambers JP (2011) Detection of *Mycobacterium avium* subsp. *paratuberculosis* in skeletal muscle and blood of ewes from a sheep farm in New Zealand. NZ Vet J 59:240–243
10. Reddacliff LA, Beh K, McGregor H, Whittington RJ (2005) A preliminary study of possible genetic influences on the susceptibility of sheep to Johne's disease. Aust Vet J 83:435–441
11. Koets AP, Adugna G, Janss LL, van Weering HJ, Kalis CH, Wentink GH, Rutten VP, Schukken YH (2000) Genetic variation of susceptibility to *Mycobacterium avium* subsp. *paratuberculosis* infection in dairy cattle. J Dairy Sci 83:2702–2708
12. Mortensen H, Nielsen SS, Berg P (2004) Genetic variation and heritability of the antibody response to *Mycobacterium avium* subspecies *paratuberculosis* in Danish Holstein cows. J Dairy Sci 87:2108–2113
13. Sorge US, Lissemore K, Godkin A, Hendrick S, Wells S, Kelton D (2011) Associations between *paratuberculosis* milk ELISA result, milk production, and breed in Canadian dairy cows. J Dairy Sci 94:754–761
14. Shephard R, Sergeant E, Citer L (2014) Technical validation of the Australian Johne's disease market assurance program for sheep, 12th international colloquium on *Paratuberculosis*. Parma, Italy
15. Begg DJ, de Silva K, Di Fiore L, Taylor DL, Bower K, Zhong L, Kawaji S, Emery D, Whittington RJ (2010) Experimental infection model for Johne's disease using a lyophilised, pure culture, seedstock of *Mycobacterium avium* subspecies *paratuberculosis*. Vet Microbiol 141:301–311
16. Pérez V, García Marín JF, Badiola JJ (1996) Description and classification of different types of lesion associated with natural *paratuberculosis* infection in sheep. J Comp Pathol 114:107–122
17. Plain KM, Waldron AM, Begg DJ, de Silva K, Purdie AC, Whittington RJ (2015) Efficient, validated method for detection of mycobacterial growth in liquid culture media by use of bead beating, magnetic-particle-based nucleic acid isolation, and quantitative PCR. J Clin Microbiol 53:1121–1128
18. Whittington RJ, Whittington AM, Waldron A, Begg DJ, de Silva K, Purdie AC, Plain KM (2013) Development and validation of a liquid medium (M7H9C) for routine culture of *Mycobacterium avium* subsp. *paratuberculosis* to replace modified Bactec 12B medium. J Clin Microbiol 51:3993–4000
19. Plain KM, Marsh IB, Waldron AM, Galea F, Whittington AM, Saunders VF, Begg DJ, de Silva K, Purdie AC, Whittington RJ (2014) High-throughput direct fecal PCR assay for detection of *Mycobacterium avium* subsp. *paratuberculosis* in sheep and cattle. J Clin Microbiol 52:745–757
20. Begg DJ, de Silva K, Bosward K, Di Fiore L, Taylor DL, Jungersen G, Whittington RJ (2009) Enzyme-linked immunospot: an alternative method for the detection of interferon gamma in Johne's disease. J Vet Diagn Invest 21:187–196
21. Oehlert GW (1992) A note on the delta method. Am Stat. 46:27–29
22. Begg DJ, Whittington RJ (2008) Experimental animal infection models for Johne's disease, an infectious enteropathy caused by *Mycobacterium avium* subsp. *paratuberculosis*. Vet J 176:129–145
23. Begg DJ, de Silva K, Plain KM, Purdie AC, Dhand N, Whittington RJ (2015) Specific faecal antibody responses in sheep infected with *Mycobacterium avium* subspecies *paratuberculosis*. Vet Immunol Immunopathol 166:125–131
24. Bower KL, Begg DJ, Whittington RJ (2011) Culture of *Mycobacterium avium* subspecies *paratuberculosis* (MAP) from blood and extra-intestinal tissues in experimentally infected sheep. Vet Microbiol 147:127–132
25. Sweeney RW, Uzonna J, Whitlock RH, Habecker PL, Chilton P, Scott P (2006) Tissue predilection sites and effect of dose on *Mycobacterium avium* subs. *paratuberculosis* organism recovery in a short-term bovine experimental oral infection model. Res Vet Sci 80:253–259
26. Clarke CJ (1997) The pathology and pathogenesis of *paratuberculosis* in ruminants and other species. J Comp Pathol 116:217–261
27. de Silva K, Begg DJ, Plain KM, Purdie AC, Kawaji S, Dhand NK, Whittington RJ (2013) Can early host responses to mycobacterial infection predict eventual disease outcomes? Prev Vet Med 112:203–212
28. de Silva K, Begg D, Carter N, Taylor D, Di Fiore L, Whittington R (2010) The early lymphocyte proliferation response in sheep exposed to *Mycobacterium avium* subsp. *paratuberculosis* compared to infection status. Immunobiology 215:12–25
29. de Silva K, Plain KM, Begg DJ, Purdie AC, Whittington RJ (2015) CD4(+) T-cells, γδ T-cells and B-cells are associated with lack of vaccine protection in *Mycobacterium avium* subspecies *paratuberculosis* infection. Vaccine 33:149–155
30. Elzo MA, Rae DO, Lanhart SE, Wasdin JG, Dixon WP, Jones JL (2006) Factors associated with ELISA scores for *paratuberculosis* in an Angus-Brahman multibreed herd of beef cattle. J Anim Sci 84:41–48
31. Clarke CJ, Patterson IA, Armstrong KE, Low JC (1996) Comparison of the absorbed ELISA and agar gel immunodiffusion test with clinicopathological findings in ovine clinical *paratuberculosis*. Vet Rec 139:618–621
32. Pérez V, Tellechea J, Badiola JJ, Gutiérrez M, García Marín JF (1997) Relation between serologic response and pathologic findings in sheep with naturally acquired *paratuberculosis*. Am J Vet Res 58:799–803
33. Nielsen SS, Toft N (2008) Ante mortem diagnosis of *paratuberculosis*: a review of accuracies of ELISA, interferon-gamma assay and faecal culture techniques. Vet Microbiol 129:217–235
34. Nhamoyebonde S, Leslie A (2014) Biological differences between the sexes and susceptibility to tuberculosis. J Infect Dis 209(Suppl 3):S100–S106
35. Shah SK, Dogar OF, Siddiqi K (2015) Tuberculosis in women from Pashtun region: an ecological study in Pakistan. Epidemiol Infect 143:901–909
36. Guerra-Silveira F, Abad-Franch F (2013) Sex bias in infectious disease epidemiology: patterns and processes. PLoS One 8:e62390
37. Mackintosh CG, Clark RG, Tolentino B, de Lisle GW, Liggett S, Griffin JF (2011) Immunological and pathological responses of red deer resistant or susceptible genotypes, to experimental challenge with *Mycobacterium avium* subsp. *paratuberculosis*. Vet Immunol Immunopathol 143:131–142

11

Helicobacter suis induces changes in gastric inflammation and acid secretion markers in pigs of different ages

C. De Witte[1][*] , B. Devriendt[2], B. Flahou[1], I. Bosschem[1], R. Ducatelle[1], A. Smet[3][†] and F. Haesebrouck[1][†]

Abstract

Gastric mRNA expression of markers for acid secretion and inflammation and presence of gastric ulceration was studied in naturally *Helicobacter suis*-infected and non-infected 2–3 months old, 6–8 months old and adult pigs. In *H. suis*-infected 2–3 months old pigs, IL-8 and IL-1β transcript levels were upregulated in the pyloric gland zone, indicating an innate immune response. A similar response was demonstrated in the fundic gland zone of adult pigs, potentially due to a shift of *H. suis* colonization from the pyloric to the fundic gland zone. A Treg response in combination with decreased expressions of IL-8, IL-17A and IFN-γ was indicated to be present in the *H. suis*-infected 6–8 months old pigs, which may have contributed to persistence of *H. suis*. In *H. suis*-infected adult pigs, a Treg response accompanied by a Th17 response was indicated, which may have played a role in the decreased number of *H. suis* bacteria in the stomach of this age group. The decreased G-cell mass and upregulated expression of somatostatin indicated decreased acid secretion in *H. suis*-infected 6–8 months old pigs. In *H. suis*-infected adult pigs, upregulation of most markers for gastric acid secretion and increased G-cell mass was detected. Presence of severe hyperkeratosis and erosions in the non-glandular part of the stomach were mainly seen in the *H. suis*-positive groups. These results show that *H. suis* infection affects the expression of markers for acid secretion and inflammation and indicate that these effects differ depending on the infection phase.

Introduction

Gastric ulceration is a common disease entity of pigs worldwide, with prevalences of up to 93% [1]. Although the disease outcome is often subclinical, animal welfare issues as well as economic losses due to decreased daily weight gain, decreased feed intake and sudden death, are of major importance [1]. The etiology seems to be multifactorial. Indeed, several factors, including diet particle size [2], management [3], gastric microbiota composition, infection with *Helicobacter suis* [4, 5], and hormonal changes [6] have been hypothesized to be involved. The pathogenesis of porcine gastric ulceration, however, remains largely unknown [1]. What we do know is that, in contrast to other animal species, in pigs gastric ulcers

develop almost exclusively in the *Pars œsophagea*, a small area around the opening of the œsophagus which does not contain glands. Since this stomach region is not protected by mucus, it is highly susceptible to irritation with for instance hydrochloric acid, produced in the fundic gland zone of the porcine stomach [1]. Chronic insult of the *Pars œsophagea* results in hyperkeratosis, erosion and finally ulceration.

Pigs are commonly infected with the zoonotic pathogen *H. suis* [1]. This pathogen mainly colonizes the fundic and pyloric gland zone of the porcine stomach, inducing inflammation and a decreased daily weight gain [5]. It has been hypothesized that alterations in hydrochloric acid production in the glandular region of the stomach, associated with chronic *H. suis* infections, may play a role in the pathogenesis of swine gastric ulceration [1, 4, 5]. Hellemans et al. [4] demonstrated a tropism of *H. suis* for the gastric acid producing parietal cells. Histological analysis of the stomach of *H. suis*-infected pigs at slaughter age,

*Correspondence: chloe.dewitte@ugent.be
[†]A. Smet and F. Haesebrouck shared senior authorship
[1] Department of Pathology, Bacteriology and Avian Diseases, Faculty of Veterinary Medicine, Ghent University, Merelbeke, Belgium
Full list of author information is available at the end of the article

has revealed that these bacteria are often found in close vicinity of parietal cells and even inside the canaliculi of these cells [4]. In addition, *H. suis* can cause degenerative changes and necrosis of parietal cells in porcine, human and rodent models of gastric disease [7, 8]. Recent reports indicated that *H. suis* may disturb homeostasis of porcine parietal cells and affect their expression of genes encoding H+/K+ ATPase [9]. The latter is an enzyme typically associated with parietal cells and is involved in gastric acid production by these cells. Not only parietal cells, but also gastrin producing G-cells and somatostatin producing D-cells can be altered during *H. suis* infection [10]. Gastrin stimulates and somatostatin suppresses gastric acid production through their association with CCK-B and SST2 receptors on parietal cells, respectively, suggesting that *H. suis* infection may indeed affect gastric acid secretion through different mechanisms.

The main objectives of this study were to obtain further insights in the mechanisms involved in persistence of *H. suis* in the porcine stomach and in its effects on gastric acid secretion and lesion development. This was studied in naturally *H. suis* infected pigs during the acute and chronic phases of infection. Therefore, the mRNA expression of different cytokines, chemokines and markers for gastric acid secretion was studied, the parietal cell, D-cell and G-cell mass was analyzed and the severity of *Pars œsophageal* lesions was determined in *H. suis* infected and non-infected 2–3 months old pigs, 6–8 months old pigs and adult sows.

Materials and methods
Sampling of porcine stomachs
Sixty-eight stomachs of 6–8 months old pigs and 60 stomachs of adult sows (1–3 years old) were collected over a period of 10 months from 2 slaughterhouses in Flanders, Belgium. The pigs originated from different herds. The stomachs of the 6–8 months old pigs had also been used in a previous study [11]. In addition, stomachs of 34, 2–3 months old pigs were collected from 2 different pig herds (17 samples from each herd). The stomachs were transported immediately to the laboratory and stored at 4 °C until further examination within 2 h. The stomachs were opened along the greater curvature and rinsed with sterile tap water. Based on the method of Hessing [12], mucosal lesions of the *Pars œsophagea* were scored as follows: score 0 for normal mucosa, score 1 for mild hyperkeratosis covering less than 50% of the surface, score 2 for severe hyperkeratosis covering more than 50% of the surface, score 3 for hyperkeratosis with few erosions, score 4 for hyperkeratosis with several erosions and score 5 for hyperkeratosis with many erosions or ulceration. Using autoclaved tweezers and scalpels, biopsies of 40–50 mg consisting of mucosa and submucosa

were taken from the *Pars œsophagea* as well as from the cardiac, fundic and pyloric gland zone for quantification of *H. suis* DNA by qPCR. In addition, biopsies consisting of mucosa and submucosa were taken from the fundic and pyloric gland zones to determine mRNA expression levels of genes encoding host factors (markers) involved in gastric acid secretion and inflammation. In order to correlate altered markers with gastritis and the number of parietal cells, D-cells and G-cells, biopsies consisting of mucosa, submucosa and tunica muscularis were taken from fundic and pyloric gland zones, fixed in 10% phosphate-buffered formalin and used for histopathology and immunohistochemistry.

H. suis quantification
DNA was extracted from the biopsies of each stomach region, using the Isolate II Genomic DNA Kit® (Bioline, Taunton, USA), according to the instructions of the manufacturer. The presence of *H. suis* DNA was determined using a species-specific, real time quantitative (RT)-PCR based on the *ureA* gene [13]. The copy number of the obtained amplicons was calculated and converted to the number of *H. suis* bacteria per mg gastric tissue, by including tenfold dilutions of an external standard consisting of a 1236 bp segment of the *ureAB* gene cluster from *H. suis* strain HS5 [14].

Histopathology and immunohistochemistry
The biopsies were embedded in paraffin, sectioned at 5 μm, rehydrated, deparaffinized, stained with hæmatoxylin and eosin, dehydrated and finally mounted with a coverslip for light microscopic evaluation. The severity of gastritis was scored according to the Updated Sydney System with some modifications [5, 15]. Both diffuse infiltration with inflammatory cells and the presence of lymphoid aggregates and lymphoid follicles in the mucosa and submucosa were taken into consideration. The infiltration of mononuclear and polymorphonuclear cells was scored as follows: score 0 for absence of infiltration, score 1 for mild infiltration, score 2 for moderate infiltration and score 3 for marked infiltration. In addition, the formation of lymphoid follicle formation was scored as follows: score 0 for absence of lymphoid aggregates, score 1 for presence of a small number of lymphoid aggregates ($n < 5$), score 2 for a large number of lymphoid aggregates ($n \geq 5$) and/or the presence of 1 organized lymphoid follicle and score 3 for the presence of at least 2 organized lymphoid follicles. Based on the scoring of the diffuse infiltration with inflammatory cells and the presence of lymphoid aggregates and lymphoid follicles, an overall gastritis score was obtained. Therefore, the average score was calculated for each *H. suis*-negative and *H. suis*-positive age group and this for the pyloric and fundic

gland zone. When an overall score of $0 \leq n \leq 1$; $1 < n \leq 2$ or $2 < n \leq 3$ was obtained, the gastritis was considered as mild, moderate and severe, respectively.

To determine the number of parietal cells, D-cells and G-cells, 3 consecutive sections of 5 µm were cut from the paraffin embedded tissues. After rehydration and deparaffinization, heat-induced antigen retrieval was performed in citrate buffer (pH 6.0) using a microwave oven. Slides were incubated with 3% H_2O_2 in methanol (5 min) to block endogenous peroxidase activity and with 30% goat serum (30 min) to block non-specific reactions. Parietal cells were identified by immunohistochemical staining for the H+/K+ ATPase using a mouse monoclonal antibody (1/200; Abcam Ltd, Cambridge, United Kingdom) and a biotinylated goat anti-mouse IgG antibody (1/200; Agilent Technologies, Santa Clara, California, USA) [9]. D-cells and G-cells were identified by immunohistochemical staining using a rabbit polyclonal anti-somatostatin and anti-gastrin antibody, respectively (1/600; Agilent Technologies, Santa Clara, California, USA) and a biotinylated goat anti-rabbit IgG antibody (1/600; Agilent Technologies, Santa Clara, California, USA). After rinsing, the sections were incubated with a streptavidin–biotin-HRP complex (Agilent Technologies, Santa Clara, California, USA) [10]. The color was developed with diaminobenzidine tetrahydrochloride (DAB) and H_2O_2. Finally, positive D-cells and G-cells were counted in five randomly chosen high power fields (magnification: ×400), both in the fundic and pyloric gland zone. The average number of positive cells per high power field was then calculated for each pig in both stomach regions. As a positive control for the parietal cell staining, the fundic gland zone of a non-*H. suis* infected pig was used, as this zone is known to contain large numbers of these cells [10]. The pyloric gland zone of this pig was used as a positive control for D-cells and G-cells staining. This zone indeed contains large numbers of these cell types [10]. Negative controls to confirm the specificity of the secondary antibodies were obtained by incubating the sections without the primary antibodies. In addition, the cardiac gland zone was also used as a negative control, as this stomach region is known to contain only mucus and bicarbonate producing cells [10].

Expression analysis of markers for inflammation and gastric acid secretion

RNA was extracted from the gastric biopsies using the RNeasy Mini Kit® (Qiagen, Hilden, Germany) according to the manufacturer's instructions. The obtained RNA concentrations were measured using a NanoDrop® spectrophotometer (Isogen Life Science, Utrecht, The Netherlands), after which the concentration of all samples was adjusted to 1 µg/µL, followed by cDNA synthesis using

the iScript™ cDNA Synthesis Kit (Bio-Rad, Hercules, California, USA). Expression of genes encoding host factors involved in gastric acid secretion (H+/K+ ATPase, Sonic Hedgehog, KCNQ1, gastrin, the cholinergic muscarinic M3 receptor, somatostatin, the histamine H2 receptor and the gastrin CCK-B receptor), mucosal integrity (claudin 18) and inflammation (IL-4, IL-8, IL-10, IL-17A, IL-1β, IFN-γ and CXCL13) was analyzed. HPRT, Cyc5 and ACTB have been shown to have a stable mRNA expression and were therefore included as reference genes [9]. All primer sequences are shown in the Additional file 1. The mRNA expression levels of the reference and target genes were quantified using RT-qPCR, as described earlier [16]. No-template control reaction mixtures were included and all samples were run in duplicate. The threshold cycle (Ct)-values were first normalized to the geometric mean of the Ct-values of the reference genes. Fold changes were calculated using ΔΔCT method with the means of Ct-values from the *H. suis* negative pigs. Finally, for each target gene, the results were expressed as fold changes of the mRNA expression of *H. suis* positive pigs relative to mRNA expression levels of *H. suis* negative pigs and this for each age group separately.

Statistical analysis

Statistical analysis was performed using SPSS statistics 24® (IBM, New York, USA). Differences in severity of *Pars œsophageal* lesions, severity of gastritis, number of parietal cells, D-cells and G-cells and fold changes of the markers for gastric acid secretion and inflammation between the *H. suis*-negative and *H. suis*-positive groups were investigated using the non-parametric Kruskal-Wallis H test with Bonferroni correction. A p value ≤ 0.05 was considered to be significant. Correlations between mucosal lesions, severity of gastritis, number of parietal cells, D-cells and G-cells, fold changes and the number of *H. suis* bacteria were examined using the Pearson correlation coefficient. Differences were considered statistically significant at $p \leq 0.05$.

Results

H. suis prevalence and association with mucosal lesions, gastritis and number of parietal cells, D-cells and G-cells
Two–3 months old pigs
The prevalence of *H. suis* was 47% and the average number of *H. suis* bacteria per mg tissue was higher in the pyloric gland zone than in the other stomach regions ($p < 0.001$) (Additional file 2). Almost all pigs had *H. suis* DNA in the fundic and pyloric gland zone (=15/16). On gross examination, all pigs showed an intact mucosa or mild hyperkeratosis of the *Pars œsophagea* (Table 1), with moderate gastritis in the fundic and pyloric gland zone

Table 1 General overview of the score distribution of lesions (%) in the *Pars œsophagea* of pigs of different ages

Age group	Pars œsophagea—lesion score					
	0 (%)	1 (%)	2 (%)	3 (%)	4 (%)	5 (%)
2–3 months old (*n* = 34)	38	44	18	0	0	0
H. suis positive (*n* = 16)	37	44	19	0	0	0
H. suis negative (*n* = 18)	39	44	17	0	0	0
6–8 months old (*n* = 68)	2	27	50	13	3	5
H. suis positive (*n* = 55)	0	13	61	17	4	6
H. suis negative (*n* = 13)	8	92	0	0	0	0
Adult sows (*n* = 60)	0	5	20	15	10	50
H. suis positive (*n* = 55)	0	5	20	13	9	53
H. suis negative (*n* = 5)	0	0	20	40	20	20

Score 0 = normal mucosa, 1 = mild hyperkeratosis covering less than 50% of the surface, 2 = severe hyperkeratosis covering more than 50% of the surface, 3 = hyperkeratosis with few erosions, 4 = hyperkeratosis with several erosions, 5 = hyperkeratosis with many erosions or ulceration, *n* = total number of investigated pigs' stomachs per age group. The data are shown as the percentage of pigs showing a certain lesion score.

(Additional file 3). The scores for *Pars œsophageal* lesions and gastritis were not significantly different between the *H. suis*-negative and *H. suis*-positive pigs. Similarly, the number of G-cells and D-cells in the pyloric gland zone did not differ between the *H. suis*-negative and *H. suis*-positive group (Figures 1A and B). A small number of G-cells and D-cells was detected in the fundic gland zone of the pigs, varying from 0 to 3 per high power field and independent from the *H. suis* status (data not shown). In the fundic gland zone of both *H. suis*-infected and non-infected pigs, the number of parietal cells was high in each high power field (> 800/field), making the counting impossible. A small number of parietal cells was detected in the pyloric gland zone of the pigs, varying from 0 to 2 per high power field and independent from the *H. suis*

status (data not shown). For the *H. suis*-positive pigs, statistical analysis did not reveal significant correlations between mucosal lesions, gastritis and the number of *H. suis* bacteria. Analysis of gene expression, histopathology and immunohistochemistry was done on samples from all pigs in this age category (see below).

Six–8 months old pigs

Helicobacter suis was detected in 81% of the investigated stomachs. The average number of *H. suis* bacteria per mg tissue was similar for the fundic and pyloric gland zone (Additional file 2). *H. suis* DNA was detected in the fundic and pyloric gland zone of all *H. suis*-infected pigs. Severe hyperkeratosis and erosions were only seen in the *H. suis*-positive group (Table 1). The number of

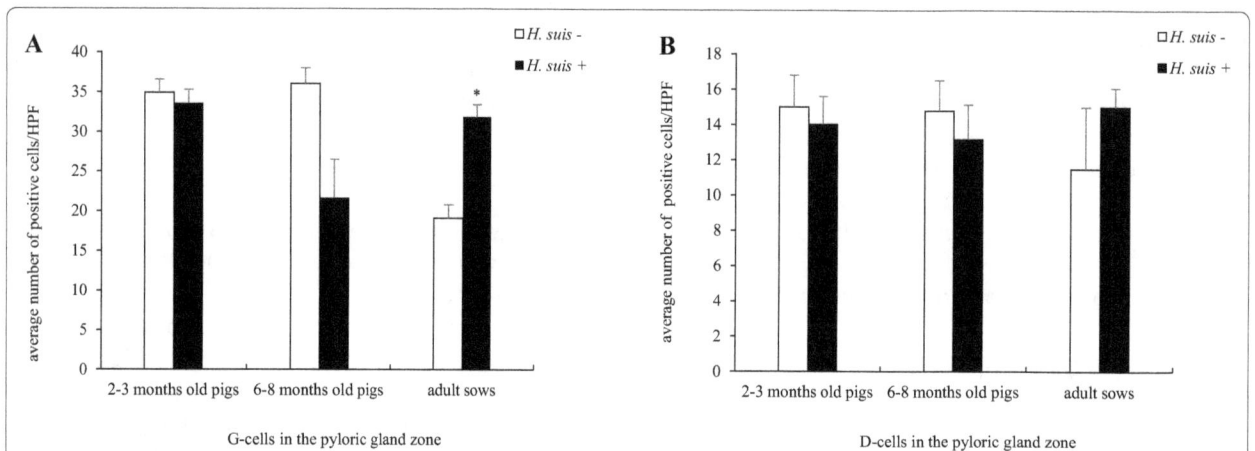

Figure 1 A, B The number of G-cells (A) and D-cells (B) present in the pyloric gland zone of *H. suis*-negative (−) and *H. suis*-positive (+) pigs of different ages. Data are shown as the average number of G-positive and D-positive cells of each age group with standard deviation. Statistical differences were calculated using the non-parametric Kruskal–Wallis H test. * Significant differences between the *H. suis*-negative and *H. suis*-positive pigs ($p < 0.01$); HPF, high power field.

D-cells did not differ between the *H. suis*-negative and *H. suis*-positive group, whereas the number of G-cells was decreased in the *H. suis*-positive group ($p = 0.054$) (Figures 1A and B). A small number of G-cells and D-cells was detected in the fundic gland zone of the pigs, varying from 0 to 3 per high power field and independent from the *H. suis* status (data not shown). In the fundic gland zone of both *H. suis*-infected and non-infected pigs, the number of parietal cells was high in each high power field (> 800/field), making the counting impossible. A small number of parietal cells was detected in the pyloric gland zone of the pigs, varying from 0 to 2 per high power field and independent from the *H. suis* status (data not shown). No significant correlations were detected between the number of *H. suis* bacteria and severity of gastritis. All *H. suis*-negative pigs ($n = 13$), 5 pigs with > 1000 *H. suis* bacteria/mg tissue in the fundic gland zone, 5 pigs with > 1000 *H. suis* bacteria/mg tissue in the pyloric gland zone and 5 pigs with < 100 *H. suis* bacteria/mg tissue in both the fundic and pyloric gland zone were selected for analysis of gene expression, histopathology and immunohistochemistry.

Adult sows

Helicobacter suis was detected in the stomach of 55/60 sows (92%). In contrast with the other age groups, the average number of *H. suis* bacteria per mg tissue was higher in the fundic gland zone than in the other stomach regions ($p < 0.01$) (Additional file 2). All *H. suis*-infected sows had *H. suis* DNA in the fundic and pyloric gland zone. Ulceration was mainly found in the *H. suis*-positive sows, although this was not significantly different from the *H. suis*-negative group (Table 1). No significant differences were detected in the severity of gastritis between the *H. suis*-negative and *H. suis*-positive pigs (Additional file 3). A significant positive correlation was found, however, between the number of *H. suis* bacteria per mg gastric tissue and lymphoid infiltration in the fundic gland zone ($p < 0.001$). The number of D-cells did not differ between the *H. suis*-negative and *H. suis*-positive group, while the number of G-cells was increased in the *H. suis*-positive group ($p = 0.002$) (Figures 1A and B; Additional file 4). A small number of G-cells and D-cells was detected in the fundic gland zone of the pigs, varying from 0 to 3 per high power field and independent from the *H. suis* status (data not shown). In the fundic gland zone of both *H. suis*-infected and non-infected pigs, the number of parietal cells was high in each high power field (> 800/field), making the counting impossible. A small number of parietal cells was detected in the pyloric gland zone of the pigs, varying from 0 to 2 per high power field and independent from the *H. suis* status (data not shown). All *H. suis*-negative sows ($n = 5$) were selected

for gene expression, histopathological and immunohistochemical analysis. From the *H. suis*-positive group, these analyses were performed on 20 stomachs, selected as follows: 5 sows with > 1000 *H. suis* bacteria/mg tissue in both the fundic and pyloric gland zone, 5 sows with > 1000 *H. suis* bacteria/mg tissue in the fundic gland zone, 5 sows with > 1000 *H. suis* bacteria/mg tissue in the pyloric gland zone and 5 sows with < 100 *H. suis* bacteria/mg tissue in both the fundic and pyloric gland zone.

Comparison of the different age groups

The scores given for *Pars œsophageal* lesions were significantly different between each age group ($p < 0.001$), with more severe lesions in adult sows, followed by 6–8 months old pigs. In contrast, the scores for lymphoid infiltration and lymphoid follicle formation did not differ significantly between the age groups, nor did the number of parietal cells, G-cells and D-cells (Figures 1A and B; Additional file 3). Although the prevalence of *H. suis* progressively increased with age, the number of *H. suis* bacteria per mg tissue decreased with age, especially in the pyloric gland zone ($p < 0.05$; Figure 2). Significantly higher scores for lymphoid infiltration and lymphoid follicle formation were found in the pyloric gland zone compared to the fundic gland zone ($p < 0.005$), independent from the *H. suis* status, and this in all age groups.

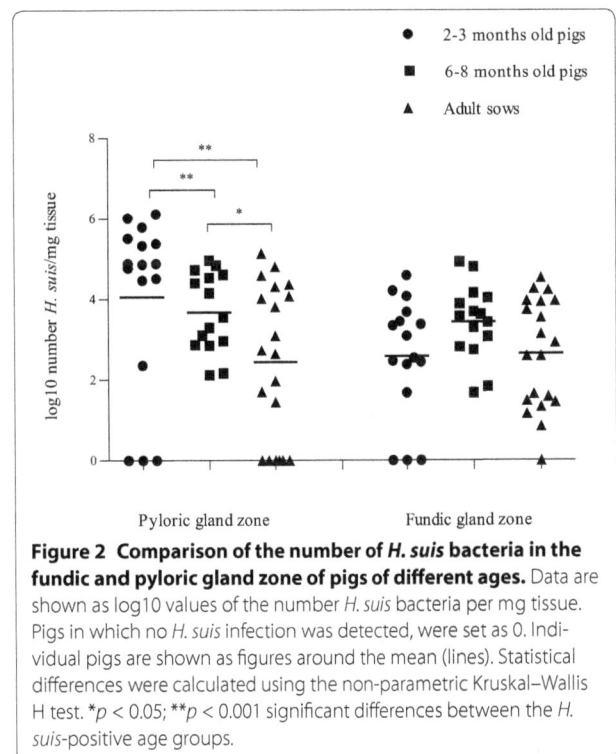

Figure 2 Comparison of the number of *H. suis* bacteria in the fundic and pyloric gland zone of pigs of different ages. Data are shown as log10 values of the number *H. suis* bacteria per mg tissue. Pigs in which no *H. suis* infection was detected, were set as 0. Individual pigs are shown as figures around the mean (lines). Statistical differences were calculated using the non-parametric Kruskal–Wallis H test. *$p < 0.05$; **$p < 0.001$ significant differences between the *H. suis*-positive age groups.

Gene expression analysis of markers for inflammation
Two–3 months old pigs
Compared to the non-infected group, the mRNA expression of CXCL13 was significantly upregulated in the fundic and pyloric gland zones of the *H. suis*-infected group

($p = 0.027$ and < 0.001, respectively), as well as the IL-8 and IL-1β transcript levels in the pyloric gland zone ($p = 0.001$ and 0.034, respectively). In contrast, IL-17A was significantly downregulated in the pyloric gland zone ($p = 0.039$) (Figures 3A and B; Additional file 5). Since

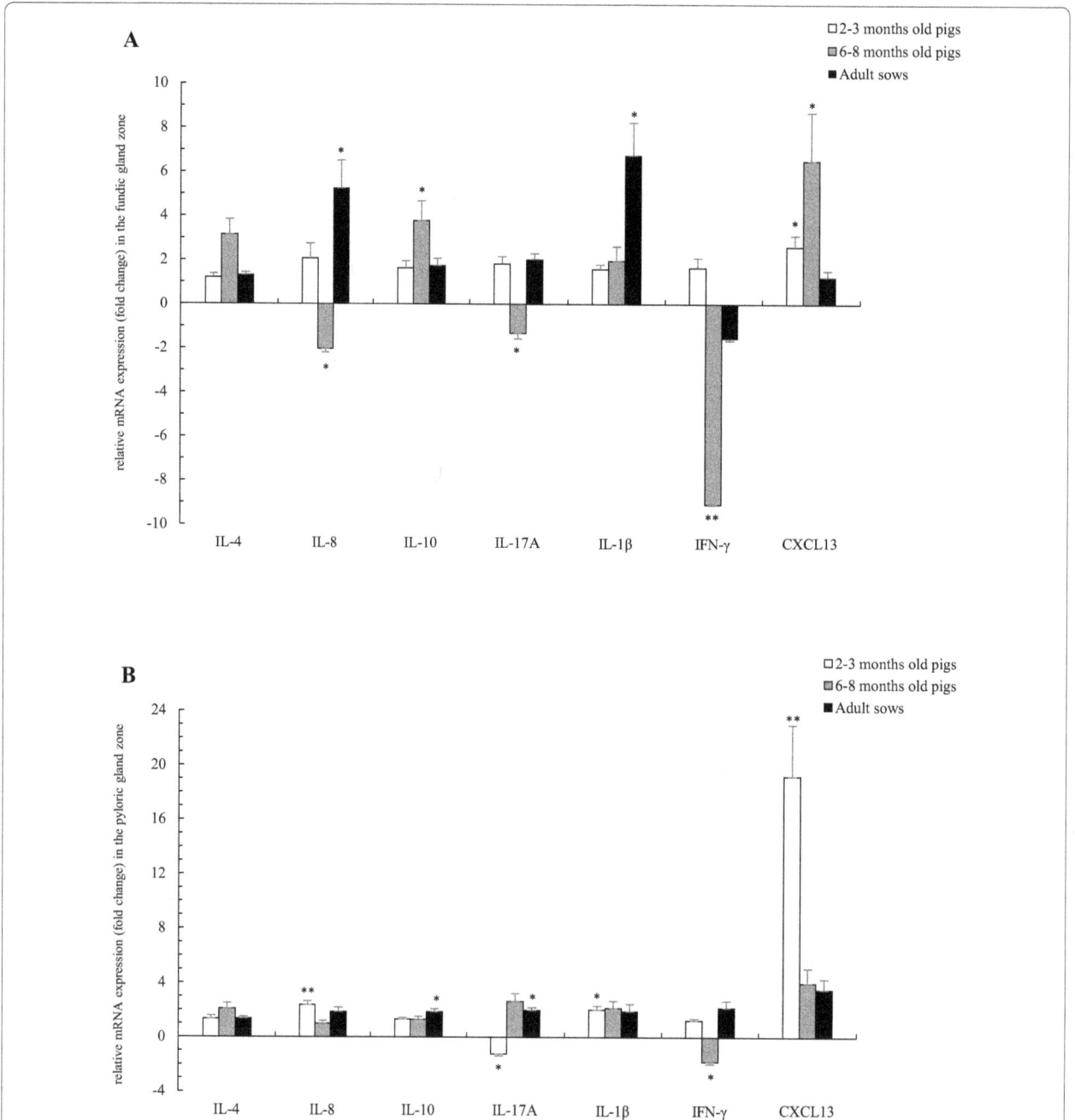

Figure 3 A, B General overview of gene expression analysis of markers for inflammation in the fundic (A) and pyloric (B) gland zone of *H. suis*-infected pigs of different ages. The data are presented as fold changes in gene expression normalized to 3 reference genes and relative to a *H. suis*-negative control group which is considered as 1. The fold changes are shown as means with the standard error of the mean. Statistical differences were calculated using the non-parametric Kruskal–Wallis H test. *$p < 0.05$; **$p < 0.001$ significant differences between the *H. suis*-positive pigs and *H. suis*-negative pigs.

significant correlations were found between both, the altered fold changes of IL-8, IL-17A, IL-1β and CXCL13 were more pronounced in pigs with a high number of *H. suis* bacteria per mg gastric tissue (Additional file 6).

Six–8 months old pigs

Upregulated expression of inflammatory cytokines was as described in the study of Bosschem et al. [11]. In brief, compared to the non-infected group, in the *H. suis*-positive group, significant upregulations of IL-10 and CXCL13 were detected in the fundic gland zone ($p = 0.047$ and 0.011, respectively). The expressions of IL-4 in the fundic gland zone and that of IL-4, IL-17A and CXCL13 in the pyloric gland zone were also upregulated, although not significantly. A significant downregulation of IL-8 and IL-17A was detected in the fundic gland zone ($p = 0.040$ and 0.029, respectively), while IFN-γ was significantly downregulated in both fundic and pyloric gland zone ($p < 0.001$ and $= 0.005$, respectively) (Figures 3A and B; Additional file 5). Since significant correlations were found between both, the altered fold changes of IL-4, IL-8, IL-10, IL-17A, IFN-γ and CXCL13 were more pronounced in pigs with > 1000 *H. suis* bacteria/mg gastric tissue (Additional file 6).

Adult sows

Compared to the non-infected sows, in the *H. suis*-infected adult sows, the mRNA expression of IL-8 and IL-1β was significantly upregulated in the fundic gland zone ($p = 0.018$ for IL-8 and 0.037 for IL-1β), while IL-10 and IL-17A were upregulated in the pyloric gland zone of *H. suis*-infected sows ($p = 0.019$ and 0.042, respectively). Although not significantly, increased IL-10 and IL-17A mRNA expression was also detected in the fundic gland zone and in the pyloric gland zone for IFN-γ and CXCL13 (Figures 3A and B; Additional file 5). Since significant correlations were found between both, the altered fold changes of IL-8, IL-10, IL-17A, IL-1β, IFN-γ and CXCL13 were more distinct in pigs with > 1000 *H. suis* bacteria/mg gastric tissue (Additional file 6).

Gene expression analysis of markers for gastric acid secretion

Two–3 months old pigs

Compared to the non-infected group, in the *H. suis*-infected 2–3 months old pigs, the majority of the markers for gastric acid secretion were not altered, except for a significant downregulated expression of the M3-receptor in the pyloric gland zone ($p = 0.027$). The expression of KCNQ1 was upregulated in the fundic gland zone, while somatostatin was downregulated in the pyloric gland zone, although not significantly (Figures 4A and B; Additional file 7). Since significant correlations were

found between both, the altered fold changes of KCNQ1, M3-receptor and somatostatin were more pronounced in pigs with > 1000 *H. suis* bacteria/mg per mg gastric tissue (Additional file 8). In addition, since significant correlations were found between both markers, the altered fold change of somatostatin was more pronounced in pigs with a high expression of CXCL13 and IL-1β (Additional file 9).

Six–8 months old pigs

Compared to the non-infected group, in the *H. suis*-infected group claudin 18, gastrin, M3 receptor and CCK-B receptor were significantly downregulated in the fundic gland zone ($p = 0.022$, 0.040, 0.002 and 0.004, respectively), whereas Sonic Hedgehog and somatostatin mRNA levels were significantly upregulated in the pyloric gland zone ($p = 0.048$ and 0.007, respectively). The H+/K+ ATPase expression in the pyloric gland zone was upregulated as well, although not significantly. In the pyloric gland zone of 9 *H. suis*-infected pigs, the expression of gastrin was upregulated (Figures 4A and B; Additional file 7), while for 6 *H. suis*-infected pigs the expression was not altered. Since significant correlations were found between both, the altered fold changes of H+/K+ ATPase, Sonic Hedgehog, claudin 18, gastrin, M3 receptor, somatostatin and CCK-B receptor were more pronounced in pigs with > 1000 *H. suis* bacteria/mg gastric tissue (Additional file 8). In addition, since significant correlations were found between both markers, the altered fold changes of claudin 18, M3 receptor, somatostatin and CCK-B receptor were more pronounced in pigs with lower expressions of IL-8, IL-17A and IFN-γ (Additional file 9).

Adult sows

Compared to the non-infected sows, most markers for gastric acid secretion were upregulated in the *H. suis*-infected sows. The expression of genes encoding H+/K+ ATPase, claudin 18, H2 receptor and CCK-B receptor were significantly upregulated in the fundic and pyloric gland zone of the *H. suis*-infected sows ($p = 0.049$, 0.002, 0.019, 0.049, 0.002, 0.012, 0.015 and 0.012, respectively). In addition, KCNQ1 and gastrin transcript levels were significantly upregulated in the fundic gland zone ($p = 0.012$ and < 0.001, respectively), whereas a significant downregulated mRNA expression of the M3 receptor in the pyloric gland zone was noticed ($p = 0.049$). An upregulated expression of Sonic Hedgehog was also detected in the fundic and pyloric gland zone, although not significant (Figures 4A and B; Additional file 7). Since significant correlations were found between both, the altered fold changes of genes encoding H+/K+ ATPase, Sonic Hedgehog, claudin 18, KCNQ1 and CCK-B

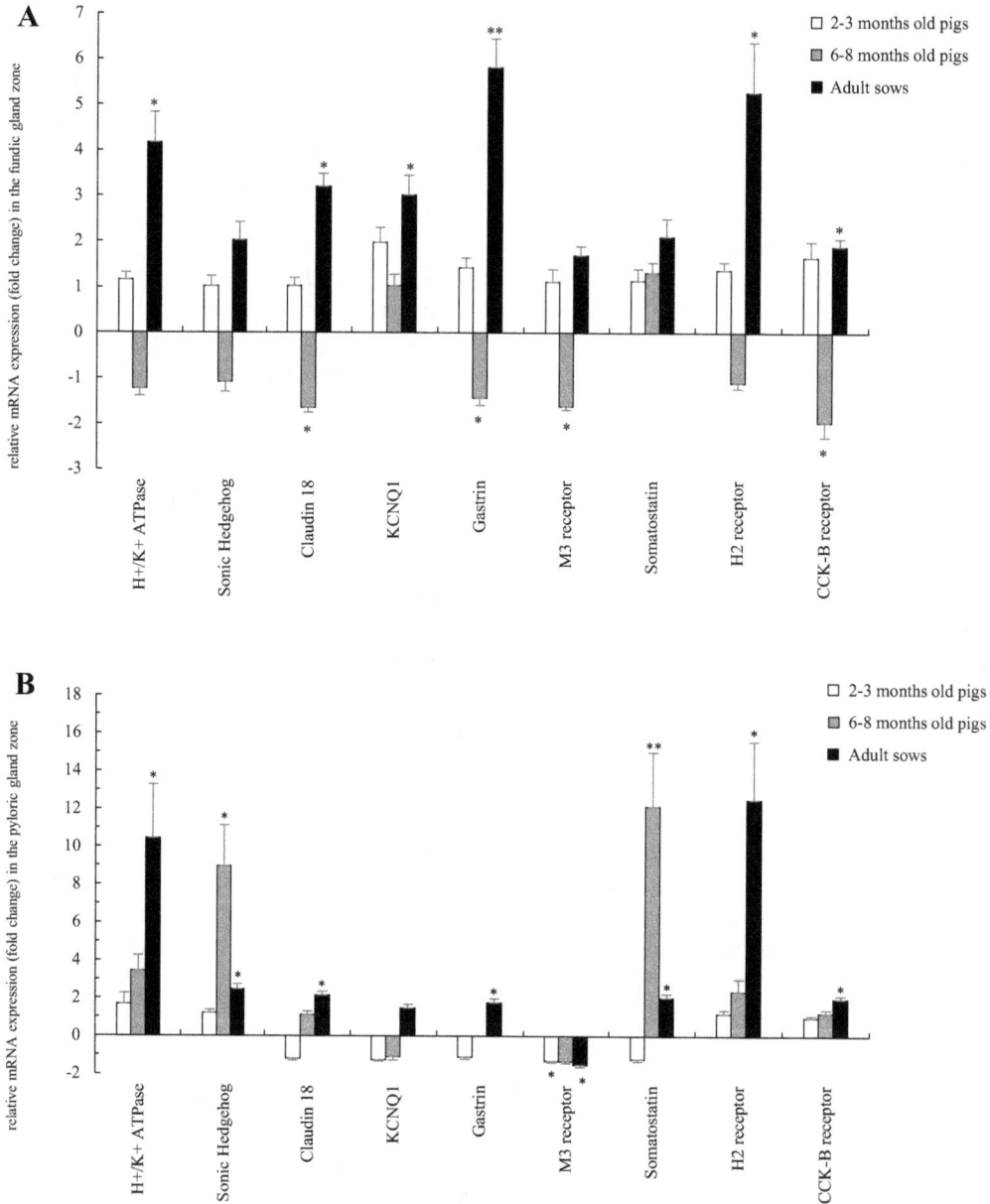

Figure 4 A, B General overview of gene expression analysis of markers for gastric acid secretion in the fundic (A) and pyloric (B) gland zone of *H. suis*-infected pigs of different ages. The data are presented as fold changes in gene expression normalized to 3 reference genes and relative to a *H. suis*-negative control group which is considered as 1. The fold changes are shown as means with the standard error of the mean. The average fold change of gastrin in the pyloric gland zone of 6–8 months old pigs is not shown, since these values were too high (231.97 ± 64.63). Statistical differences were calculated using the non-parametric Kruskal–Wallis H test. *$p < 0.05$; **$p < 0.001$ significant differences between the *H. suis*-positive pigs and *H. suis*-negative pigs.

receptor were more pronounced in pigs with > 1000 *H. suis* bacteria/mg gastric tissue (Additional file 8). In addition, since significant correlations were found between both markers, the altered fold changes of genes encoding H+/K+ ATPase, Sonic Hedgehog, claudin 18, gastrin and CCK-B receptor were more pronounced in pigs with high expressions of IL-10, IL-17A and IFN-γ (Additional file 9). Furthermore, since significant positive correlations were found between both, an increased G-cell number may have contributed to the increased expression of gastrin in both fundic and pyloric gland zone ($r = 0.562$, $p = 0.003$; $r = 0.465$, $p = 0.022$, respectively).

Discussion

In the present study, the prevalence of *H. suis* was 47% in 2–3 months old pigs and increased to 81% in pigs at slaughter age, which is in line with the results of previous studies [17–19].

The prevalence of *H. suis* was very high in adult animals, indicating that the host immune response is not able to clear the infection. In a recent study, Bosschem et al. [11] showed that *H. suis* induces a semimaturation of porcine monocyte-derived dendritic cells, characterized by increased expression of CD25, CD80/86 and CD40, but impaired expression of MHC class II molecules on the surface of these cells. It was suggested that this impaired dendritic cell response may elicit the expansion of Treg cells, which may help to establish a chronic infection as Treg cells are immune-suppressive and tolerogenic [20]. Indeed, a tolerogenic immune response was indicated to be present in this study, since the Treg cell-associated cytokine IL-10 was upregulated in both *H. suis*-infected 6–8 months old pigs and adult sows. In addition, the downregulated expressions of IL-8, IL-17A and especially IFN-γ indicated presence of an immune-suppressive environment in the *H. suis*-infected 6–8 months old pigs, which may have contributed to the establishment of a chronic infection. In the *H. suis*-infected adult sows, however, the mRNA expression of the Th17 cell-associated IL-17A was upregulated. We also found a shift in colonization of *H. suis* from the pyloric gland zone during the more acute phase of the infection (2–3 months old pigs) to the fundic gland zone in the more chronic phase of the infection (adults sows) in combination with upregulated expressions of IL-8 and IL-1β. Taken together, these findings suggest that shortly after colonization, the immune response is suboptimal, contributing to the persistence of *H. suis* infection. Later a more pronounced immune response is seen, which may result in lower numbers of *H. suis* bacteria in that stomach region. Indeed, although the prevalence of *H. suis* was highest in adult sows, the average number of *H. suis* bacteria per mg tissue decreased with age, as was also

observed in other studies [8]. The presence of a specific Treg/Th17 response should be confirmed in future studies, where the expansion of Treg and Th17 cells is directly assessed by the use of staining or flow cytometry.

Interestingly, the expression of CXCL13 was upregulated in *H. suis*-infected pigs of each age group. Since this chemokine attracts B-lymphocytes, its upregulation may be important for the development of a specific local immune response towards *H. suis*, but this requires further research [11]. The upregulation of CXCL13 has also been demonstrated in *H. suis* infected mice [21] and has been linked with the development of mucosa associated lymphoid tissue (MALT)-lymphomas in *Helicobacter* sp. infected human patients [21]. MALT-lymphoma lesions were not detected in the present study and, as far as we know, have not been described in pigs.

In 2–3 months old pigs, the average number of *H. suis* bacteria was the highest in the pyloric gland zone, indicating that *H. suis* colonization starts in this stomach region, as already suggested by others [22]. In adult sows, the average number of *H. suis* bacteria was the highest in the fundic gland zone, indicating a shift in colonization to that region in animals infected during longer periods of time, which is similar to the findings of Hellemans et al. [22]. It appears that when *H. suis* colonizes the stomach epithelium, it triggers an innate immune response in that region, characterized by upregulated expression of the pro-inflammatory cytokines IL-8 and IL-1β in the pyloric gland zone of 2–3 months old pigs and in the fundic gland zone of adult sows.

Severe hyperkeratosis and erosions were only seen in the *H. suis* infected 6–8 months old pigs and not in non-infected pigs of this age group. In adult sows, ulceration was also mainly found in the *H. suis*-positive animals, although this was not significantly different from the *H. suis*-negative group, which may be due to the low number of non-infected sows available. In this field study, interpretation of results is further complicated by variation between herds of other factors that may play a role in development of gastric pathologies such as diet, feeding strategy and management [1]. Nevertheless, our findings provide further evidence that *H. suis* may be one of the factors playing a role in the pathogenesis of gastric ulceration in pigs. A similar conclusion was drawn from results of an experimental infection study in pigs [5]. Interestingly, severe lesions in the *Pars œsophagea* were more frequently found in adult sows compared to the other age groups, indicating that ulceration is a long-term process which may affect the majority of the adult pigs.

It is not yet clear how exactly *H. suis* might influence ulcer development in the *Pars œsophagea*, but alterations in gastric acid secretion might be involved. No clear effects on the markers for gastric acid secretion or number of parietal cells, D-cells and G-cells, and no lesions in the *Pars œsophagea* were detected in the *H. suis*-infected 2–3 months old pigs (acute phase of infection). In a later phase of infection (6–8 months *H. suis* infected pigs), markers for gastric acid secretion were downregulated, genes encoding somatostatin were upregulated and the number of G-cells was decreased, indicating inhibition of gastric acid secretion. In this age group, lesions in the *Pars œsophagea* were present in several animals. The prevalence of severe lesions was extremely high in *H. suis* infected adult sows (chronic phase of infection). Markers for gastric acid secretion were upregulated and the number of G-cells was increased in this age group, indicating increased gastric acid secretion. We hypothesize that decreased gastric acid secretion in the glandular part of the stomach may affect the composition of the *Pars œsophageal* microbiota which may affect development of lesions in this non-glandular part of the stomach. Indeed, higher numbers of a recently described *Fusobacterium* species, designated *F. gastrosuis*, were detected in the *Pars œsophagea* of *H. suis*-infected 6–8 months old pigs than in non-infected pigs of the same age group [23]. Increased production of gastric acid during the chronic phase of infection might further aggravate severity of lesions in this stomach region, which is not protected by mucus. Further studies in which for instance the gastric microbiota and pH are determined in *H. suis*-infected and non-infected pigs, are necessary to confirm or reject this hypothesis.

Several mechanisms might be involved in altered gastric acid secretion in *H. suis* infected animals. A clear parietal cell loss, as described in *H. suis*-infected Mongolian gerbils and mice [9, 24], was not seen in the *H. suis*-infected pigs, although small differences in the number of these cells between the infected and non-infected animals cannot be excluded since counting was impossible in the fundic gland zone. The expression of genes encoding H+/K+ ATPase was, however, altered. As this enzyme is typically associated with gastric acid production by parietal cells, this shows that the function of these cells was affected. This is also indicated by altered expression of H2-, M3- and CCK-B receptors, although these receptors are also found on

enterochromaffin cells, which were not studied here. The exact mechanism behind the effect of a *H. suis* infection on gastric acid secretion by parietal cells is not clear and requires further studies. Since *H. suis* is often found in close proximity to these host cells, a direct effect of this bacterium on the parietal cells might be involved. Indirect effects probably also play a role since the number of G-cells and/or the expression of gastrin was decreased or enhanced in pigs with downregulated and upregulated expression of H+/K+ ATPase, respectively. In *H. pylori* infections, increased gastric acid secretion has been associated with increased expression of genes encoding IL-8 and IL-1β [25–29]. Expression of genes encoding these cytokines was upregulated in the fundic gland zone of adult sows with upregulated expression of genes encoding H+/K+ ATPase. Literature dealing with the effect of IL-1β is, however, controversial as Beales and Calam [30] demonstrated that IL-1β inhibits acid secretion in cultured parietal cells.

In *H. suis* infected 6–8 months old pigs and adult sows, expression of genes encoding Sonic Hedgehog was upregulated in the fundic and pyloric gland zone. Since Sonic Hedgehog is involved in the regeneration of damaged epithelium [31], this may indicate a compensation for epithelial loss induced by *H. suis* in these gastric regions. Disruption of the gastric epithelium, followed by regeneration was further suggested by the downregulated expression of genes encoding claudin 18, an important tight junction protein of the stomach [32], in *H. suis*-infected 6–8 months old pigs and its upregulation in adult sows. The increased IL-10 and IL-17A transcript levels in *H. suis*-infected adult sows may have promoted the regeneration of the gastric epithelium as well, as both cytokines are associated with intestinal barrier restoration [33].

To summarize, we revealed an increased prevalence of *H. suis* and a shift of colonization towards the fundic gland zone in adult sows, while the number of *H. suis* bacteria per mg tissue decreased with age. Gastric erosion and ulceration were more frequently detected in *H. suis*-infected pigs. During the more acute phase of the infection, an innate immune response was indicated to be present, followed by a Treg and Th17 response in pigs colonized during longer periods of time. While no clear alterations in the markers for gastric acid secretion were detected in 2–3 months old pigs, a decrease and increase were found in 6–8 months old pigs and adult sows, respectively. These results indicate that *H. suis* affects the expression of markers for gastric acid secretion and inflammation and indicate that these effects

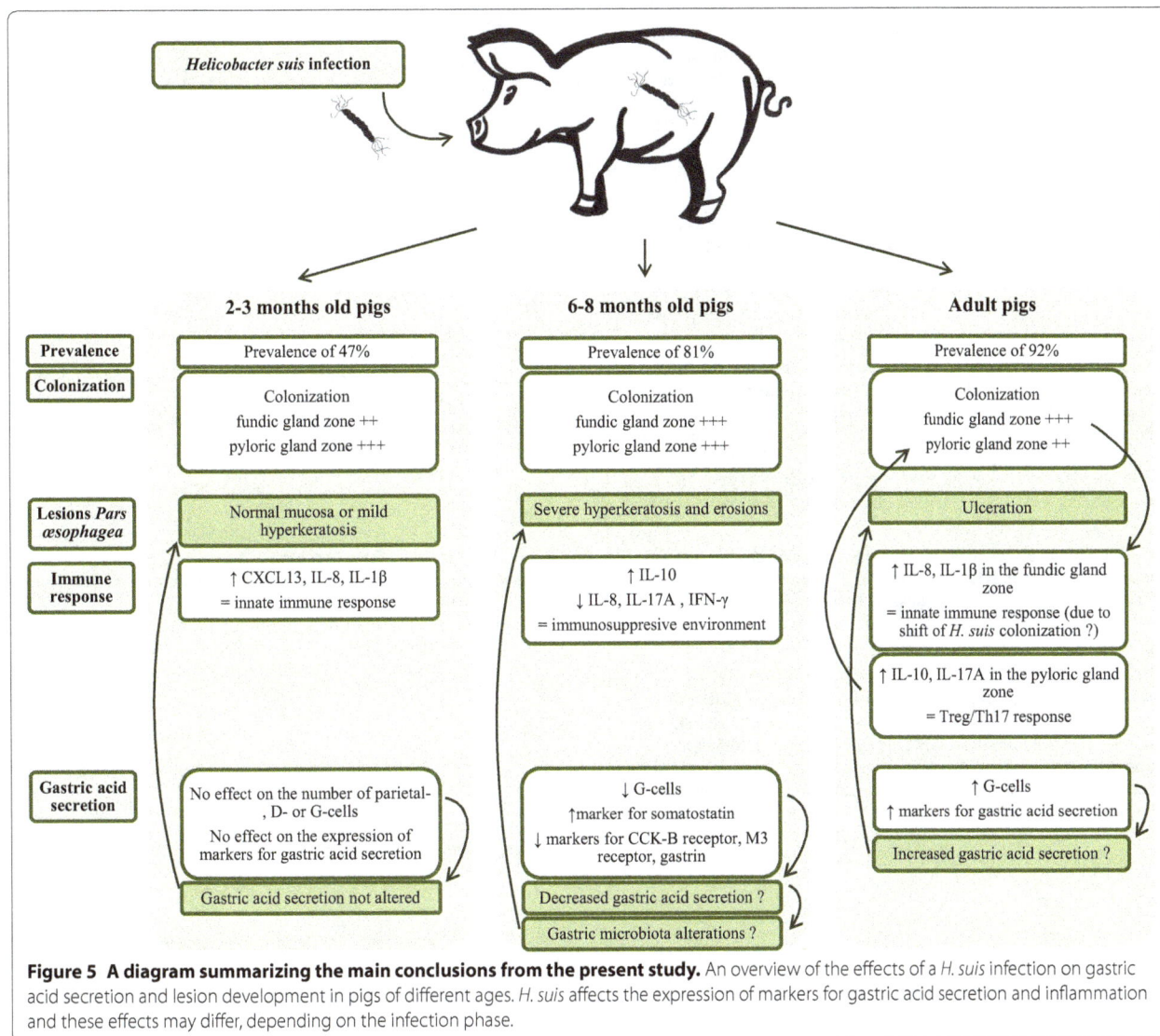

Figure 5 A diagram summarizing the main conclusions from the present study. An overview of the effects of a *H. suis* infection on gastric acid secretion and lesion development in pigs of different ages. *H. suis* affects the expression of markers for gastric acid secretion and inflammation and these effects may differ, depending on the infection phase.

differ, depending on the infection phase. An overview of the main results and conclusions of the present study is presented in Figure 5.

Additional files

Additional file 1. List of primers used in quantitative RT-PCR for gene expression analysis of markers for gastric acid secretion and inflammation.

Additional file 2. The number of *H. suis* bacteria in the different stomach regions of 2–3 months old pigs (A), 6–8 months old pigs (B) and adult sows (C). Data are shown as log10 values of the average number of *H. suis* bacteria per mg tissue with standard deviation. Statistical differences were calculated using the non-parametric Kruskal–Wallis H test. *, $p < 0.01$; **, $p < 0.001$ significant differences between the stomach regions.

Additional file 3. General overview of the average scores of infiltration with inflammatory cells and lymphoid follicle formation in

the fundic and pyloric gland zone of pigs of different ages. Gastritis was scored based on infiltration with inflammatory cells/lymphoid follicle formation, with score 0 = absence of infiltration/absence of lymphoid aggregates, 1 = mild infiltration/small number of lymphoid aggregates ($n < 5$), 2 = moderate infiltration/large number of lymphoid aggregates ($n > 5$) or presence of 1 organized lymphoid follicle, 3 = marked infiltration/at least 2 organized lymphoid follicles, n = total number of investigated pigs' stomachs per age group. The data are shown as the average of the administered scores with standard deviation.

Additional file 4. Microscopic visualization of the parietal cells (A), D-cells (B) and G-cells (C–D) in the porcine stomach using immunohistochemistry. (A) H+/K+ ATPase staining of the fundic gland zone of a *H. suis*-positive adult sow, showing parietal cells (brown). No clear parietal cell loss was detected. Original magnification ×100. (B) Somatostatin staining of the pyloric gland zone of a *H. suis*-positive adult sow, showing D-cells (brown). Original magnification ×200. (C) Gastrin staining of the pyloric gland zone of a *H. suis*-positive adult sow, showing G-cells (brown). Original magnification ×200. (D) Gastrin staining of the pyloric gland zone of a *H. suis*-negative sow, showing G-cells (brown). Original magnification ×200. The number of G-cells in the *H. suis*-negative sow (D) is lower than observed in the *H. suis*-positive sow (C).

Additional file 5. Overview of the relative fold changes of altered markers for inflammation in *H. suis* infected pigs of different ages. The data are presented as fold changes in gene expression normalized to 3 reference genes and relative to the *H. suis*-negative control group which is considered as 1. The fold changes are shown as means with the standard error of the mean. Statistical differences were calculated using the non-parametric Kruskal–Wallis H test. A *p* value lower than 0.05 is considered to be significant.

Additional file 6. Overview of important correlations between markers for inflammation and the number of *H. suis* bacteria in pigs of different ages. *r* = Pearson correlation coefficient, calculated using SPSS Statistics 24®. A *r*-value close to 1 indicates a strong, positive correlation, whereas a *r*-value of −1 indicates a strong, negative correlation. A *p*-value lower than 0.05 is considered to be significant.

Additional file 7. Overview of relative fold changes of altered markers for gastric acid secretion in *H. suis*-infected pigs of different ages. The data are presented as fold changes in gene expression normalized to 3 reference genes and relative to the *H. suis*-negative control group which is considered as 1. The fold changes are shown as means with the standard error of the mean. Statistical differences were calculated using the non-parametric Kruskal–Wallis H test. A *p*-value lower than 0.05 is considered to be significant.

Additional file 8. Overview of important correlations between markers for gastric acid secretion and the number of *H. suis* bacteria in pigs of different ages. *r* = Pearson correlation coefficient, calculated using SPSS Statistics 24®. A *r*-value close to 1 indicates a strong, positive correlation, whereas a *r*-value of -1 indicates a strong, negative correlation. *P*-values lower than 0.05 are considered to be significant.

Additional file 9. Correlations of altered markers for gastric acid secretion with the number of *H. suis* bacteria and with the altered markers for inflammation in *H. suis*-infected pigs of different age groups. *r* = Pearson correlation coefficient, calculated using SPSS Statistics 24®. A *r*-value close to 1 indicates a strong, positive correlation, whereas a *r*-value of −1 indicates a strong, negative correlation. *P*-values lower than 0.05 are considered to be significant./= no clear correlation, yes = correlation with *H. suis* colonization rate (see Additional files 6, 8 for the *r* and *p*-values).

Competing interests
The authors declare that they have no competing interests.

Authors' contributions
CDW, FH and BF participated in the design of the study. CDW carried out the experiments, analyzed the data and drafted the manuscript. FH, AS and BF coordinated the study and participated in the design of the study, analysis of the data and drafting of the manuscript. All authors read and approved the final manuscript.

Acknowledgements
This work was supported by a grant from the Special Research Fund of Ghent University (BOF), Ghent, Belgium (Grant No. 01D20414). We thank Marjan Steppe and Christian Puttevils for their excellent technical support with the tissue staining.

Author details
[1] Department of Pathology, Bacteriology and Avian Diseases, Faculty of Veterinary Medicine, Ghent University, Merelbeke, Belgium. [2] Department of Virology, Parasitology, Immunology, Faculty of Veterinary Medicine, Ghent University, Merelbeke, Belgium. [3] Laboratory of Experimental Medicine and Pediatrics, Faculty of Medicine and Health Sciences, Antwerp University, Antwerp, Belgium.

References
1. Haesebrouck F, Pasmans F, Flahou B, Chiers K, Baele M, Meyns T, Decostere A, Ducatelle R (2009) Gastric helicobacters in domestic animals and nonhuman primates and their significance for human health. Clin Microbiol Rev 22:202–223
2. Ayles HL, Friendship RM, Ball RO (1996) Effect of dietary particle size on gastric ulcers, assessed by endoscopic examination, and relationship between ulcer severity and growth performance of individually fed pigs. Swine Health Prod 4:211–216
3. Herskin MS, Jensen HE, Jespersen A, Forkman B, Jensen MB, Canibe N, Pedersen LJ (2016) Impact of the amount of straw provided to pigs kept in intensive production conditions on the occurrence and severity of gastric ulceration at slaughter. Res Vet Sci 104:200–206
4. Hellemans A, Chiers K, Decostere A, De Bock M, Haesebrouck F, Ducatelle R (2007) Experimental infection of pigs with "Candidatus Helicobacter suis". Vet Res Commun 31:385–395
5. De Bruyne E, Flahou B, Chiers K, Meyns T, Kumar S, Vermoote M, Pasmans F, Millet S, Dewulf J, Haesebrouck F, Ducatelle R (2012) An experimental *Helicobacter suis* infection causes gastritis and reduced daily weight gain in pigs. Vet Microbiol 160:449–454
6. Bubenik GA, Ayles HL, Friendship RM, Brown GM, Ball RO (1998) Relationship between melatonin levels in plasma and gastrointestinal tissues and the incidence and severity of gastric ulcers in pigs. J Pineal Res 24:62–66
7. Joo M, Ji EK, Sun HC, Kim H, Chi JG, Kim KA, Jeon HY, June SL, Moon YS, Kim KM (2007) *Helicobacter heilmannii*-associated gastritis: clinicopathologic findings and comparison with *Helicobacter pylori*-associated gastritis. J Korean Med Sci 22:63–69
8. Flahou B, Haesebrouck F, Pasmans F, D'Herde K, Driessen A, Van Deun K, Smet A, Duchateau L, Chiers K, Ducatelle R (2010) *Helicobacter suis* causes severe gastric pathology in mouse and mongolian gerbil models of human gastric disease. PLoS One 5:e14083
9. Zhang G, Ducatelle R, Mihi B, Smet A, Flahou B, Haesebrouck F (2016) *Helicobacter suis* affects the health and function of porcine gastric parietal cells. Vet Res 47:101
10. Sapierzyński R, Fabisiak M, Kizerwetter-Swida M, Cywińska A (2007) Effect of *Helicobacter* sp. infection on the number of antral gastric endocrine cells in swine. Pol J Vet Sci 10:65–70
11. Bosschem I, Flahou B, Van Deun K, De Koker S, Volf J, Smet A, Ducatelle R, Devriendt B, Haesebrouck F (2017) Species-specific immunity to *Helicobacter suis*. Helicobacter. doi:10.1111/hel.12375
12. Hessing MJC, Geudeke MJ, Scheepens CJM, Tielen MJM, Schouten WGP, Wiepkema PR (1992) Mucosal lesion sin the *Pars œsophagea* in pigs — prevalence and influence of stress. Tijdschr Diergeneeskd 117:445–450
13. Blaecher C, Smet A, Flahou B, Pasmans F, Ducatelle R, Taylor D, Weller C, Bjarnason I, Charlett A, Lawson AJ, Dobbs RJ, Dobbs SM, Haesebrouck F (2013) Significantly higher frequency of *Helicobacter suis* in patients with idiopathic parkinsonism than in control patients. Aliment Pharmacol Ther 38:1347–1353
14. O'Rourke JL, Solnick JV, Neilan BA, Seidel K, Hayter R, Hansen LM, Lee A (2004) Description of "Candidatus Helicobacter heilmannii" based on DNA sequence analysis of 16S rRNA and urease genes. Int J Syst Evol Microbiol 54:2203–2211
15. Dixon MF, Genta RM, Yardley JH, Correa P (1996) Classification and grading of gastritis. The updated Sydney system. International workshop on the histopathology of gastritis, Houston 1994. Am J Surg Pathol 20:1161–1181
16. Flahou B, Deun KV, Pasmans F, Smet A, Volf J, Rychlik I, Ducatelle R, Haesebrouck F (2012) The local immune response of mice after *Helicobacter suis* infection: strain differences and distinction with *Helicobacter pylori*. Vet Res 43:1
17. Roosendaal R, Vos JH, Roumen T, van Vugt R, Cattoli G, Bart A, Klaasen HL, Kuipers EJ, Vandenbroucke-Grauls CM, Kusters JG (2000) Slaughter pigs are commonly infected by closely related but distinct gastric ulcerative lesion-inducing gastrospirilla. J Clin Microbiol 38:2661–2664
18. Choi YK, Han JH, Joo HS (2001) Identification of novel *Helicobacter* species in pig stomachs by PCR and partial sequencing. J Clin Microbiol 39:3311–3315
19. Park JH, Seok SH, Cho SA, Baek MW, Lee HY, Kim DJ, Park JH (2004) The high prevalence of *Helicobacter* sp. in porcine pyloric mucosa and its histopathological and molecular characteristics. Vet Microbiol 104:219–225

20. Kao JY, Zhang M, Miller MJ, Mills JC, Wang B, Liu M, Eaton KA, Zou W, Berndt BE, Cole TS, Takeuchi T, Owyang SY, Luther J (2010) *Helicobacter pylori* immune escape is mediated by dendritic cell–induced treg skewing and Th17 suppression in mice. Gastroenterology 138:1046–1054

21. Zhang G, Ducatelle R, De Bruyne E, Joosten M, Bosschem I, Smet A, Haesebrouck F, Flahou B (2015) Role of γ-glutamyltranspeptidase in the pathogenesis of *Helicobacter suis* and *Helicobacter pylori* infections. Vet Res 46:31

22. Hellemans A, Chiers K, De Bock M, Decostere A, Haesebrouck F, Ducatelle R, Maes D (2007) Prevalence of *"Candidatus Helicobacter suis"* in pigs of different ages. Vet Rec 161:189–192

23. De Witte C, Flahou B, Ducatelle R, Smet A, De Bruyne E, Cnockaert M, Taminiau B, Daube G, Vandamme P, Haesebrouck F (2017) Detection, isolation and characterization of *Fusobacterium gastrosuis* sp. nov. colonizing the stomach of pigs. Syst Appl Microbiol 40:42–50

24. Joosten M, Blaecher C, Flahou B, Ducatelle R, Haesebrouck F, Smet A (2013) Diversity in bacterium-host interactions within the species *Helicobacter heilmannii* sensu stricto. Vet Res 44:65

25. Calam J (1999) *Helicobacter pylori* modulation of gastric acid. Yale J Biol Med 72:195–202

26. Calam J (1996) *Helicobacter pylori* and hormones. Yale J Biol Med 69:39–49

27. Haruma K, Kawaguchi H, Kohmoto K, Okamoto S, Yoshihara M, Sumii K, Kajiyama G (1995) *Helicobacter pylori* infection, serum gastrin, and gastric acid secretion in teen-age subjects with duodenal ulcer, gastritis, or normal mucosa. Scand J Gastroenterol 30:322–326

28. Lehmann FS, Golodner EH, Wang J, Chen MC, Avedian D, Calam J, Walsh JH, Dubinett S, Soll AH (1996) Mononuclear cells and cytokines stimulate gastrin release from canine antral cells in primary culture. Am J Physiol 270:G783–G788

29. Beales I, Calam J, Post L, Srinivasan S, Yamada T, DelValle J (1997) Effect of transforming growth factor alpha and interleukin 8 on somatostatin release from canine fundic D cells. Gastroenterology 112:136–143

30. Beales IL, Calam J (1998) Interleukin 1 beta and tumour necrosis factor alpha inhibit acid secretion in cultured rabbit parietal cells by multiple pathways. Gut 42:227–234

31. Feng R, Xiao C, Zavros Y (2012) The role of Sonic Hedgehog as a regulator of gastric function and differentiation. Vitam Horm 88:473–489

32. Caron TJ, Scott KE, Fox JG, Hagen SJ (2015) Tight junction disruption: *Helicobacter pylori* and dysregulation of the gastric mucosal barrier. World J Gastroenterol 21:11411–11427

33. Lee SH (2015) Intestinal permeability regulation by tight junction: implication on inflammatory bowel diseases. Intest Res 13:11–18

12

Infectivity, transmission and pathogenicity of H5 highly pathogenic avian influenza clade 2.3.4.4 (H5N8 and H5N2) United States index viruses in Pekin ducks and Chinese geese

Mary J. Pantin-Jackwood* ⓘ, Mar Costa-Hurtado, Kateri Bertran, Eric DeJesus, Diane Smith and David E. Swayne

Abstract

In late 2014, a H5N8 highly pathogenic avian influenza (HPAI) virus, clade 2.3.4.4, spread by migratory waterfowl into North America reassorting with low pathogenicity AI viruses to produce a H5N2 HPAI virus. Since domestic waterfowl are common backyard poultry frequently in contact with wild waterfowl, the infectivity, transmissibility, and pathogenicity of the United States H5 HPAI index viruses (H5N8 and H5N2) was investigated in domestic ducks and geese. Ducks infected with the viruses had an increase in body temperature but no or mild clinical signs. Infected geese did not show increase in body temperature and most only had mild clinical signs; however, some geese presented severe neurological signs. Ducks became infected and transmitted the viruses to contacts when inoculated with high virus doses [(10^4 and 10^6 50% embryo infective dose (EID$_{50}$)], but not with a lower dose (10^2 EID$_{50}$). Geese inoculated with the H5N8 virus became infected regardless of the virus dose given, and transmitted the virus to direct contacts. Only geese inoculated with the higher doses of the H5N2 and their contacts became infected, indicating differences in infectivity between the two viruses and the two waterfowl species. Geese shed higher titers of virus and for a longer period of time than ducks. In conclusion, the H5 HPAI viruses can infect domestic waterfowl and easily transmit to contact birds, with geese being more susceptible to infection and disease than ducks. The disease is mostly asymptomatic, but infected birds shed virus for several days representing a risk to other poultry species.

Introduction

The Asian-origin H5N1 A/goose/Guangdong/1/1996 (Gs/GD) lineage of highly pathogenic avian influenza (HPAI) viruses has spread across several continents affecting wild birds, poultry and humans. Despite great efforts to control H5N1 HPAI viruses, these viruses continue to circulate and evolve, which has led to the emergence of multiple genotypes or sublineages and the generation of reassortant H5 strains with novel gene constellations. Subclade 2.3.4.4 H5N1 viruses have mixed with several neuraminidase subtypes to generate widely circulating H5N2, H5N5, H5N6, and H5N8 subtypes of H5 HPAI viruses [1–6]. In early 2014, outbreaks of H5N8 HPAI virus were reported in South Korea and Japan in poultry and wild aquatic birds, with migratory aquatic birds strongly suspected in playing a key role in the spread of the virus [7, 8]. In late autumn 2014, H5N8 HPAI viruses were detected in Siberia, several countries in Europe, in South Korea, and in Japan [3, 4]. Concurrently, this virus was detected in the United States (U.S.) in captive falcons, wild birds, and backyard aquatic and gallinaceous poultry [5]. In addition, another novel reassortant H5 HPAI clade 2.3.4.4 virus (H5N2) was identified as the cause of an outbreak in poultry farms in

*Correspondence: mary.pantin-jackwood@ars.usda.gov
Exotic and Emerging Avian Viral Diseases Research Unit, Southeast Poultry Research Laboratory, U.S. National Poultry Research Center, Agricultural Research Service, U.S. Department of Agriculture, 934 College Station Rd, Athens, GA 30605, USA

British Columbia, Canada, during November 2014 [9], and was subsequently detected in the U.S. in wild waterfowl, raptors, and backyard poultry, including domestic ducks and geese [10]. From March to June 2015, this H5N2 virus predominated in the U.S., with extensive inter-farm transmission occurring in the Midwestern region. Over 7.5 million turkeys and 42.1 million chickens died or were depopulated in the USA during this outbreak which ended in June 2015 [11].

Wild and domestic waterfowl have played an important role in the maintenance and spread of Gs/GD lineage H5 HPAI viruses. Infected migratory waterfowl contributed to the spread of H5N1 and H5N8 HPAI viruses from Asia to other parts of the world [4, 8, 12, 13]. In 2016, H5N8 viruses of the same Gs/GD H5 lineage (HA clade 2.3.4.4) have been again detected in wild waterfowl in Russia, Europe, Middle East and Africa, these viruses causing outbreaks in poultry in many countries [14–16]. Domestic waterfowl have an important role in the maintenance and spread of H5N1 HPAI viruses, and have been shown to serve as intermediaries in the transmission of these viruses between wild waterfowl and other poultry species [17–19]. Wild waterfowl and domestic ducks are also important in the emergence and maintenance of H5N8 HPAI [3]. Hill et al. [20] found that wild waterfowl migration and domestic duck density were important factors in the epidemiology of H5N8 in the Republic of Korea. During the U.S. outbreak, H5N8 and H5N2 HPAI viruses were detected in backyard poultry including waterfowl [21], with possible contact with wild waterfowl or ponds reported in some cases [22]. H5N8 HPAI viruses have also affected commercial duck facilities in Europe and in the U.S. [16, 23, 24]. Recently, non-Gs/GD lineage H5 HPAI viruses (H5N1, H5N2, H5N9) have also caused outbreaks in domestic ducks in France in [25].

H5N1 Gs/GD lineage HPAI viruses are highly lethal to chickens; however, in domestic ducks these viruses can produce a range of clinical outcomes from asymptomatic infections to severe disease with mortality [26]. Both sick and asymptomatic infected ducks can shed high virus quantities into the environment favoring increased risk of transmission and potential outbreaks in commercial poultry. Naturally or experimentally, mortality in ducks caused by HPAI viruses had been infrequently reported before the Gs/GD H5N1 HPAI outbreaks in Asia [27, 28]. However, many Gs/GD lineage H5N1 HPAI viruses, and recently other Gs/GD-derived H5 viruses, have caused disease and death in domestic ducks (reviewed in [26]) [15, 16, 23, 24, 29]. Similarly, in domestic geese, outcome of infection with H5N1 HPAI viruses depends on the virus strain and the geese species. Domestic geese, naturally or experimentally infected with H5N1 viruses, showed from no clinical signs to neurological signs with

or without mortality [30–35]. H5N8 and H5N2 HPAI viruses have also been detected in wild geese [16, 36]. In Taiwan, H5 clade 2.3.4.4 viruses (H5N2, H5N3 and H5N8) produced a severe epidemic in the domestic geese population in 2015, and more than 2.2 million geese died or were culled [37]. Recently, infections with H5N8 HPAI viruses have also been reported in domestic geese in Europe [16].

The recent emergence and recurrence of outbreaks of H5NX Gs/GD lineage HPAI in poultry underscore the need to better understand the pathobiology of these viruses in domestic waterfowl. In this study, in order to improve early detection of H5 HPAI viruses in domestic waterfowl, the infectivity, transmissibility and pathogenicity of the index H5N8 and H5N2 clade 2.3.4.4 HPAI viruses from the U.S. outbreak, was investigated in Pekin ducks and Chinese geese.

Materials and methods

Virus

The highly pathogenic avian influenza (HPAI) viruses A/gyrfalcon/Washington/40188-6/2014 H5N8 (GF/WA/14 H5N8) and A/Northern Pintail/Washington/40964/2014 H5N2 (NP/WA/14 H5N2) were used as challenge viruses. These were the first two Gs/GD H5 HPAI isolates, HA clade 2.3.4.4, from the U.S. outbreak and are considered representative of both the wholly Eurasian H5N8 lineage viruses and reassortant Eurasian/North American lineage H5N2 viruses, respectively [5]. The viruses were propagated and titrated in specific pathogen free (SPF) embryonating chicken eggs (ECE) using standard methods [38]. Stocks were diluted to the target dose with brain–heart infusion (BHI) broth (Becton, Dickinson and Company, Sparks, MD, USA). The experiments were performed in biosecurity level-3 enhanced (BSL-3E) facilities in accordance with procedures approved by the U.S. National Poultry Research Center (USNPRC) Institutional Biosecurity Committee.

Animals and housing

Pekin ducks (*Anas platyrhynchos var. domestica*) and White Chinese geese (*Anser cygnoides*) were obtained at 2 days of age from a commercial hatchery and reared in USNPRC facilities. At 2 weeks of age, birds were transferred to ABSL-3 enhanced facilities for virus challenge. Serum samples were collected from ten birds from each species prior to challenge to ensure that the birds were serologically negative for AI viruses by ELISA (Flock-Check Avian Influenza MultiS-Screen Antibody Test®, IDEXX Laboratories, Westbrook, ME, USA). Each experimental group was housed separately in self-contained isolation units ventilated under negative pressure with inlet and exhaust HEPA-filtered air within the animal

BSL-3 enhanced facilities at Southeast Poultry Research Laboratory. This study and associated procedures were reviewed and approved by the USNPRC Institutional Animal Care and Use Committee (IACUC).

Experimental design and sampling

Similar experiments were conducted with each bird species to evaluate the mean bird infectious dose (BID_{50}), transmissibility, and pathogenicity of the 2014 H5 HPAI index viruses. The 2-week-old ducks and geese were separated into virus-inoculated groups (4–5 birds for each species) as shown in Table 1. Non-inoculated control groups were included for each species. Groups containing 4–5 Pekin ducks were challenged with the appropriate dose per bird (10^2 50% egg infectious doses [EID_{50}] per bird [low dose], 10^4 EID_{50} per bird [medium dose], or 10^6 EID_{50} per bird [high dose]), administered in 0.1 mL by the intrachoanal route. To examine pathogenesis, two additional birds were challenged with the high dose of the viruses. Sham-inoculated control ducks were inoculated with 0.1 mL of sterile allantoic fluid diluted 1:300 in BHI. To assess transmission by contact, three naïve ducks were introduced in the isolators with virus-inoculated ducks at one day post-inoculation (dpi). Groups containing four Chinese geese were challenged by intrachoanal inoculation with sham inoculum or with a dose of 10^2,

10^4, or 10^6 EID_{50}/bird in 0.1 mL of either virus (Table 1). Two additional geese were challenged with the high dose of the viruses. Two naïve geese were introduced in the isolators with virus-inoculated geese at 1 dpi. The inoculum titers were subsequently verified by back titration in ECE as 1.7–1.9 (low dose), 3.5–3.9 (medium dose), and 5.7–6.1 (high dose) $\log_{10} EID_{50}$/0.1 mL.

Clinical signs were monitored daily for 10 days in the duck experiment and for 11 days in the geese experiment. Oropharyngeal (OP) and cloacal (CL) swabs were collected from all birds at days 2, 4, 7 and 10, 11 to determine virus shed. Body temperatures were taken at 2 and 4 dpi from birds inoculated with the high dose of the viruses and from the sham inoculated control birds. Significant difference for body temperatures between groups was analyzed using Kruskal–Wallis test (GraphPad Prism™ Version 5 software). A p value of < 0.05 was considered to be significant. For each species, the two additional birds challenged with the high dose of the viruses were euthanized and necropsied at 4 dpi to evaluate gross lesions. A full set of tissues were collected from each bird and fixed in 10% neutral buffered formalin solution, paraffin-embedded, sectioned, and stained with hematoxylin-and-eosin for histopathologic evaluation. Duplicate sections were stained by immunohistochemical (IHC) methods to determine influenza viral antigen distribution

Table 1 Mortality, number of birds infected, 50% bird infectious doses, and seroconversion of 2-week-old Pekin ducks and Chinese geese inoculated by the intrachoanal route and contact-exposed to A/gyrfalcon/WA/40188-6/2014 (H5N8) and A/Northern pintail/WA/40964/2014 (H5N2) HPAI viruses

Species	Virus	Inoculated birds					Contact-exposed birds		
		Virus dose ($\log_{10} EID_{50}$)	# of infected birds/total[a]	BID_{50}[b] ($\log_{10}$ EID_{50})	Mortality[c] (dpi[d])	Serology[d] (range of antibody titers, $\log_2$)	# of infected birds/total	Mortality (dpe[e])	Serology (range of antibody titers, $\log_2$)
Pekin ducks	H5N8	2	0/5	3.0	0/5	0/5	0/3	0/3	0/3
		4	5/5		0/5	5/5 (4–5)	1/3	0/3	1/3 (4)
		6	5/5		0/5	5/5 (4–5)	2/3	0/3	2/3 (4)
	H5N2	2	0/5	3.0	0/5	0/5	0/3	0/3	0/3
		4	5/5		0/5	5/5 (3)	2/3	0/3	1/3 (3)
		6	4/4		0/4	4/4 (3–4)	3/3	0/3	3/3 (3–5)
Chinese geese	H5N8	2	4/4	< 2	0/4	1/4 (4)	2/2	0/2	0/2
		4	4/4		0/4	0/4	2/2	0/2	1/2 (3)
		6	4/4		0/4	2/4 (3)	2/2	1/2 (11)	0/2
	H5N2	2	0/4	3.0	0/4	0/4	0/2	0/2	0/4
		4	4/4		0/4	1/4 (3)	2/2	1/2 (10)	0/1
		6	4/4		1/4 (8)	1/3 (3)	2/2	0/2	0/2

[a] Number of birds infected/total number of birds inoculated; determined by qRRT-PCR and serology.

[b] BID_{50}, mean bird infectious dose.

[c] Number of dead birds/total number of birds inoculated (days post-inoculation).

[d] Number of birds with positive antibody titers/total number of birds inoculated.

[e] Days post-exposure.

in individual tissues [39]. Portions of lung, heart, brain, muscle and spleen were also collected and stored at −80 °C for subsequent virus detection and quantification. Sera were collected from all surviving birds at the end of the experiments to evaluate infection status by antibody levels using hemagglutination inhibition (HI) assay. HI assays were performed using standard methods and homologous antigen [40]. The virus infectious dose was calculated by the Reed–Muench method [41], using the criteria that birds were considered infected if they shed detectable levels of virus at any time and/or were positive for antibody at the end of the study.

Viral RNA quantification in swabs and tissues

OP and CL swabs were collected in 1 mL of BHI broth with a final concentration of 10 µg/mL of gentamicin, 100 units/mL of penicillin G, and 56 µg/mL of amphotericin B, and kept frozen at −80 °C until processed. RNA was extracted using MagMAX™-96 AI/ND Viral RNA Isolation Kit® (Ambion, Inc.) following the manufacturer's instructions. qRRT-PCR reactions targeting the influenza virus M gene [42] were conducted using AgPath-ID one-step RT-PCR Kit (Ambion, Austin, TX, USA) and the ABI 7500 Fast Real-Time PCR system (Applied Biosystem, Carlsbad, CA, USA). Viral RNA was extracted from tissues using Trizol LS reagent (Invitrogen, Carlsbad, CA, USA) and the Qiagen RNeasy Mini Kit (Qiagen Corp, Valencia, CA, USA). In tissue homogenates, and in order to standardize the amount of nonspecific RNA from the tissue, the resulting viral RNA extracts were quantified by NanoDrop™ 1000 Spectrophotometer (Thermo Fisher Scientific) following the manufacturer's

instructions and accordingly diluted with phosphate buffered saline to obtain 50 ng/µL. For virus quantification, a standard curve was established with RNA extracted from dilutions of the same titrated stock of the challenge virus. Results were reported as EID_{50}/mL or EID_{50}/g equivalents and the lower limit of detection was was $10^{1.8}$ EID_{50}/mL for both viruses. For statistical purposes, qRRT-PCR negative samples were given a numeric value of 1.7 $\log_{10}$ EID_{50}/mL (1.7 $\log_{10}$ EID_{50}/g).

Results

Infectivity, transmission and pathogenicity of the H5N8 and H5N2 HPAI viruses in domestic ducks

No ducks were infected in the groups inoculated with the lowest dose (10^2 EID_{50}) of each virus (Table 1). Birds were considered infected if they had detectable virus or seroconverted. All ducks inoculated with the medium (10^4 EID_{50}) or high (10^6 EID_{50}) dose of the viruses were infected but no mortality occurred. The 50% bird infectious dose (BID_{50}) for both viruses was 3 $\log_{10}$ EID_{50}. One or 2 of 3 contact ducks in the groups inoculated with the medium dose for both viruses were infected, and 2 or 3 of 3 contact ducks in the high dose groups were infected. No mortality was observed in these ducks either.

A significant difference in body temperature was observed at 2 dpi, but not at 4 dpi, between sham-inoculated control ducks and H5N8-inoculated ducks (high dose group) (Figure 1). Four of six ducks inoculated with the H5N2 virus also showed high body temperatures. Conjunctivitis, tearing of the eyes, and diarrhea was observed intermittently in a low percentage of ducks in each group (1–2 ducks). One duck in the H5N2 high dose

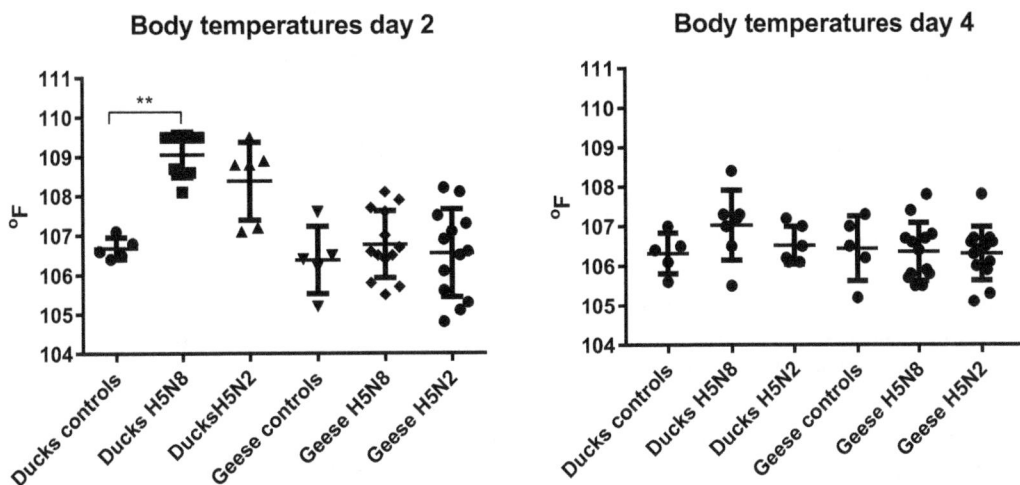

Figure 1 Mean body temperatures of 2-week-old Pekin ducks and Chinese geese inoculated by the intrachoanal route with 10^6 EID_{50} of H5N8 and H5N2 HPAI viruses, at 2 and 4 days post-inoculation. Bars represent the standard deviation of the mean. Significant difference in body temperature compared to controls (**$p < 0.01$).

group presented mild ataxia starting at 2 dpi. At the end of the study (10 dpi) one duck from the H5N8 medium dose group and a second duck from the H5N2 high dose group also had mild ataxia. No other clinical signs were observed in the virus-inoculated and contact ducks. At 4 dpi, two ducks inoculated with the high dose of the viruses were euthanized for gross examination. One of the ducks inoculated with the H5N8 virus had airsacculitis and marbled spleen. No gross lesions were observed in the three other ducks.

Infectivity, transmission and pathogenicity of the H5N8 and H5N2 HPAI viruses in domestic geese

All geese inoculated with the H5N8 virus were infected regardless of the dose given (BID_{50} was less than 2 $\log_{10}$ EID_{50}) (Table 1). No geese were infected in the group inoculated with the lowest dose of the H5N2 virus, but the virus did infect all geese at the medium and high doses (BID_{50} was 3 $\log_{10}$ EID_{50}). No differences in body temperature were found among virus-inoculated geese (high dose groups) at 2 and 4 dpi when compared to sham-inoculated controls (Figure 1). In the groups of geese inoculated with the H5N8 virus, no or mild clinical signs (conjunctivitis) were observed during the study, but at 11 dpi one goose from the high dose group had mild tremors and incoordination, and one of the contacts from the same group was found dead. In the groups of geese inoculated with the H5N2 virus, one goose and a contact goose from the high and medium dose groups presented severe ataxia and torticollis, at 8 and 10 days respectively, and were euthanized and necropsied. At 11 dpi, one goose from each of the medium and high dose groups had mild ataxia. The rest of the geese inoculated with H5N2 showed no or mild clinical signs (conjunctivitis). No gross lesions were observed in the two geese that were euthanized and examined at 4 dpi from the H5N8 pathogenesis group. The two geese from the H5N2 pathogenesis group had multifocal areas of necrosis in the pancreas. The goose from the H5N2 high dose group euthanized at 8 dpi due to severe neurological signs had nasal discharge and empty intestines. The contact goose from the H5N2 medium dose group euthanized at 10 dpi had a pale spleen, enlarged heart, hemorrhagic thymus, malacic brain, and nasal discharge.

Microscopic lesions and viral antigen distribution

In order to evaluate microscopic lesions and sites of virus replication, tissues collected from ducks and geese necropsied at 4 dpi were examined, and immunohistochemical staining for AI virus nucleoprotein antigen was performed (Table 2; Figure 2). Tissues from the two geese that were euthanized at 8 and 10 dpi were also examined.

In all ducks and geese examined at 4 dpi, mild catarrhal rhinitis and sinusitis was observed. The tracheas had mild degenerative changes of the overlying epithelium and mild lymphocytic infiltration in the submucosa. Also present: mild to moderate interstitial pneumonia, mild airsacculitis, focal necrosis of the epithelia of the Harderian glands, mild proliferation of gut-associated lymphoid tissues, and mild to moderate lymphoid depletion in cloacal bursa, thymus and spleen. Remaining organs lacked significant histopathologic changes. The two geese from the H5N2 pathogenesis group had, in addition, multifocal areas of necrosis in the pancreas, and the two geese examined at 8 and 10 dpi had individual cell necrosis of myofibers and focal mononuclear inflammation in the heart and thigh skeletal muscle (Figures 2A and B), and in the brain, randomly scattered foci of malacia, gliosis and perivascular cuffing (Figure 2C). Viral antigen staining was present in multiple tissues from ducks and geese infected with the H5 HPAI viruses indicating systemic infection (results in Table 2; Figures 2C–G). Viral antigen was present in epithelial cells and infiltrating phagocytes in the nasal turbinates, trachea, bronchus, lung air capillaries, air sac, Harderian glands, cloacal bursa, and in resident and infiltrating phagocytes of the spleen. Viral antigen staining was also present in pancreatic acinar epithelial cells, hepatocytes, neurons and glial cells of the brain, fragmented cardiac and skeletal myofibers of geese infected with the H5N2 virus.

Replication of H5N8 and H5N2 HPAI viruses in Pekin ducks and Chinese geese

Quantitation of viral shed was performed by qRRT-PCR using extrapolation of a standard curve generated with the challenge viruses via virus isolation and titration. OP and CL viral shed was examined at 2, 4, 7 and 10 dpi in ducks (Figures 3A, C, E and G) and at 2, 4, 7 and 11 dpi in geese (Figures 4A, C, E and G). To evaluate viral shed in contact birds, naïve birds were introduced in the isolator with inoculated birds at 1 dpi and sampled at 1, 3, 6 and 9 or 10 days post-exposure (dpe) (Figures 3 and 4B, D, F and H).

Ducks inoculated with the low dose of either the H5N8 or H5N2 virus did not shed virus and virus was not transmitted to contacts. Ducks inoculated or contact-exposed in the medium and high dose groups shed virus mostly through the OP route (Figures 3A, B, E and F); few ducks (including the contacts) shed through the CL route and, if so, at very low titers (Figures 3C, D, G and H). Ducks from the medium and high dose groups shed virus by the OP route up to 7 dpi (6 dpe for contacts). Ducks inoculated with the high doses of the viruses were able to transmit to 3–4 of the 6 contacts, but higher titers were shed by the H5N2 contacts (Figures 3F and H).

All geese inoculated with H5N8 virus shed virus through the OP and CL routes at high titers regardless of

Table 2 AI virus antigen immunohistochemical staining in tissues from Pekin ducks and Chinese geese inoculated by the intrachoanal route or contact-exposed to H5N8 and H5N2 HPAI viruses

Species	Virus	Detection of AI virus antigen in tissues													
		Nasal ep.	Trachea	Lung	Air sacs	Brain	Heart	Spleen	Liver	Skeletal muscle	Pancreas	Cloacal bursa	Cecal tonsils	Harderian gland	Thymus
Pekin ducks 4 dpi	H5N8	++/+	+/++	+/++	+++/+	+/+	+/+	++/+	-/-	+/+	-/-	+/-	-/-	++/+++	-/-
	H5N2	+/+	+/+	+/-	+/+	-/+	-/-	-/-	-/-	+/-	-/-	+/-	-/-	-/-	+/-
Chinese geese 4 dpi	H5N8	+/++	+/-	+/++	+/-	+/+	+/++	++/+	-/+	+/-	-/-	-/-	-/-	-/+++	-/+
	H5N2	++/+++	+/+	++/++	+/na	++/++	++/+++	++/+++	+/+	+/-	+/+	+/++	++/++	-/-	++/+++
Chinese geese 8 and 10 dpi	H5N2	+/+	+/+	++/++	na/na	+++/++++	++/++	++/+	+/+	+/+	+/+	+/++	+/+	na/na	+/-

Birds were euthanized at 4, 8 or 10 dpi (bird 1/bird 2).

Kidney, adrenal glands, and intestine were negative for virus antigen staining.

– no positive cells, + single positive cells, ++ scattered groups of positive cells, +++ widespread positivity, *na* not available.

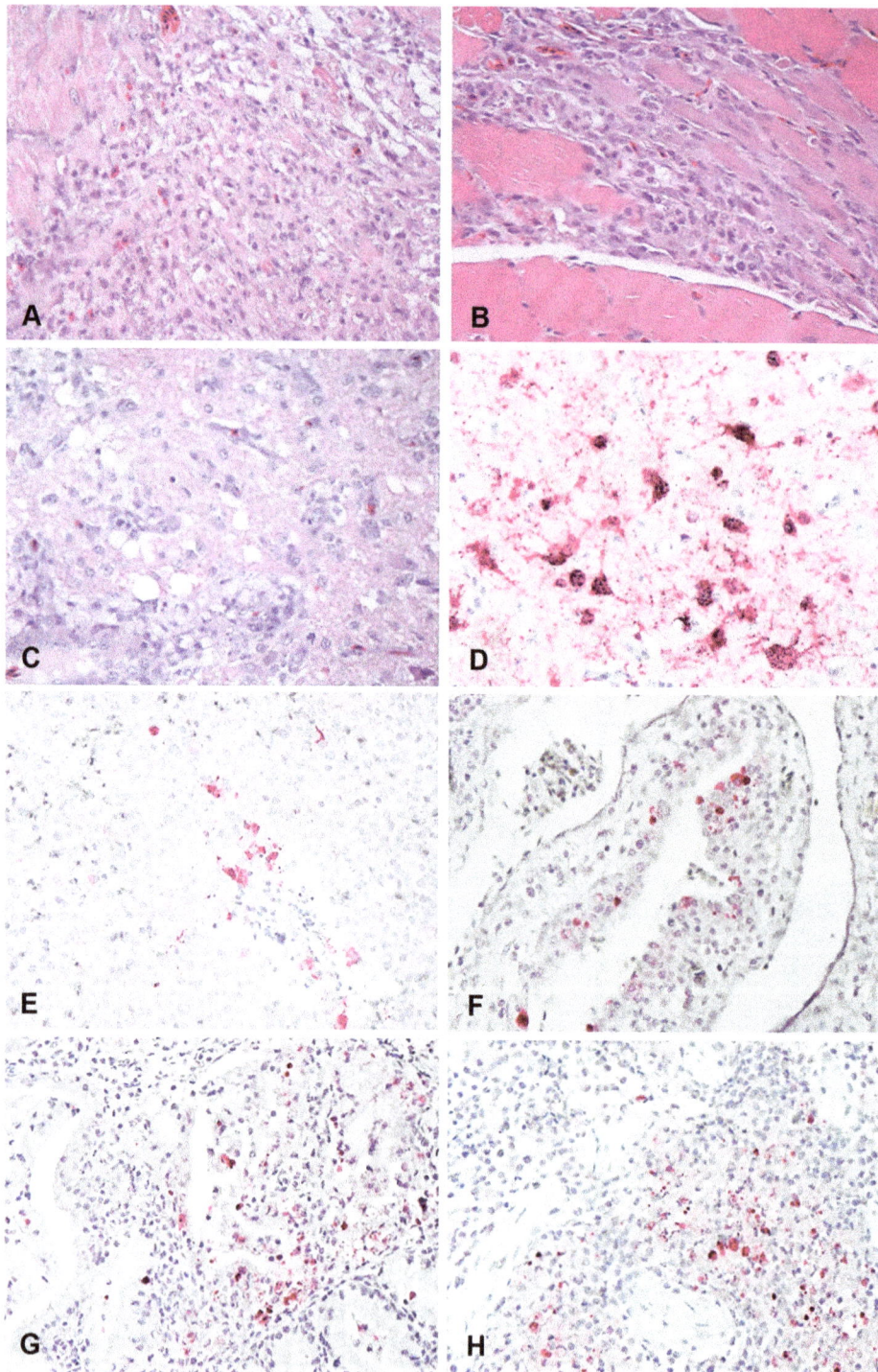

Figure 2 Histological lesions and immunohistochemical detection of viral antigen in 2-week old Pekin ducks and Chinese geese inoculated by the intrachoanal route with H5N8 and H5N2 HPAI viruses. 40×; viral antigen staining in red. A Heart. Goose inoculated with H5N2, 8 dpi; lymphoplasmacytic inflammation. **B** Skeletal muscle. Goose inoculated with H5N2, 10 dpi; lymphoplasmacytic inflammation. **C** Cerebrum. Goose inoculated with H5N2, 8 dpi; foci of malacia, and gliosis. **D** Cerebrum. Goose inoculated with H5N2, 10 dpi; viral antigen in neurons and glial cells. **E** Spleen. Goose inoculated with H5N2, 8 dpi; viral antigen in necrotic cells and mononuclear cells. **F** Airsac. Pekin duck inoculated with H5N8, 4 dpi; viral antigen present in epithelial cells. **G** Harderian gland. Pekin duck inoculated with H5N8, 4 dpi; viral antigen present in epithelial cells and infiltrating monocytes. **H** Lung. Pekin duck inoculated with H5N8, 4 dpi; viral antigen in epithelium of air capillaries and infiltrating monocytes.

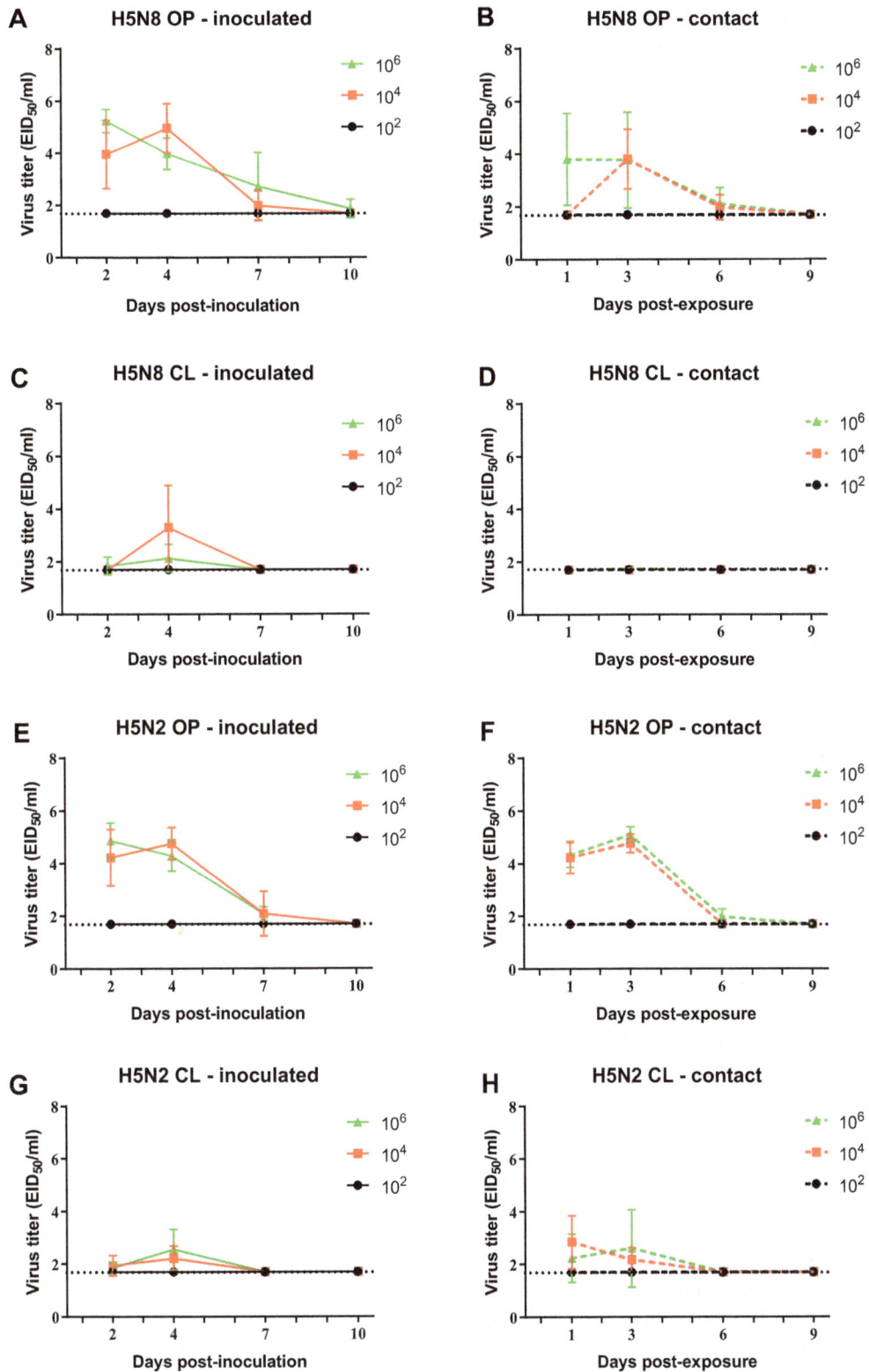

Figure 3 Mean oropharyngeal (OP) and cloacal (CL) viral shed from 2-week-old Pekin ducks directly inoculated (A, C, E, G) or contact-exposed (B, D, F, H) with H5N8 and H5N2 HPAI viruses. Ducks were inoculated with 10^2, 10^4 and 10^6 EID_{50} of either virus and titers determined by qRRT-PCR. Bars represent the standard deviation of the mean. Swabs from which virus was not detected were given a numeric value of $10^{1.7}$ EID_{50}/mL.

the inoculation dose (Figures 4A and C). H5N8 and H5N2 contact exposed geese became infected and showed a similar virus shedding pattern as the directly inoculated geese (Figures 4B and D). Only geese inoculated with the medium and high dose of the H5N2 virus shed virus (Figure 2E, G). Contact geese in these groups also shed virus similar to the inoculated birds (Figures 4F and H). H5N2 OP viral titers were similar to those observed with the H5N8 virus, but H5N2 virus was shed for longer by the CL route. Overall, the Pekin ducks shed lower virus titers and for a shorter period of time (7 days vs 11 days) than the Chinese geese. The peak of viral shedding for both viruses in both species was between 3 and 5 dpi.

To evaluate systemic replication of H5N8 and H5N2 HPAI viruses in ducks and geese, viral titers were determined in brain, heart, spleen, lung and muscle. Tissues were collected from 2 birds of each 10^6 EID_{50} inoculated groups at 4 dpi (Figure 5). Ducks and geese showed moderate to high H5N8 and H5N2 HPAI virus titers in all tissues examined, with the highest titers found in tissues of geese inoculated with the H5N2 virus. Tissues were also collected from the two geese exposed to H5N2 virus and showing neurological signs; both birds also presenting high virus titers in all tissues, especially in brain.

Serology

Serum samples were examined for detectable titers of antibodies against the corresponding challenge virus at 10 or 11 dpi, for Pekin ducks or geese respectively. All Pekin ducks inoculated with the medium and high dose of either virus seroconverted (Table 1); 1 of 3 contacts placed in the medium dose groups and 2 or 3 of 3 in the highest dose groups seroconverted. Only one goose inoculated with the low dose, two geese inoculated with the high dose and one contact goose in the medium dose group seroconverted to the H5N8 virus. Two geese, one from the medium dose and one from the high dose group seroconverted to the H5N2 virus.

Discussion

In this study we describe the pathogenesis and transmission dynamics of the U.S. index H5N8 and H5N2 HPAI viruses (Gs/GD lineage, HA clade 2.3.4.4) in domestic ducks and geese with the objective of better understanding the infection process in order to improve strategies for early detection of HPAI viruses in domestic waterfowl. Based on viral shed and serology results, only ducks inoculated with the medium and high doses of the viruses (10^4 and 10^6 EID_{50}, respectively) were infected and were able to efficiently transmit to contacts, resulting in a BID_{50} of 3 $\log_{10}$ EID_{50} for both viruses. Similarly, geese inoculated with the medium and high doses of the H5N2 HPAI virus and the contact birds in these groups

were infected, resulting also in a BID_{50} of 3 $\log_{10}$ EID_{50}. In contrast to ducks, all geese inoculated with the low, medium and high doses of the H5N8 HPAI virus were infected and transmitted the virus to contacts, with a resulting BID_{50} of < 2 $\log_{10}$ EID_{50}. These findings support the conclusion that geese were more susceptible than ducks to infection by the H5N8 virus.

Although most ducks and geese in this study survived virus infection and showed only minimal clinical signs, occasionally neurological signs were present in both species but were more common and severe in geese. Virus was detected by qRRT-PCR and IHC in the brain of both ducks and geese, but virus titers were higher and presence of viral antigen was more common in the brain of infected geese, especially in geese infected with the H5N2 virus. In general, virus replication in tissues was higher in the geese than in the ducks. This higher virus replication and more severe clinical signs in geese compared to ducks has been also observed in other studies comparing H5N1 HPAI virus infections side by side using these species [31, 32]. In addition, geese shed both viruses for longer times and in higher titers, especially by the CL route, than ducks, indicating that the viruses tested in this study replicated better in this species.

The Gs/GD H5N1 HPAI viruses developed the unique capacity among HPAI viruses to infect and cause disease in domestic waterfowl and wild birds producing a range of syndromes from asymptomatic infections to systemic disease and death [31]. The pathogenicity of Gs/GD lineage H5N1 HPAI viruses in waterfowl is associated with the efficiency of virus replication [43]. Viral dissemination to the brain, leading to severe neurological dysfunction, is considered one of the causes of the high virulence of H5N1 viruses in ducks, but lesions to other important organs could lead to multi-organ failure and death [44–47]. In addition to the virus strain, the susceptibility of wild and domestic waterfowl to H5N1 HPAI virus infection and the presentation of disease vary depending on other factors, including the age and species of the birds and management practices [19, 48]. In wild geese, neurological disease along with systemic virus replication and mortality was observed following experimental inoculation with Gs/GD lineage H5N1 HPAI viruses [49, 50]. Canada geese (*Branta canadiensis*) experienced sporadic deaths in natural H5N1 HPAI virus outbreaks [51–54], and have shown high susceptibility to the virus as evidenced by systemic replication and high mortality rates after experimental infection [34, 50, 55], although age-related differences in susceptibility were described [56]. Similar findings have been reported for other species of wild geese, including bar-headed geese (*Anser indicus*) and cackling geese (*B. utchinsii*) [49, 57]. Domestic geese naturally infected with H5N1 HPAI virus showed severe

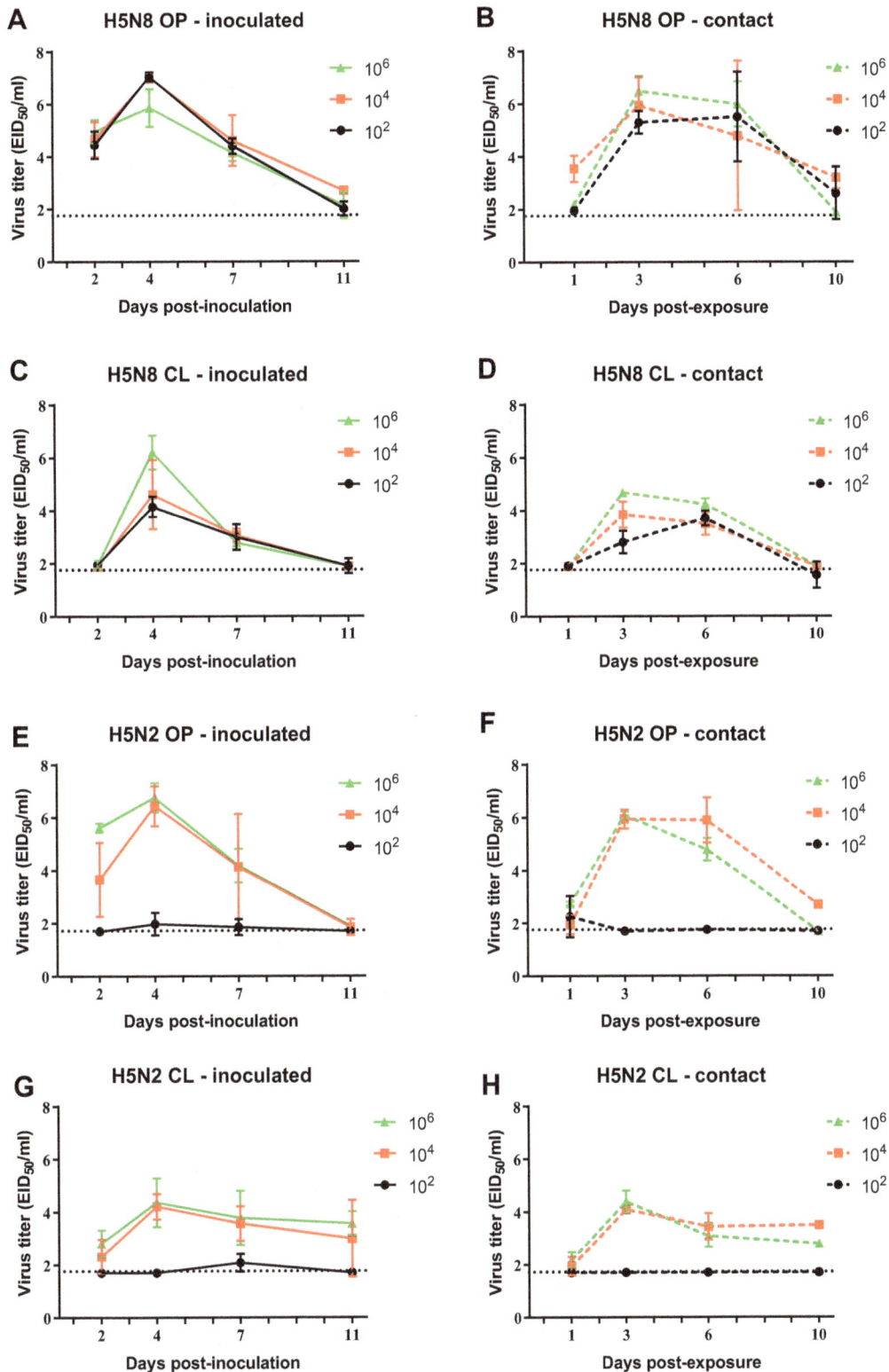

Figure 4 Mean oropharyngeal (OP) and cloacal (CL) viral shed from 2-week-old Chinese geese directly inoculated (A, C, E, G) or contact-exposed (B, D, F, H) with H5N8 and H5N2 HPAI viruses. Geese were inoculated with 10^2, 10^4 and 10^6 EID_{50} of either virus and titers determined by qRRT-PCR. Bars represent the standard deviation of the mean. Swabs from which virus was not detected were given a numeric value of $10^{1.7}$ EID_{50}/mL.

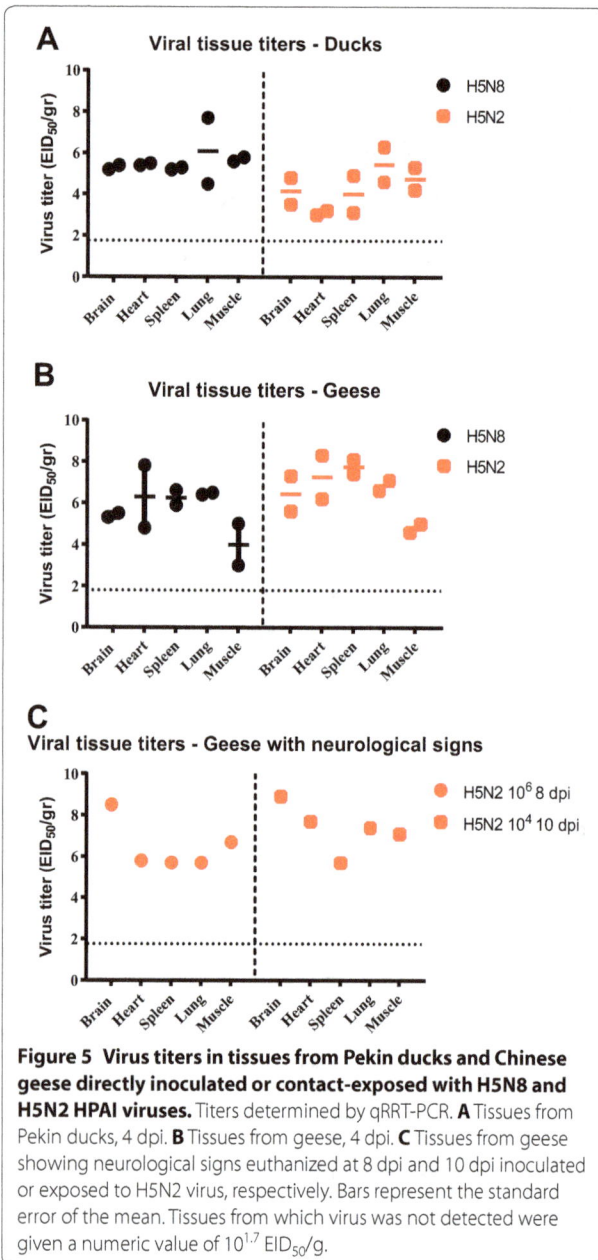

Figure 5 Virus titers in tissues from Pekin ducks and Chinese geese directly inoculated or contact-exposed with H5N8 and H5N2 HPAI viruses. Titers determined by qRRT-PCR. **A** Tissues from Pekin ducks, 4 dpi. **B** Tissues from geese, 4 dpi. **C** Tissues from geese showing neurological signs euthanized at 8 dpi and 10 dpi inoculated or exposed to H5N2 virus, respectively. Bars represent the standard error of the mean. Tissues from which virus was not detected were given a numeric value of $10^{1.7}$ EID_{50}/g.

clinical signs including neurological signs [33]. Domestic geese (*Anser anser var. domestica*) experimentally infected with H5N1 viruses presented neurological signs and 40–50% mortality [34]. Similarly, domestic White Chinese geese (*Anser cygnoides*) showed high mortality when experimentally infected [30]. However, Embden geese (*Anser anser var. domestica*) and Graylag geese (*Anser anser*) inoculated with different H5N1 HPAI viruses developed neurological signs, but lacked mortality [31, 32]. These observations indicate that both the virus strain and waterfowl species affect the outcome of

infection with Gs/GD lineage H5 viruses, similar to what was observed in our study.

Most Pekin ducks infected with either of the H5 viruses examined in this study had high body temperatures at 2 dpi when compared to controls, but this difference was only significant in the H5N8 group. An increase in body temperature after infection with the same H5N8 virus was seen in our previous studies with mallards [58, 59], and it has also been reported with H5N1 virus infections in several breeds of *Anas platyrrhynchs var. domestica* ducks (Pekin, Mallards, Black Runners, Rouen, Khaki Campbell), but not in Muscovy ducks (*Cairina moschata*) [60, 61]. Similar to Muscovy ducks, no increase in body temperature was observed in the geese, indicating differences in the innate immune response between Pekin ducks and geese, which could also explain the differences in disease severity. Most surviving geese examined at 11 dpi did not have antibodies against the challenge virus, contrary to most ducks, also indicating differences in humoral immune responses between these two species. This low seroconversion rate in geese after AI virus infection was also reported in our previous study examining the pathogenesis of a H7N9 virus in different avian species [62]. The immunological differences observed between waterfowl species could affect virus infection, replication, tissue tropism, and virus clearing, consequently affecting the severity of the pathogenic outcome observed.

When comparing the present study with our previous studies examining the pathobiology of the same H5N8 and H5N2 HPAI viruses in mallards, we observe that both viruses are more infectious for mallards (BID_{50} of < 2 $\log_{10}$ EID_{50}) than for Pekin ducks (3 $\log_{10}$ EID_{50}) [58, 59]. Similar to Pekin ducks, infected mallards showed minimal clinical signs and transmitted the viruses to all contacts; however, mallards shed virus for longer than Pekin ducks. Interestingly, when examining two H5N2 HPAI viruses isolated later in the U.S. outbreak from commercial poultry, both had a similar high infectivity as the index H5N2 virus in mallards, but one of the viruses showed lower replication and one caused some mortality when given at high doses [58]. These results show that individual H5N2 Gs/GD clade 2.3.4.4 viruses have different pathobiology in infected ducks, and that the duck type can also affect the pathogenic outcome of infection.

Likewise, a range of pathobiological outcomes, from no clinical signs to severe disease including neurological signs, were observed in wild and domestic ducks experimentally inoculated with H5N8 viruses of the same Gs/GD lineage (clade 2.3.4.4), with mortality rates varying from 0 to 20% [1, 29, 58, 59, 63–68], and the viruses transmitting efficiently to naïve contacts [63–65, 67, 68]. A study describing the pathobiologic characteristics of a H5N1 virus isolated in Canada also belonging to HA clade 2.3.4.4, found that the virus was highly pathogenic to juvenile Muscovy ducks and adult Chinese geese causing systemic infections with neurological signs and mortality (36 and 22% respectively) in both species [69]. The virus was also efficiently transmitted and caused mortality (40 and 80% respectively) in naïve contact ducks and geese of the same species.

Natural infections of domestic ducks with H5N8 HPAI viruses have been associated with disease and mortality, but such mortality is typically low. Hungary reported a H5N8 HPAI outbreak during late winter of 2015 at a Pekin duck fattening facility [70]. In addition to increased mortality in the flock and respiratory symptoms, the affected birds showed lethargy and neurological signs. The H5N8 HPAI outbreak in Korea in 2014 mostly resulted in drops in egg production [63], and the outbreak in the United Kingdom in 2014 showed a gradual reduction in egg production and mild increased mortality over a 7-day period [24]. Similarly, an outbreak with H5N8 HPAI virus in commercial Pekin ducks in California in early 2015 resulted in decreased feed consumption, moderate increase in mortality and severe neurological signs in 2% of the ducks [23]. In these natural infections other factors could have increased the severity of disease presentation. In line with this, fungal and bacterial lesions probably exacerbated the mortality and clinical presentation in the outbreak in the UK, motivating disease investigation [24]. If concurrent infections with other pathogens or added stress under intensive conditions do not prompt an avian notifiable disease investigation, the virus can continue to circulate with mild clinical signs or asymptomatically in domestic waterfowl and potentially spread to other holdings, resulting in a more extensive outbreak of HPAI.

As the Gs/GD H5 HPAI viruses continue to evolve and reassort, antigenic and genetic divergent strains have emerged, many expressing distinct pathobiological features and increased virulence for waterfowl. New H5N8 reassortants recently detected in Europe have caused disease and death in both domestic and wild ducks [15, 16], these viruses appearing to be more pathogenic for waterfowl and other wild bird species than the 2014–2015 H5N8 HPAI viruses.

In conclusion, the results of the present study indicate that infection of naïve domestic Pekin ducks and Chinese geese with clade 2.3.4.4 H5 HPAI viruses resulted in efficient virus replication and transmission to contacts. Mortality was low and clinical signs were uncommon, consisting mostly of mild neurological signs. In the field, clinical signs could be exacerbated by other infectious and non-infectious factors. Our findings emphasize the need to implement and improve active surveillance in domestic waterfowl (backyard and commercial), and increase biosecurity compliance to reduce direct and indirect contact between poultry and wild waterfowl in order to detect, prevent and control AI in poultry.

Abbreviations
AI: avian influenza; Gs/GD: A/goose/Guangdong/1/1996; dpi: day post-inoculation; dpe: days post-exposure; ECE: embryonating chicken eggs; HA: hemagglutinin; HI: hemagglutination inhibition; HPAI: highly pathogenic avian influenza; LPAI: low pathogenic avian influenza; BID_{50}: mean bird infectious dose; MDT: mean death time; EID_{50}: mean egg infectious dose; na: not applicable; qRRT-PCR: quantitative real-time RT-PCR; SPF: specific pathogen free.

Competing interests
The authors declare that they have no competing interests.

Authors' contributions
MPJ conceived this project. MPJ, MCH, EDJ, and DS conducted the animal experiments and sample processing. MPJ, MCH, DS, KB analyzed the data. MPJ, MCH, EDJ, DS, KB, and DES help write and reviewed the manuscript. All authors read and approved the final manuscript.

Acknowledgements
The authors appreciate the technical assistance provided by Scott Lee and Nikolai Lee, and the animal care provided by Roger Brock, Keith Crawford, and Gerald Damron in conducting these studies.

Funding
This research was supported by the USDA/ARS CRIS Project 6612-32000-063-00D and by Center of Research in Influenza Pathogenesis (CRIP) an NIAID funded Center of Excellence in Influenza Research and Surveillance (CEIRS, Contract HHSN272201400008C). Its contents are solely the responsibility of the authors and do not necessarily represent the official views of the USDA or NIH. Mention of trade names or commercial products in this publication is solely for the purpose of providing specific information and does not imply recommendation or endorsement by the USDA. USDA is an equal opportunity provider and employer.

References
1. Zhao K, Gu M, Zhong L, Duan Z, Zhang Y, Zhu Y, Zhao G, Zhao M, Chen Z, Hu S, Liu W, Liu X, Peng D, Liu X (2013) Characterization of three H5N5 and one H5N8 highly pathogenic avian influenza viruses in China. Vet Microbiol 163:351–357
2. Wong FY, Phommachanh P, Kalpravidh W, Chanthavisouk C, Gilbert J, Bingham J, Davies KR, Cooke J, Eagles D, Phiphakhavong S, Shan S, Stevens V, Williams DT, Bounma P, Khambounheuang B, Morrissy C, Douangngeun B, Morzaria S (2015) Reassortant highly pathogenic influenza A(H5N6) virus in Laos. Emerg Infect Dis 21:511–516
3. Verhagen JH, Herfst S, Fouchier RA (2015) Infectious disease. How a virus travels the world. Science 347:616–617
4. Lee DH, Torchetti MK, Winker K, Ip HS, Song CS, Swayne DE (2015) Intercontinental spread of Asian-origin H5N8 to North America through Beringia by migratory birds. J Virol 89:6521–6524

5. Ip HS, Torchetti MK, Crespo R, Kohrs P, DeBruyn P, Mansfield KG, Baszler T, Badcoe L, Bodenstein B, Shearn-Bochsler V, Killian ML, Pedersen JC, Hines N, Gidlewski T, DeLiberto T, Sleeman JM (2015) Novel Eurasian highly pathogenic avian influenza A H5 viruses in wild birds, Washington, USA, 2014. Emerg Infect Dis 21:886–890

6. Wu H, Peng X, Xu L, Jin C, Cheng L, Lu X, Xie T, Yao H, Wu N (2014) Novel reassortant influenza A(H5N8) viruses in domestic ducks, eastern China. Emerg Infect Dis 20:1315–1318

7. Lee YJ, Kang HM, Lee EK, Song BM, Jeong J, Kwon YK, Kim HR, Lee KJ, Hong MS, Jang I, Choi KS, Kim JY, Lee HJ, Kang MS, Jeong OM, Baek JH, Joo YS, Park YH, Lee HS (2014) Novel reassortant influenza A(H5N8) viruses, South Korea. Emerg Infect Dis 20:1087–1089

8. Jeong J, Kang HM, Lee EK, Song BM, Kwon YK, Kim HR, Choi KS, Kim JY, Lee HJ, Moon OK, Jeong W, Choi J, Baek JH, Joo YS, Park YH, Lee HS, Lee YJ (2014) Highly pathogenic avian influenza virus (H5N8) in domestic poultry and its relationship with migratory birds in South Korea during 2014. Vet Microbiol 173:249–257

9. Pasick J, Berhane Y, Joseph T, Bowes V, Hisanaga T, Handel K, Alexandersen S (2015) Reassortant highly pathogenic influenza A H5N2 virus containing gene segments related to Eurasian H5N8 in British Columbia, Canada, 2014. Sci Rep 5:9484

10. United States Department of Agriculture, Animal and Plant Health Inspection Service. Highly pathogenic H5 avian influenza confirmed in wild birds in Washington State H5N2 found in Northern pintail ducks and H5N8 found in captive Gyrfalcons. https://www.usda.gov/wps/portal/usda/usdahome?contentid=2014/12/0273.xml&contentidonly=true. Accessed 15 Jan 2017

11. United States Department of Agriculture, animal and plant health inspection service. Animal disease information, avian influenza, HPAI 2014/2015 confirmed detections. https://www.aphis.usda.gov/aphis/ourfocus/animalhealth/animal-disease-information/avian-influenza-disease/sa_detections_by_states/hpai-2014-2015-confirmed-detections. Accessed 15 Jan 2017

12. Cattoli G, Monne I, Fusaro A, Joannis TM, Lombin LH, Aly MM, Arafa AS, Sturm-Ramirez KM, Couacy-Hymann E, Awuni JA, Batawui KB, Awoume KA, Aplogan GL, Sow A, Ngangnou AC, El Nasri Hamza IM, Gamatié D, Dauphin G, Domenech JM, Capua I (2009) Highly pathogenic avian influenza virus subtype H5N1 in Africa: a comprehensive phylogenetic analysis and molecular characterization of isolates. PLoS One 4:e4842

13. Keawcharoen J, van Riel D, van Amerongen G, Bestebroer T, Beyer WE, van Lavieren R, Osterhaus AD, Fouchier RA, Kuiken T (2008) Wild ducks as long-distance vectors of highly pathogenic avian influenza virus (H5N1). Emerg Infect Dis 14:600–607

14. Lee DH, Sharshov K, Swayne DE, Kurskaya O, Sobolev I, Kabilov M, Alekseev A, Irza V, Shestopalov A (2017) Novel reassortant clade 2.3.4.4 avian influenza A(H5N8) virus in wild aquatic birds, Russia, 2016. Emerg Infect Dis 23:359–360

15. Pohlmann A, Starick E, Harder T, Höper D, Globig A, Staubach C, Dietze K, Grund C, Strebelow G, Ulrich RG, Schinköthe J, Teifke JP, Conraths FJ, Mettenleiter TC, Beer M (2017) Outbreaks among wild birds and domestic poultry caused by reassorted influenza A(H5N8) clade 2.3.4.4 viruses, Germany, 2016. Emerg Infect Dis 23:633–636

16. Food and Agricultural Organization of the United Nations. Animal Production and Health. H5N8 HPAI Global situation update. http://www.fao.org/ag/againfo/programmes/en/empres/H5N8/situation_update.html. Accessed 15 Jan 2017

17. Gilbert M, Chaitaweesub P, Parakamawongsa T, Premashthira S, Tiensin T, Kalpravidh W, Wagner H, Slingenbergh J (2006) Free-grazing ducks and highly pathogenic avian influenza, Thailand. Emerg Infect Dis 12:227–234

18. Henning J, Wibawa H, Morton J, Usman TB, Junaidi A, Meers J (2010) Scavenging ducks and transmission of highly pathogenic avian influenza, Java, Indonesia. Emerg Infect Dis 16:1244–1250

19. Songserm T, Jam-on R, Sae-Heng N, Meemak N, Hulse-Post DJ, Sturm-Ramirez K, Webster RG (2006) Domestic ducks and H5N1 influenza epidemic, Thailand. Emerg Infect Dis 12:575–581

20. Hill SC, Lee YJ, Song BM, Kang HM, Lee EK, Hanna A, Gilbert M, Brown IH, Pybus OG (2015) Wild waterfowl migration and domestic duck density shape the epidemiology of highly pathogenic H5N8 influenza in the Republic of Korea. Infect Genet Evol 34:267–277

21. United States Department of Agriculture. HPAI 2014-2015 Infected premises. https://www.aphis.usda.gov/animal_health/animal_dis_spec/poultry/downloads/hpai-positive-premises-2014-2015.pdf. Accessed 15 Jan 2017

22. United States Department of Agriculture, animal and plant health inspection service. Stakeholder announcement. H5N8 found in backyard poultry in Oregon https://www.aphis.usda.gov/publications/animal_health/2014/SA_H5N8_Oregon.pdf. Accessed 15 Jan 2017

23. Shivaprasad HSS, Carnaccini S, Crossley B, Senties-Cue G, Chin R (2016) An overview of outbreaks of LPAI and HPAI H5N8 in commercial poultry in California. In: Sixty-fifth Western poultry disease conference, Vancouver, Canada April 24–27:261

24. Nuñez A, Brookes SM, Reid SM, Garcia-Rueda C, Hicks DJ, Seekings JM, Spencer YI, Brown IH (2016) Highly pathogenic avian influenza H5N8 clade 2.3.4.4 virus: equivocal pathogenicity and implications for surveillance following natural infection in Breeder ducks in the United Kingdom. Transbound Emerg Dis 63:5–9

25. HPAI outbreaks continue in France (2016) Vet Rec 179:158

26. Pantin-Jackwood MJ, Swayne DE (2009) Pathogenesis and pathobiology of avian influenza virus infection in birds. Rev Sci Tech 28:113–136

27. Alexander DJ, Allan WH, Parsons DG, Parsons G (1978) The pathogenicity of four avian influenza viruses for fowls, turkeys and ducks. Res Vet Sci 24:242–247

28. Capua I, Mutinelli F (2001) Mortality in Muscovy ducks (Cairina moschata) and domestic geese (Anser anser var. domestica) associated with natural infection with a highly pathogenic avian influenza virus of H7N1 subtype. Avian Pathol 30:179–183

29. Lee DH, Kwon JH, Noh JY, Park JK, Yuk SS, Erdene-Ochir TO, Lee JB, Park SY, Choi IS, Lee SW, Song CS (2016) Pathogenicity of the Korean H5N8 highly pathogenic avian influenza virus in commercial domestic poultry species. Avian Pathol 45:208–211

30. Webster RG, Guan Y, Peiris M, Walker D, Krauss S, Zhou NN, Govorkova EA, Ellis TM, Dyrting KC, Sit T, Perez DR, Shortridge KF (2002) Characterization of H5N1 influenza viruses that continue to circulate in geese in Southeastern China. J Virol 76:118–126

31. Kwon YK, Thomas C, Swayne DE (2010) Variability in pathobiology of South Korean H5N1 high-pathogenicity avian influenza virus infection for 5 species of migratory waterfowl. Vet Pathol 47:495–506

32. Perkins LE, Swayne DE (2002) Pathogenicity of a Hong Kong-origin H5N1 highly pathogenic avian influenza virus for emus, geese, ducks, and pigeons. Avian Dis 46:53–63

33. Szeredi L, Dán A, Pálmai N, Ursu K, Bálint A, Szeleczky Z, Ivanics E, Erdélyi K, Rigó D, Tekes L, Glavits R (2010) Tissue tropism of highly pathogenic avian influenza virus subtype H5N1 in naturally infected mute swans (Cygnus Olor), domestic geese (Aser Anser var. domestica), pekin ducks (Anas platyrhynchos) and mulard ducks (Cairina moschata x anas platyrhynchos). Acta Vet Hung 58:133–145

34. Smietanka K, Minta Z, Reichert M, Olszewska M, Wyrostek K, Jóźwiak M, van den Berg T (2013) Experimental infection of juvenile domestic and Canada geese with two different clades of H5N1 high pathogenicity avian influenza virus. Vet Microbiol 163:235–241

35. Yuan R, Cui J, Zhang S, Cao L, Liu X, Kang Y, Song Y, Gong L, Jiao P, Liao M (2014) Pathogenicity and transmission of H5N1 avian influenza viruses in different birds. Vet Microbiol 168:50–59

36. United States Department of Agriculture. Wild bird highly pathogenic avian influenza cases in the United States. https://www.aphis.usda.gov/wildlife_damage/downloads/DEC%202014%20-%20JUNE%202015%20WILD%20BIRD%20POSITIVE%20HIGHLY%20PATHOGENIC%20AVIAN%20INFLUENZA%20CASES%20IN%20THE%20UNITED%20STATES.pdf. Accessed 15 Jan 2017

37. Lee MS, Chen LH, Chen YP, Liu YP, Li WC, Lin YL, Lee F (2016) Highly pathogenic avian influenza viruses H5N2, H5N3, and H5N8 in Taiwan in 2015. Vet Microbiol 187:50–57

38. Spackman E, Killian ML (2014) Avian influenza virus isolation, propagation, and titration in embryonated chicken eggs. Methods Mol Biol 1161:125–140

39. Pantin-Jackwood MJ (2014) Immunohistochemical staining of influenza virus in tissues. Methods Mol Biol 1161:51–58

40. Pedersen JC (2014) Hemagglutination-inhibition assay for influenza virus subtype identification and the detection and quantitation of serum antibodies to influenza virus. Methods Mol Biol 1161:11–25

41. Reed LJ, Muench H (1938) A simple method for estimating fifty percent endpoints. Am J Epidemiol 27:493–497

42. Spackman E, Senne DA, Bulaga LL, Myers TJ, Perdue ML, Garber LP, Lohman K, Daum LT, Suarez DL (2003) Development of real-time RT-PCR for the detection of avian influenza virus. Avian Dis 47:1079–1082

43. Wasilenko JL, Arafa AM, Selim AA, Hassan MK, Aly MM, Ali A, Nassif S, Elebiary E, Balish A, Klimov A, Suarez DL, Swayne DE, Pantin-Jackwood MJ (2012) Pathogenicity of two Egyptian H5N1 highly pathogenic avian influenza viruses in domestic ducks. Arch Virol 156:37–51

44. Kajihara M, Sakoda Y, Soda K, Minari K, Okamatsu M, Takada A, Kida H (2013) The PB2, PA, HA, NP, and NS genes of a highly pathogenic avian influenza virus A/whooper swan/Mongolia/3/2005 (H5N1) are responsible for pathogenicity in ducks. Virol J 10:45

45. Bingham J, Green DJ, Lowther S, Klippel J, Burggraaf S, Anderson DE, Wibawa H, Hoa DM, Long NT, Vu PP, Middleton DJ, Daniels PW (2009) Infection studies with two highly pathogenic avian influenza strains (Vietnamese and Indonesian) in Pekin ducks (*Anas platyrhynchos*), with particular reference to clinical disease, tissue tropism and viral shedding. Avian Pathol 38:267–278

46. Löndt BZ, Nunez A, Banks J, Nili H, Johnson LK, Alexander DJ (2008) Pathogenesis of highly pathogenic avian influenza A/turkey/Turkey/1/2005 H5N1 in Pekin ducks (*Anas platyrhynchos*) infected experimentally. Avian Pathol 37:619–627

47. Hulse-Post DJ, Sturm-Ramirez KM, Humberd J, Seiler P, Govorkova EA, Krauss S, Scholtissek C, Puthavathana P, Buranathai C, Nguyen TD, Long HT, Naipospos TS, Chen H, Ellis TM, Guan Y, Peiris JS, Webster RG (2005) Role of domestic ducks in the propagation and biological evolution of highly pathogenic H5N1 influenza viruses in Asia. Proc Natl Acad Sci USA 102:10682–10687

48. Pantin-Jackwood MJ, Smith DM, Wasilenko JL, Cagle C, Shepherd E, Sarmento L, Kapczynski DR, Afonso CL (2012) Effect of age on the pathogenesis and innate immune responses in Pekin ducks infected with different H5N1 highly pathogenic avian influenza viruses. Virus Res 167:196–206

49. Brown JD, Stallknecht DE, Swayne DE (2008) Experimental infection of swans and geese with highly pathogenic avian influenza virus (H5N1) of Asian lineage. Emerg Infect Dis 14:136–142

50. Pasick J, Berhane Y, Embury-Hyatt C, Copps J, Kehler H, Handel K, Babiuk S, Hooper-McGrevy K, Li Y, Le Mai Q, Lien Phuong S (2007) Susceptibility of Canada geese (*Branta canadensis*) to highly pathogenic avian influenza virus (H5N1). Emerg Infect Dis 13:1821–1827

51. Ellis TM, Bousfield RB, Bissett LA, Dyrting KC, Luk GS, Tsim ST, Sturm-Ramirez K, Webster RG, Guan Y, Malik Peiris JS (2004) Investigation of outbreaks of highly pathogenic H5N1 avian influenza in waterfowl and wild birds in Hong Kong in late 2002. Avian Pathol 33:492–505

52. Teifke JP, Klopfleisch R, Globig A, Starick E, Hoffmann B, Wolf PU, Beer M, Mettenleiter TC, Harder TC (2007) Pathology of natural infections by H5N1 highly pathogenic avian influenza virus in mute (*Cygnus olor*) and whooper (*Cygnus cygnus*) swans. Vet Pathol 44:137–143

53. Liu J, Xiao H, Lei F, Zhu Q, Qin K, Zhang XW, Zhang XL, Zhao D, Wang G, Feng Y, Ma J, Liu W, Wang J, Gao GF (2005) Highly pathogenic H5N1 influenza virus infection in migratory birds. Science 309:1206

54. Chen H, Smith GDJ, Zhang SY, Qin K, Wang J, Li KS, Webster RG, Peiris JSM, Guan Y (2005) Avian flu: H5N1 virus outbreak in migratory waterfowl. Nature 436:191–192

55. Berhane Y, Embury-Hyatt C, Leith M, Kehler H, Suderman M, Pasick J (2014) Pre-exposing Canada Geese (*Branta canadensis*) to a low-pathogenic H1N1 avian influenza virus protects them against H5N1 HPAI virus challenge. J Wildl Dis 50:84–97

56. Neufeld JL, Embury-Hyatt C, Berhane Y, Manning L, Ganske S, Pasick J (2009) Pathology of highly pathogenic avian influenza virus (H5N1) infection in Canada geese (*Branta canadensis*): preliminary studies. Vet Pathol 46:966–970

57. Nemeth NM, Brown JD, Stallknecht DE, Howerth EW, Newman SH, Swayne DE (2013) Experimental infection of bar-headed geese (*Anser indicus*) and ruddy shelducks (*Tadorna ferruginea*) with a clade 2.3.2 H5N1 highly pathogenic avian influenza virus. Vet Pathol 50:961–970

58. DeJesus E, Costa-Hurtado M, Smith D, Lee DH, Spackman E, Kapczynski DR, Torchetti MK, Killian ML, Suarez DL, Swayne DE, Pantin-Jackwood MJ (2016) Changes in adaptation of H5N2 highly pathogenic avian influenza H5 clade 2.3.4.4 viruses in chickens and mallards. Virology 499:52–64

59. Pantin-Jackwood MJ, Costa-Hurtado M, Shepherd E, DeJesus E, Smith D, Spackman E, Kapczynski DR, Suarez DL, Stallknecht D, Swayne DE (2016) Pathogenicity and transmission of H5 and H7 highly pathogenic avian influenza viruses in mallards. J Virol 90:9967–9982

60. Pantin-Jackwood M, Swayne DE, Smith D, Shepherd E (2013) Effect of species, breed and route of virus inoculation on the pathogenicity of H5N1 highly pathogenic influenza (HPAI) viruses in domestic ducks. Vet Res 44:62

61. Cagle C, To TL, Nguyen T, Wasilenko J, Adams SC, Cardona CJ, Spackman E, Suarez DL, Pantin-Jackwood MJ (2011) Pekin and Muscovy ducks respond differently to vaccination with a H5N1 highly pathogenic avian influenza (HPAI) commercial inactivated vaccine. Vaccine 29:6549–6557

62. Pantin-Jackwood MJ, Miller PJ, Spackman E, Swayne DE, Susta L, Costa-Hurtado M, Suarez DL (2014) Role of poultry in the spread of novel H7N9 influenza virus in China. J Virol 88:5381–5390

63. Kang HM, Lee EK, Song BM, Jeong J, Choi JG, Jeong J, Moon OK, Yoon H, Cho Y, Kang YM, Lee HS, Lee YJ (2015) Novel reassortant influenza A(H5N8) viruses among inoculated domestic and wild ducks, South Korea, 2014. Emerg Infect Dis 21:298–304

64. Kim YI, Pascua PNQ, Kwon HI, Lim GJ, Kim EH, Yoon SW, Park SJ, Kim SM, Choi EJ, Si YJ, Lee OJ, Shim WS, Kim SW, Mo IP, Bae Y, Lim YT, Sung MH, Kim CJ, Webby RJ, Webster RG, Choi YK (2014) Pathobiological features of a novel, highly pathogenic avian influenza A(H5N8) virus. Emerg Microbes Infect 3:e75

65. Sun H, Pu J, Hu J, Liu L, Xu G, Gao GF, Liu X, Liu J (2016) Characterization of clade 2.3.4.4 highly pathogenic H5 avian influenza viruses in ducks and chickens. Vet Microbiol 182:116–122

66. Kanehira K, Uchida Y, Takemae N, Hikono H, Tsunekuni R, Saito T (2015) Characterization of an H5N8 influenza A virus isolated from chickens during an outbreak of severe avian influenza in Japan in April 2014. Arch Virol 160:1629–1643

67. Kang HM, Lee EK, Song BM, Heo GB, Jung J, Jang I, Bae YC, Jung SC, Lee YJ (2017) Experimental infection of mandarin duck with highly pathogenic avian influenza A (H5N8 and H5N1) viruses. Vet Microbiol 198:59–63

68. Li J, Gu M, Liu D, Liu B, Jiang K, Zhong L, Liu K, Sun W, Hu J, Wang X, Hu S, Liu X, Liu X (2016) Phylogenetic and biological characterization of three K1203 (H5N8) like avian influenza A virus reassortants in China in 2014. Arch Virol 161:289–302

69. Berhane Y, Kobasa D, Embury-Hyatt C, Pickering B, Babiuk S, Joseph T, Bowes V, Suderman M, Leung A, Cottam-Birt C, Hisanaga T, Pasick J (2016) Pathobiological haracterization of a novel reassortant highly pathogenic H5N1 virus isolated in British Columbia, Canada, 2015. Sci Rep 6:23380

70. Banyái K, Bistyák AT, Thuma A, Gyuris E, Ursu K, Marton S, Farkas SL, Hortobágyi E, Bacsadi Á, Dán Á (2016) Neuroinvasive influenza virus A(H5N8) in fattening ducks, Hungary, 2015. Infect Genet Evol 43:418–423

13

Genotyping and investigating capsular polysaccharide synthesis gene loci of non-serotypeable *Streptococcus suis* isolated from diseased pigs in Canada

Han Zheng[1†], Xiaotong Qiu[1†], David Roy[2], Mariela Segura[2], Pengchen Du[3], Jianguo Xu[1] and Marcelo Gottschalk[2*]

Abstract

Streptococcus suis (*S. suis*) is an important swine pathogen and an emerging zoonotic agent. Most clinical *S. suis* strains express capsular polysaccharides (CPS), which can be typed by antisera using the coagglutination test. In this study, 79 *S. suis* strains recovered from diseased pigs in Canada and which could not be typed using antisera were further characterized by capsular gene typing and sequencing. Four patterns of *cps* locus were observed: (1) fifteen strains were grouped into previously reported serotypes but presented several mutations in their *cps* loci, when compared to available data from reference strains; (2) seven strains presented a complete deletion of the *cps* locus, which would result in an inability to synthesize capsule; (3) forty-seven strains were classified in recently described novel *cps* loci (NCLs); and (4) ten strains carried novel NCLs not previously described. Different virulence gene profiles (based on the presence of *mrp*, *epf*, and/or *sly*) were observed in these non-serotypeable strains. This study provides further insight in understanding the genetic characteristics of *cps* loci in non-serotypeable *S. suis* strains recovered from diseased animals. When using a combination of the previously described 35 serotypes and the complete NCL system, the number of untypeable strains recovered from diseased animals in Canada would be significantly reduced.

Introduction

Streptococcus suis is recognized as one of the most important causes of bacterial disease in post-weaned piglets worldwide, generating important economic losses to the swine industry. In addition, it is an important emerging zoonotic agent [1–3]. Clinical strains of *S. suis* generally have a capsule (capsular polysaccharide or CPS), which is the basis of the serotyping traditionally used for epidemiological studies. Thirty-five serotypes of *S. suis* (serotype 1 through 34 and serotype 1/2) were identified in the 1980s and the 1990s [4–7]. More recently, serotypes 20, 22, 26, 32, 33 and 34 have been suggested as

belonging to a species different from *S. suis* [8, 9]. Strains isolated from diseased pigs primarily belong to serotype 2 in most countries, followed by serotypes 3, 4, 5, 7, 8 and 1/2 [10–12]. In some European countries, serotype 9 is also one of the most frequently recovered capsular types from diseased animals [12, 13]. Traditionally, *S. suis* is routinely serotyped by the coagglutination test using serotype-specific antisera. However, non-serotypeable *S. suis* strains are frequently reported in many studies [12, 14–18]. Given that strains not expressing the CPS cannot be serotyped using antisera, serotyping based on molecular techniques has been proposed. Since the *S. suis* CPS is synthesized by the Wzx/Wzy pathway in the CPS locus, *wzy* genes have been demonstrated to be serotype-specific [19]. Thus, high-throughput capsular gene typing systems based on serotype-specific *wzy* genes have become attractive alternatives/complement to the existing serological tests [18, 20, 21]. However, even with the

*Correspondence: marcelo.gottschalk@umontreal.ca
†Han Zheng and Xiaotong Qiu contributed equally to this work
2 Faculty of Veterinary Medicine, Swine and Poultry Infectious Diseases Research Center, University of Montreal, Quebec, Canada
Full list of author information is available at the end of the article

use of multiplex PCR tests, non-serotypeable strains are still commonly isolated from both clinically healthy and diseased animals [18, 22, 23].

In recent years, 17 novel *cps* loci (NCLs) were identified from non-serotypeable *S. suis* and were designated as NCL1 to 16 and serotype Chz [22–24]. Meanwhile, an 18-plex Luminex assay was also developed to detect these 17 NCLs and nearly 60% of non-serotypeable strains from healthy pigs carried one of these NCLs [22]. However, little is known about the distribution and characteristics of the *cps* loci of potentially virulent non-serotypeable strains recovered from diseased animals.

In this study, the *cps* loci of 79 Canadian non-serotypeable *S. suis* strains (as determined by the coagglutination test) recovered from diseased pigs were studied using two capsular gene typing systems [20, 22] and the genetic characteristics of the NCLs were analyzed. To elucidate the non-serotypeable mechanisms of strains grouped into previously described serotypes, the study was extended to compare their *cps* sequence to that of corresponding reference strains. Furthermore, the prevalence of minimum core genome (MCG) sequence typing group and virulence gene profile were also investigated in all 79 strains.

Materials and methods
Bacterial strains and chromosomal DNA preparation
A total of 79 *S. suis* strains isolated from diseased pigs on non-related farms in Canada were used in this study (Additional file 1). All strains have been isolated from primary affected organs of clinically diseased pigs, including brain (meningitis; $n = 18$), heart (endocarditis; $n = 18$), multiple organs (septicemia; $n = 14$), pleura (polyserositis; $n = 9$), lungs (pneumonia; $n = 9$) and joints (arthritis; $n = 1$). For a very few isolates, the information was not available, but they were all recovered from diseased animals with a primary diagnosis of *S. suis* infection. All isolates were serotyped using the coagglutination test [25]. Chromosomal DNA was prepared from all strains as previously described [21]. The species identity of the 79 strains was determined to be *S. suis* by amplification of the 16S rRNA, *recN*, *gdh*, and *thrA* genes [20, 26–28].

Capsular gene typing
The *cps* locus type of the 79 strains was identified by the 32-plex and 18-plex Luminex assays previously reported [20, 22]. The subtypes of known NCLs were determined based on the arrangement of subtype-specific homology groups (HGs) and transposases [22, 23].

Sequencing *cps* loci and bioinformatics analyses
Seventeen strains which could not be grouped using the 32- and 18-plex Luminex assays and 3 strains which could not be grouped into known subtypes, as well as 15 strains which were grouped into reference serotypes, were sequenced by Illumina sequencing as previously described [23]. Each *cps* locus sequence was extracted from the draft genome sequence and was analyzed using the same bioinformatics methods described in previous studies [19, 22, 23]. The products of the *cps* genes were assigned to novel HGs if both of the global match regions and identity of the amino acid or nucleotide sequences were below 50% when compared to the 420 currently known HGs of the 35 reference serotypes and 17 NCLs. The novel HGs were assigned numerical values from HG421 onwards [19, 22, 23]. Novel HGs that were present in all strains of a given NCL were identified as NCL-specific HGs. The strains harboring the same *wzy* were clustered into the same NCL. The Artemis comparison tool (ACT) was used to visualize the data [29].

MCG typing and PCR assays for *mrp* (muramidase released protein), *sly* (suilysin) and *epf* (extracellular protein)
MCG sequence typing was performed using PCR amplification and DNA sequencing as previously described [30, 31]. The full-length *mrp* gene was amplified and sequenced using a previously described method [11]. Amplification of the *sly* and *epf* genes was performed according to methods previously described [32, 33].

Nucleotide sequence accession number
Sequences of *cps* loci obtained in this study were deposited in GenBank under the accession numbers KX870047–KX870056, KX870058–KX870064, KX870067–KX870072, and KX870074–KX870076. Reads of the sequenced strains were deposited in GenBank under accession number SRR5177663–SRR5177696 and SRR5177711. All accession numbers can also be found in Additional file 1.

Results
Serotyping of strains
The 79 strains used in the present study showed auto-agglutination, poly-agglutination or non-agglutination using the reference antisera and the coagglutination test and were thus considered as non-serotypeable. All strains were then typed using our previously developed capsular gene typing systems [20, 22]. Fifteen strains (18.9%) were grouped into reference serotypes while 47 (59.4%) were grouped into 17 known NCLs. The remaining 17 strains remained non-typeable (Additional file 1).

Of the 15 strains belonging to the previously described serotypes, serotype 2 or 1/2 ($n = 4$), which cannot be distinguished by capsular gene typing, was the most frequent, followed by serotypes 15 ($n = 3$), 11 ($n = 2$), and

30 ($n = 2$). Serotypes 5, 17, 27 and 29 only contained a single strain (Additional file 1).

Of the 47 strains which were assigned to previously known NCLs, NCL3 ($n = 18$) was the most prevalent, followed by NCL4 ($n = 8$), NCL7 ($n = 4$), NCL2 ($n = 3$), NCL12 ($n = 3$), and NCL13 ($n = 3$). In addition, one strain each of the NCL1, 5, 6, 10, 11, 14, 16, and Chz were also found (Additional file 1).

Identification of four new NCLs

The remaining 17 non-serotypeable strains mentioned above were sequenced by Illumina sequencing. The *cps* locus was absent from 7 strains. The *cps* loci of the remaining 10 strains were divided into four new NCLs which were named NCL17 to 20 based on their *wzy* gene sequences. NCL17 was the most prevalent ($n = 4$), followed by NCL18 ($n = 3$), NCL19 ($n = 2$), and NCL20 ($n = 1$) (Additional file 1). In addition, two types of patterns were found in the four new NCLs. NCL17 and NCL18 belonged to pattern I-a, while NCL19 and NCL20 belonged to pattern I-b [19].

The sizes of these NCLs ranged from 21.34 to 29.90 kb and the percentage of G+C content varied between 33.9 and 35.1%. Fifty-nine predicted coding sequences were designated *cps* HGs. Twenty-two HGs were also present in the *cps* loci of the reference strains of known serotypes and 17 known NCLs. An initial sugar transferase gene was located in the 5′ region and was classified into three HGs: HG6 (NCL20), HG8 (NCL17), and HG295 (NCL18 and NCL19). The 5′ regions of four NCLs were conserved, whereas the central and 3′ regions of these were highly variable (Figure 1A).

Thirty-two HGs were NCL-specific. Each NCL contained 4–11 NCL-specific genes, with 4 HGs for NCL17, 7 HGs for NCL18, 11 HGs for NCL19, and 10 HGs for NCL20. Among these, 11 HGs encoded putative glycosyl transferases and two encoded acetyltransferases. As expected, all Wzy polymerases and Wzx flippases were NCL-specific (Additional file 2).

Determining the subtypes of NCLs

NCL2, NCL3, NCL7, and NCL11 strains were found to belong to a single subtype; NCL2-4, NCL3-1, NCL7-1, and NCL11-5, respectively. Genetic heterogeneity was not found within strains of NCL12, NCL15, and NCL17 to 20 (Additional file 2).

i. NCL1: strain 1640373 could not be classified into any known NCL1 subtype and was sequenced by Illumina sequencing, named as NCL1-12. The replacement of HG293, HG294, and HG292 by the HG354 and HG355 was found in its three side regions (Figure 1B).

ii. Chz: compared to the reference strain Chz-2, the deletion of HG55 was found in strain 1232225, named as Chz-3 (Figure 1C).

iii. NCL16: compared to the reference strain YS525 (NCL16-1), the insertion of HG55 was found in strain 1093407, named NCL16-3 (Figure 1D).

Mutations in the *cps* loci of strains belonging to previously described serotypes

The 15 strains that were negative by coagglutination test but positive by multiplex Luminex assay for the reference serotypes were further analyzed. Comparing to the *cps* locus of the corresponding serotype reference strains, insertions and deletions were found in the serotype 5, 11, 15, 17 and 30 strains. The *cps* loci of four serotype 2 or 1/2 strains and one serotype 27 strain were intact and small-scale mutations were detected in these (Table 2).

i. Serotype 2 or 1/2: compared to the serotype 2 reference strain P1/7 (GenBank accession number BR001000), all four strains had a 33 bp insertion in *wxy* genes and four strains had single-nucleotide substitutions in *wzx* genes. The single-nucleotide substitutions in glycosyltransferase genes and a 27 bp deletion in the side-chain formation gene were also found in five strains (Table 2).

ii. Serotype 5: compared to the serotype 5 reference strain 11538 (GenBank accession number BR001003), the deletions of HG17 to HG19 at the 3′ end were found in strain 1218846 (Figure 2A).

iii. Serotype 11: compared to the serotype 11 reference strain 12814 (GenBank accession number AB737819), HG72 and HG73 were replaced by HG32 and HG40 in strains 1336897 and 1336915. In addition, the nucleotide substitutions (TA→CC) of the termination codon of HG32 were found in the *cpsQ* gene of strains 1336897 and 1336915, which resulted in the chimeric HG32/HG39 gene (Figure 2B).

iv. Serotype 15: two types of variations were found within this serotype. Strains 1424566 and 1449343 possessed identical *cps* sequences. A novel HG (*cpsH*, putative acetyltransferase) was inserted between HG33 and HG77, and the insertions of HG19 and HG17 at the 3′ end were found in two strains (Table 1). Moreover, the transversion (T→G) was found at the site of the termination codon of HG19, which resulted in the chimeric HG18/HG19 gene in two strains. Compared to strains 1424566 and 1449343, HG18 and HG17 were replaced by a transposase in strain 1761402 (Figure 2C).

v. Serotype 17: compared to the serotype 17 reference strain 93A (GenBank accession number

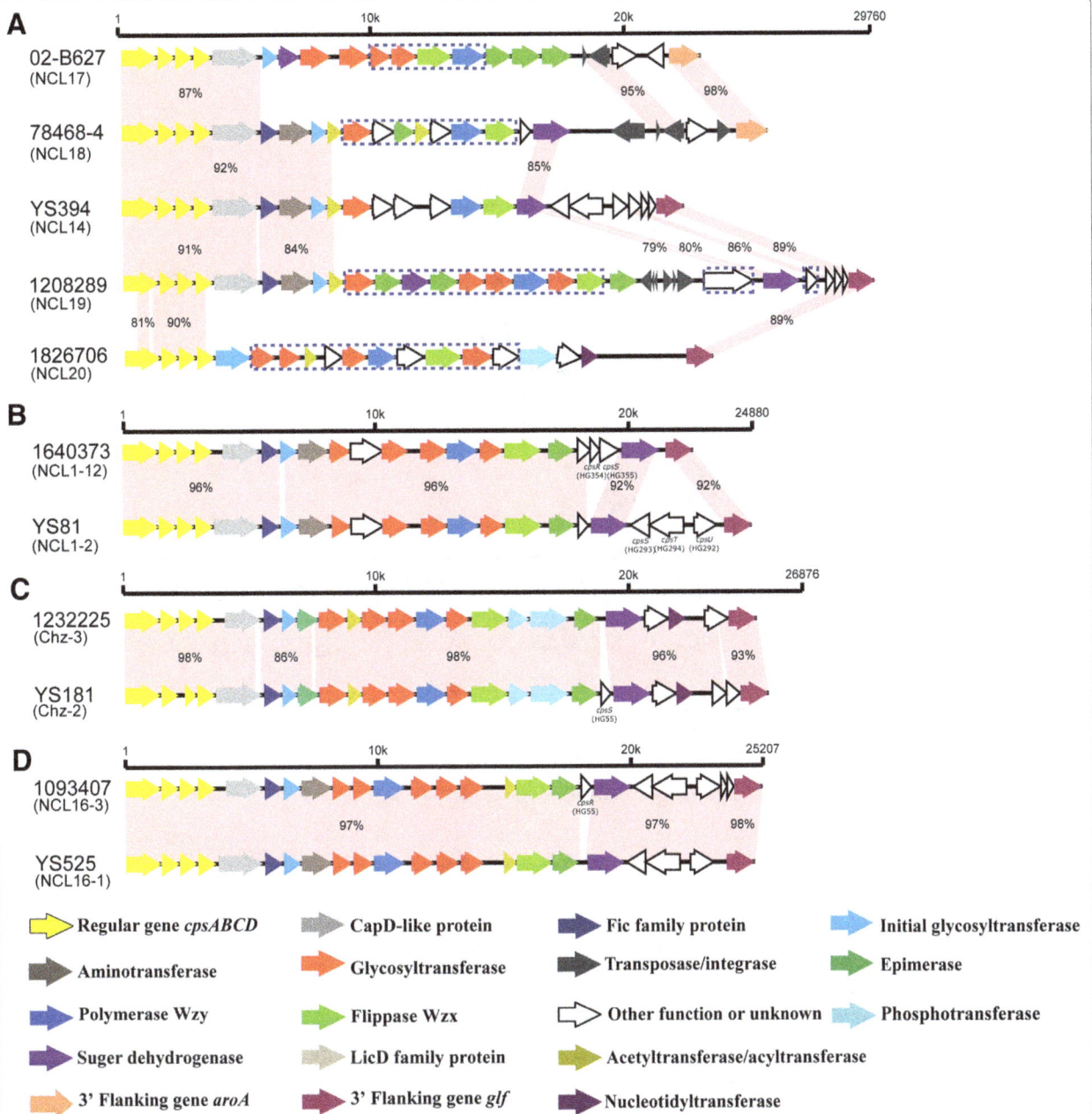

Figure 1 **Comparison of the *cps* loci among NCL17 to 20 (A) and within NCL1 (B), Chz (C) and NCL16 (D).** Each colored arrow represents the gene whose predicted function is shown in the below panel. NCL-specific genes are indicated by dotted blue lines.

AB737824), two deletions (HG21 and HG161) and two insertions (HG354 and HG355) were found. Furthermore, HG79 and HG80 were replaced by a putative phosphotransferase, a putative hypothetical protein, a putative biotin carboxylase, and a putative glycosyltransferase (initial sugar transferase), which were not assigned to any previous homology group (Table 1). Moreover, the replacement of HG48, HG17, HG18, and HG19 by

HG293, HG294, and HG292 was also found (Figure 2D).

vi. Serotype 27: compared to the serotype 27 reference strain 89–5259 (GenBank accession number AB737831), the single-nucleotide substitutions and small-scale indels in glycosyltransferase genes, *wzx* gene, and side-chain formation gene were found (Table 2).

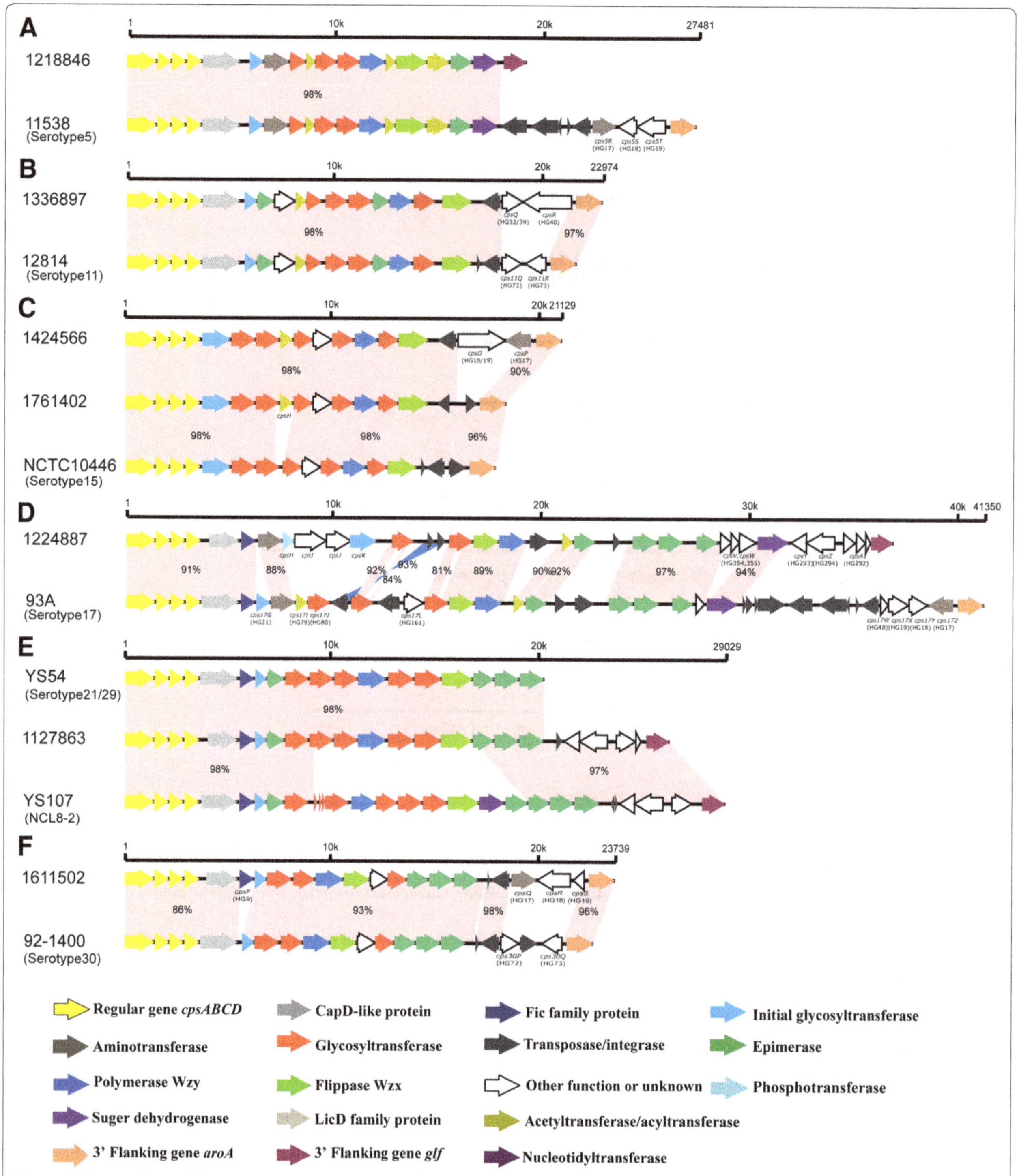

Figure 2 Comparison of the *cps* loci within serotype 5 (A), serotype 11 (B), serotype 15 (C), serotype 17 (D), serotype 21/29 (E) and Chz (F). Each colored arrow represents the gene whose predicted function is shown in the below panel.

vii. Serotype 29: compared to strain YS54 agglutinated with both serotypes 21 and 29 antisera (GenBank accession number KC537387), the insertions of a transposase gene, HG293, HG294, and HG292

on the 3′-side were found in strain 1127863 (Figure 2E).

viii. Serotype 30: compared to the serotype 30 reference strain 92–1400 (GenBank accession number

Table 1 Information of the novel HGs inserted *cps* loci of strains belonging to reference serotypes

Strain ID	*cps* locus type	Gene name	Predicted products	Similar protein, species (GenBank accession number)	Coverage/identity (%)
1424566, 1449343, 1761402	Serotype 15	*cpsH*	Acetyltransferase	Maltose O-acetyltransferase, *Lactobacillus reuteri* (CUR43586.1)	96/68
1224887	Serotype 17	*cpsH*	UDP-phosphate galactose phosphotransferase	UDP-phosphate galactose phosphotransferase, *Sphaerochaeta pleomorpha* (WP_014270310.1)	99/57
		cpsI	Hypothetical protein	Biotin carboxylase, *Sphaerochaeta pleomorpha* (WP_014270309.1)	68/48
		cpsJ	Biotin carboxylase	Biotin carboxylase, *Ruminococcus* sp. (CBL19829.1)	99/60
		cpsK	Glycosyltransferase	Glycosyltransferase family 1 protein, *Gallibacterium anatis* (WP_065231950.1)	92/58

AB737834), insertion of HG9 was found in strains 1611502 and 1839679. Moreover, HG72, transposase gene, and HG73 were replaced by HG17, HG18, and HG19 (Figure 2F).

Variations of chromosomal loci

In a previous study, the chromosomal loci of *cps* gene clusters of reference serotype 5 and 17 strains were classified into pattern I-a [19]. In the present study, strains 1218846 (serotype 5) and 1224887 (serotype 17) were classified into pattern I-b (Figures 2A and D, respectively).

MCG typing

The majority of the 79 strains were clustered in the MCG group 6 (44.3%, 35/79 strains), followed by ungroupable (24%, 19/79 strains), and group 7 (20.2%, 16/79 strains). MCG groups 4, 3, 2, and 1 also contained four, three, one, and one strains, respectively (Additional file 1).

Identifying genotypes of *mrp*, *epf*, and *sly*

Twelve strains were *mrp* positive. Frameshift mutations at 2740 bp from the reported initiator ATG codon were present in the *mrp* gene of strain 1114193, which resulted in premature stop codons. Eleven other strains contained intact full-length *mrp* gene copies and may express MRP. Based on the *mrp* subtypes reported in North America (NA) [11], the sequences of *mrp* were grouped into one of three subtypes, EU (European, $n = 3$), NA1 ($n = 7$), or NA2 ($n = 1$). Only twelve strains contained the *sly* gene and 6 strains were positive for *epf*. There were eight genotypes of *mrp*, *epf*, and *sly*, primarily based on *mrp* variation: most of the strains in this study ($n = 62$) were $mrp^-sly^-epf^-$, followed by $mrp^{NA1}sly^-epf^-$ ($n = 4$), $mrp^{NA1}sly^+epf^-$ ($n = 4$), and $mrp^{EU}sly^+epf^+$ ($n = 3$). It is noteworthy that the latter strains were serotype 2 or 1/2,

serotype 15 and serotype 30, as revealed by the 32-plex Luminex assay. In addition, $mrp^-sly^+epf^+$ ($n = 2$), $mrp^-sly^+epf^-$ ($n = 2$), $mrp^{NA2}sly^+epf^-$ ($n = 1$), and $mrp^-sly^-epf^+$ ($n = 1$) genotypes were also found (Additional file 1).

Discussion

In addition to the traditional 35 serotypes originally described for *S. suis*, 17 NCLs have recently been reported in non-serotypeable *S. suis* strains isolated from healthy animals using high-throughput typing systems and online bioinformatics [22, 23]. However, the genetic characteristics of *cps* loci in potentially virulent non-serotypeable *S. suis* strains recovered from diseased animals are still scarce.

In the present study, the *cps* loci of 79 Canadian non-serotypeable strains isolated from the internal organs of diseased pigs were analyzed. Non-serotypeable strains are frequently isolated from diseased animals in this country [34]. Based on previous gene typing and sequencing results [22, 35], the non-serotypeable phenotype may be attributed to one of three causes: (1) strains belonging to previously described serotypes harboring mutated *cps* loci causing loss of capsule expression or antigenic variation; (2) strains without *cps* locus completely losing their ability to synthesize capsule; or (3) strains with not-previously described NCL referring to novel serotypes.

In this study, 15 non-serotypeable strains could be grouped into reference serotypes by the 32-plex Luminex assay. To elucidate the lack of positive identification by the coagglutination test, we further sequenced and compared their *cps* loci to those of corresponding reference strains. Previous studies showed that replacements and large indels, as well as small-scale mutations of *cps* genes, caused phenotypical changes in agglutination tests [21,

Table 2 Mutations in glycosyltransferase, side-chain formation, *wzy* and *wzx* genes of serotype 2 or 1/2 representative strains and a serotype 27 strain

Strain	Affected gene(s)	Types of mutations	Affected nucleotide(s) [Affected amino acid]
1827702	cps2E	Missense	A61G [Thr21Ala]
	cps2I	Insertion	IS element: 33 bp
	cps2N	Deletion	27 bp
1090772	cps2E	Missense	A61G [Thr21Ala]
	cps2F	Missense	A149G [Asp50Gly]
		Missense	A1047T [Leu349Phe]
	cps2I	Insertion	IS element: 33 bp
	cps2N	Deletion	27 bp
	cps2O	Missense	C859A [Arg287Ser]
1160406	cps27E	Missense	A506G [Asp169Gly]
		Missense	T508A [Ser170Thr]
		Missense	A513T [Glu171Asp]
		Missense	A522T [Lys174Asn]
		Missense	A524T A525T [Lys175Ile]
		Missense	A541C C543G [Ile181Leu]
		Missense	A553G [Ile185Val]
		Missense	G617T T618G [Ser206Met]
		Missense	A623T [Tyr208Phe]
		Missense	T633G [Leu211Val]
		Missense	C640T A642C [Leu214Phe]
		Missense	A651T [Glu217Asp]
		Missense	C692T [Ser231Leu]
		Missense	G706A A708G [Ala236Thr]
		Missense	G874A A876T [Val292Ile]
		Missense	T905C [Val302Ala]
		Missense	A922C A924G [Lys308Gln]
		Missense	A941C G942A [Lys314Thr]
		Missense	A967G [Ile323Val]
		Missense	A997C G999C [Met333Leu]
		Missense	G1000A C1001G T1002C [Ala334Ser]
		Missense	A1174C A1175G [Lys392Arg]
		Missense	G1186A G1187T T1188G [Gly396Met]
		Missense	A1272C [Glu424Asp]
		Missense	A1279C A1280G [Lys427Arg]
		Missense	G1288T T1290A [Val430Leu]
		Missense	A1292C [Glu431Ala]
		Missense	G1324A A1326T [Val442Ile]
		Missense	A1357T T1359G [Ile453Leu]
		Missense	A1360T A1361T [Lys454Leu]
	cps27F	Deletion	27 bp
		Missense	A662T [His221Leu]
	cps27G	Insertion	IS element: 21 bp
	cps27I	Missense	G483C [Trp161Cys]
		Missense	C513A [Asp171Glu]
		Missense	A611G [Gln204Arg]
	cps27L	Deletion	57 bp
	cps27M	Missense	C1373T C1374T [Ala458Val]
		Missense	C1375T [Leu459Phe]

36–38]. We also found similar mutations in the *cps* loci of strains tested.

HG17, HG18, HG19, HG32, HG39, and HG40, which were present in the *cps* loci of the reference strains belonging to serotypes 1, 2, 4, 5, 7, 14, 17, 18, 19, 23 and 1/2, were detected in the *cps* loci of strains in the present study belonging to serotypes 11, 15, and 30. Moreover, chimeric HG18/HG19 and HG32/HG39 genes were found in serotype 11 and 15 strains. It is noteworthy that HG292, HG293, HG294, HG354, and HG355, only present in the *cps* loci of NCLs, were also detected in the *cps* locus of strain 1224889, typed herein as serotype 17. In addition, some genes which were never before assigned to any HG were found to be inserted in the *cps* loci of strains belonging to serotypes 17 and 15. The sequence differences between strains NCL8-2 and 1127863 were mainly caused by the replacement of 8 NCL-specific HGs in the center of NCL8-2 and by 6 HGs in 1127863. The replacement and insertion activities may indicate recombination events or horizontal gene transfer between the *cps* loci of *S. suis* strains, probably leading to antigenic variations that would be beneficial to *S. suis* in the course of infection or through immunity evasion.

Comparing to the *cps* loci of their corresponding reference strains, only small-scale mutations were observed in four strains typed as serotype 2 or 1/2 by the 32-plex Luminex. Previous study revealed that all serotype 2 and all serotype 14 strains had a G nucleotide at position 483 of the *cpsK* gene, while all serotype 1 and all serotype 1/2 strains (including 13 serotype 1/2 strains recovered in Canada) contained either a C or T at that nucleotide position [39]. In present study, all four strains had a G nucleotide at position 483 of the *cpsK* gene. We postulated that they were most probably non-encapsulated serotype 2 strains. A previous study reported that single-nucleotide substitutions and frameshift mutations in two glycosyltransferase genes (*cps2E* and *cps2F*) were the main causes of capsule loss in serotype 2 strains. Moreover, mutations in the genes involved in side-chain formation (*cps2J* and *cps2N*), *wzy* (*cps2I*), and *wzx* (*cps2O*) also appeared to be lethal to serotype 2 strains [36]. It may be hypothesized that the missense mutations and small scale indels found in these genes in strains of the present study also had a deleterious effect on the capsular expression. Indeed, high hydrophobic indexes have been obtained with these strains (unpublished data), which strongly suggest lack of capsule expression [15, 40]. Although non-encapsulated *S. suis* strains had originally been considered to be avirulent, they are frequently isolated from cases of endocarditis; as such, non-encapsulation could be, under certain circumstances, beneficial for *S. suis* in the course of such infections [36, 41]. In some cases, non-encapsulated strains resulting from small point mutations may switch to a capsulated phenotype in vivo [42]. Interestingly, small-scale mutations or clear deletions of *cps* loci were also found in an additional eight strains, which are also probably non-encapsulated. Finally, strains without *cps* locus completely losing their ability to synthesize capsule were also found in this study. It is possible that these strains are not able to reverse the encapsulated phenotype. The biological and pathological significance of these non-encapsulated strains need to be further evaluated. Although never described, it is not impossible that some strains lose the capsular phenotype after in vitro culture.

In this study, 60% of non-serotypeable strains carried one of the recently described NCLs. The most common NCLs were 3, 4, 7, and 17, whereas in a previous study with strains recovered from healthy pigs in China, the most common NCLs were 1, 2, 3, and 7 [22]. Differences may be due to the geographical origin of strains (Canada vs. China) and/or their virulence potential (strains from diseased or clinically healthy animals). Since many strains of NCL3 have been identified in this study, further research on its virulence potential should be performed. In addition, and similarly to a previous study [22], high diversity within the same NCL was observed. The *S. suis* species is composed of phenotypically and genetically diverse strains. Host specificity and ecological environment may contribute to this diversity. The *cps* loci could provide important information regarding the ecology of strains. The differences in dominant NCLs between clinical strains from Canada and field strains from China and the emergence of novel NCLs or subtypes in clinical strains from Canada are expected.

In this study, new NCLs (CNL17–20), distributed in 10 strains, are reported for the first time. These NCLs possess completely different Wzy and transferases from those of the previously reported serotypes and NCLs, which in turn may express unique oligosaccharide structures and antigen identities. It is noteworthy that, taking into consideration all NCLs, more than 70% of non-typeable strains could now be typed. The use of the complete serotyping and NCL typing system would considerably reduce the number of non-typeable strains recovered from diseased animals in Canada.

The presence of some genes, such as *mrp*, *epf*, and *sly*, has been associated with virulence [43, 44]. Three distinct *mrp* genotypes have been reported so far and NA1 was the dominant genotype in *S. suis* strains recovered from diseased pigs in the USA [11]. In the present study, 11 strains possessed an intact *mrp* gene and NA1 genotype whereas three strains harbored the EU genotype. One of latter strains was typed as being a serotype 2 or 1/2 by the 32-plex Luminex but, as mentioned above, it is probably a real serotype 2 as shown by the presence of a G nucleotide at position 483 of the *cpsK* gene. The fact that most

mrp^+, epf^+, and sly^+ Eurasian serotype 2 strains belong to the clonal complex 1 [12] also indicated the strain is most probably a non-encapsulated serotype 2 strain with an Eurasian profile [11] that might have been introduced to North America through the importation of animals. In fact, it has been reported that up to 5% of serotype 2 strains recovered in the United States are ST1 and probably originated from Europe [11]. Although the most prevalent virulence gene profile was $mrp^- sly^- epf^-$, 17 strains contained at least one of these three genes. The relevance of these virulence markers in strains of serotypes different from serotype 2 is still controversial.

The most prevalent MCG groups amongst the strains harboring NCLs were the groups 6 and 7, which had been described as being the most ancient groups in the *S. suis* population [30]. This indicates that their *cps* loci have existed for a long time and play important roles in the serotype diversity of *S. suis* population. The most prevalent MCG groups amongst the strains harboring mutated *cps* loci of previously described serotypes and the strains losing their *cps* loci were MCG ungroupable. These strains possibly had a more significant recombination history that prevented them from being reliably assigned; meanwhile these recombination events may facility the mutations and loss of their *cps* loci.

In conclusion, this study provides further insight in understanding the *cps* diversity of *S. suis* and may contribute to future epidemiological studies that will allow characterization of potentially virulent and previously non-serotypeable strains isolated from diseased animals. Use of the 35 serotype-based system complemented with the NCL typing system would significantly reduce the number of untypeable strains recovered from diseased animals in Canada. Further studies with *S. suis* strains isolated in other countries are needed.

Abbreviations

S. suis: *Streptococcus suis*; CPS: capsular polysaccharides; NCL: novel *cps* loci; MCG: minimum core genome; *mrp*: muramidase released protein; *sly*: suilysin; *epf*: extracellular protein factor.

Competing interests

The authors declare that they have no competing interests.

Authors' contributions

HZ, MS, JX, and MG conceived and designed this study. HZ, XQ, and DR contributed to the majority of laboratory experiments. HZ, XQ and PD interpreted the data. XQ prepared the manuscript. HZ, MS, and MG reviewed and critically revised the manuscript. All authors read and approved the final manuscript.

Funding

This work was supported by Grant (81572044) from the National Natural Science Foundation of China, "the Fundamental Research Funds for the Central Universities" from the Key Laboratory of Molecular Microbiology and Technology, Ministry of Education TEDA Institute of Biological Sciences and Biotechnology, Nankai University, and by Grants 125684 from the Canadian Institutes of Health Research (China-Canada Joint Health Research Initiative) and 154280 from the Natural Sciences and Engineering Research Council of Canada.

Author details

[1] State Key Laboratory for Infectious Disease Prevention and Control, Collaborative Innovation Center for Diagnosis and Treatment of Infectious Diseases, National Institute for Communicable Disease Control and Prevention, Chinese Center for Disease Control and Prevention, Changping, Beijing, China. [2] Faculty of Veterinary Medicine, Swine and Poultry Infectious Diseases Research Center, University of Montreal, Quebec, Canada. [3] Institute of Infectious Diseases, Beijing Ditan Hospital, Capital Medical University, Beijing Key Laboratory of Emerging Infectious Diseases, Beijing, People's Republic of China.

References

1. Gottschalk M, Segura M, Xu J (2007) *Streptococcus suis* infections in humans: the Chinese experience and the situation in North America. Anim Health Res Rev 8:29–45
2. Ye C, Zhu X, Jing H, Du H, Segura M, Zheng H, Kan B, Wang L, Bai X, Zhou Y, Cui Z, Zhang S, Jin D, Sun N, Luo X, Zhang J, Gong Z, Wang X, Wang L, Sun H, Li Z, Sun Q, Liu H, Dong B, Ke C, Yuan H, Wang H, Tian K, Wang Y, Gottschalk M, Xu J (2006) *Streptococcus suis* sequence type 7 outbreak, Sichuan, China. Emerg Infect Dis 12:1203–1208
3. Yu H, Jing H, Chen Z, Zheng H, Zhu X, Wang H, Wang S, Liu L, Zu R, Luo L, Xiang N, Liu H, Liu X, Shu Y, Lee SS, Chuang SK, Wang Y, Xu J, Yang W (2006) Human *Streptococcus suis* outbreak, Sichuan, China. Emerg Infect Dis 12:914–920
4. Gottschalk M, Higgins R, Jacques M, Beaudoin M, Henrichsen J (1991) Characterization of six new capsular types (23 through 28) of *Streptococcus suis*. J Clin Microbiol 29:2590–2594
5. Gottschalk M, Higgins R, Jacques M, Mittal KR, Henrichsen J (1989) Description of 14 new capsular types of *Streptococcus suis*. J Clin Microbiol 27:2633–2636
6. Higgins R, Gottschalk M, Boudreau M, Lebrun A, Henrichsen J (1995) Description of six new capsular types (29–34) of *Streptococcus suis*. J Vet Diagn Invest 7:405–406
7. Perch B, Pedersen KB, Henrichsen J (1983) Serology of capsulated streptococci pathogenic for pigs: six new serotypes of *Streptococcus suis*. J Clin Microbiol 17:993–996
8. le Tien HT, Nishibori T, Nishitani Y, Nomoto R, Osawa R (2013) Reappraisal of the taxonomy of *Streptococcus suis* serotypes 20, 22, 26, and 33 based on DNA-DNA homology and *sodA* and *recN* phylogenies. Vet Microbiol 162:842–849
9. Hill JE, Gottschalk M, Brousseau R, Harel J, Hemmingsen SM, Goh SH (2005) Biochemical analysis, *cpn60* and 16S rDNA sequence data indicate that *Streptococcus suis* serotypes 32 and 34, isolated from pigs, are *Streptococcus orisratti*. Vet Microbiol 107:63–69
10. Wei Z, Li R, Zhang A, He H, Hua Y, Xia J, Cai X, Chen H, Jin M (2009) Characterization of *Streptococcus suis* isolates from the diseased pigs in China between 2003 and 2007. Vet Microbiol 137:196–201
11. Fittipaldi N, Fuller TE, Teel JF, Wilson TL, Wolfram TJ, Lowery DE, Gottschalk M (2009) Serotype distribution and production of muramidase-released protein, extracellular factor and suilysin by field strains of *Streptococcus suis* isolated in the United States. Vet Microbiol 139:310–317
12. Goyette-Desjardins G, Auger JP, Xu J, Segura M, Gottschalk M (2014) *Streptococcus suis*, an important pig pathogen and emerging zoonotic agent-an update on the worldwide distribution based on serotyping and sequence typing. Emerg Microbes Infect 3:e45
13. Wisselink HJ, Smith HE, Stockhofe-Zurwieden N, Peperkamp K, Vecht U (2000) Distribution of capsular types and production of muramidase-released protein (MRP) and extracellular factor (EF) of *Streptococcus suis* strains isolated from diseased pigs in seven European countries. Vet Microbiol 74:237–248
14. Sanchez del Rey V, Fernandez-Garayzabal JF, Briones V, Iriso A, Dominguez L, Gottschalk M, Vela AI (2013) Genetic analysis of *Streptococcus suis* isolates from wild rabbits. Vet Microbiol 165:483–486

15. Gottschalk M, Lacouture S, Bonifait L, Roy D, Fittipaldi N, Grenier D (2013) Characterization of *Streptococcus suis* isolates recovered between 2008 and 2011 from diseased pigs in Quebec, Canada. Vet Microbiol 162:819–825

16. Marois C, Le Devendec L, Gottschalk M, Kobisch M (2007) Detection and molecular typing of *Streptococcus suis* in tonsils from live pigs in France. Can J Vet Res 71:14–22

17. Han DU, Choi C, Ham HJ, Jung JH, Cho WS, Kim J, Higgins R, Chae C (2001) Prevalence, capsular type and antimicrobial susceptibility of *Streptococcus suis* isolated from slaughter pigs in Korea. Can J Vet Res 65:151–155

18. Okura M, Lachance C, Osaki M, Sekizaki T, Maruyama F, Nozawa T, Nakagawa I, Hamada S, Rossignol C, Gottschalk M, Takamatsu D (2014) Development of a two-step multiplex PCR assay for typing of capsular polysaccharide synthesis gene clusters of *Streptococcus suis*. J Clin Microbiol 52:1714–1719

19. Okura M, Takamatsu D, Maruyama F, Nozawa T, Nakagawa I, Osaki M, Sekizaki T, Gottschalk M, Kumagai Y, Hamada S (2013) Genetic analysis of capsular polysaccharide synthesis gene clusters from all serotypes of *Streptococcus suis*: potential mechanisms for generation of capsular variation. Appl Environ Microbiol 79:2796–2806

20. Bai X, Liu Z, Ji S, Gottschalk M, Zheng H, Xu J (2015) Simultaneous detection of 33 *Streptococcus suis* serotypes using the luminex xTAG(R) assay. J Microbiol Methods 117:95–99

21. Liu Z, Zheng H, Gottschalk M, Bai X, Lan R, Ji S, Liu H, Xu J (2013) Development of multiplex PCR assays for the identification of the 33 serotypes of *Streptococcus suis*. PLoS One 8:e72070

22. Qiu X, Bai X, Lan R, Zheng H, Xu J (2016) Novel capsular polysaccharide loci and new diagnostic tools for high-throughput capsular gene typing in *Streptococcus suis*. Appl Environ Microbiol 82:7102–7112

23. Zheng H, Ji S, Liu Z, Lan R, Huang Y, Bai X, Gottschalk M, Xu J (2015) Eight novel capsular polysaccharide synthesis gene loci identified in nontypeable *Streptococcus suis* isolates. Appl Environ Microbiol 81:4111–4119

24. Pan Z, Ma J, Dong W, Song W, Wang K, Lu C, Yao H (2015) Novel variant serotype of *Streptococcus suis* isolated from piglets with meningitis. Appl Environ Microbiol 81:976–985

25. Gottschalk M, Higgins R, Boudreau M (1993) Use of polyvalent coagglutination reagents for serotyping of *Streptococcus suis*. J Clin Microbiol 31:2192–2194

26. Ishida S, le Tien HT, Osawa R, Tohya M, Nomoto R, Kawamura Y, Takahashi T, Kikuchi N, Kikuchi K, Sekizaki T (2014) Development of an appropriate PCR system for the reclassification of *Streptococcus suis*. J Microbiol Methods 107:66–70

27. Baker GC, Smith JJ, Cowan DA (2003) Review and re-analysis of domain-specific 16S primers. J Microbiol Methods 55:541–555

28. Okwumabua O, O'Connor M, Shull E (2003) A polymerase chain reaction (PCR) assay specific for *Streptococcus suis* based on the gene encoding the glutamate dehydrogenase. FEMS Microbiol Lett 218:79–84

29. Carver TJ, Rutherford KM, Berriman M, Rajandream MA, Barrell BG, Parkhill J (2005) ACT: the Artemis comparison tool. Bioinformatics 21:3422–3423

30. Chen C, Zhang W, Zheng H, Lan R, Wang H, Du P, Bai X, Ji S, Meng Q, Jin D, Liu K, Jing H, Ye C, Gao GF, Wang L, Gottschalk M, Xu J (2013) Mini-mum core genome sequence typing of bacterial pathogens: a unified approach for clinical and public health microbiology. J Clin Microbiol 51:2582–2591

31. Zheng H, Ji S, Lan R, Liu Z, Bai X, Zhang W, Gottschalk M, Xu J (2014) Population analysis of *Streptococcus suis* isolates from slaughtered swine by use of minimum core genome sequence typing. J Clin Microbiol 52:3568–3572

32. Staats JJ, Plattner BL, Stewart GC, Changappa MM (1999) Presence of the *Streptococcus suis* suilysin gene and expression of MRP and EF correlates with high virulence in *Streptococcus suis* type 2 isolates. Vet Microbiol 70:201–211

33. Wisselink HJ, Reek FH, Vecht U, Stockhofe-Zurwieden N, Smits MA, Smith HE (1999) Detection of virulent strains of *Streptococcus suis* type 2 and highly virulent strains of *Streptococcus suis* type 1 in tonsillar specimens of pigs by PCR. Vet Microbiol 67:143–157

34. Gottschalk M, Lacouture S (2015) Canada: distribution of *Streptococcus suis* (from 2012 to 2014) and *Actinobacillus pleuropneumoniae* (from 2011 to 2014) serotypes isolated from diseased pigs. Can Vet J 56:1093–1094

35. Salter SJ, Hinds J, Gould KA, Lambertsen L, Hanage WP, Antonio M, Turner P, Hermans PW, Bootsma HJ, O'Brien KL, Bentley SD (2012) Variation at the capsule locus, cps, of mistyped and non-typable *Streptococcus pneumoniae* isolates. Microbiology 158:1560–1569

36. Lakkitjaroen N, Takamatsu D, Okura M, Sato M, Osaki M, Sekizaki T (2014) Capsule loss or death: the position of mutations among capsule genes sways the destiny of *Streptococcus suis*. FEMS Microbiol Lett 354:46–54

37. Morona JK, Morona R, Paton JC (1999) Comparative genetics of capsular polysaccharide biosynthesis in *Streptococcus pneumoniae* types belonging to serogroup 19. J Bacteriol 181:5355–5364

38. Yun KW, Cho EY, Choi EH, Lee HJ (2014) Capsular polysaccharide gene diversity of pneumococcal serotypes 6A, 6B, 6C, and 6D. Int J Med Microbiol 304:1109–1117

39. Athey TB, Teatero S, Lacouture S, Takamatsu D, Gottschalk M, Fittipaldi N (2016) Determining *Streptococcus suis* serotype from short-read whole-genome sequencing data. BMC Microbiol 16:162

40. Bonifait L, Gottschalk M, Grenier D (2010) Cell surface characteristics of nontypeable isolates of *Streptococcus suis*. FEMS Microbiol Lett 311:160–166

41. Lakkitjaroen N, Takamatsu D, Okura M, Sato M, Osaki M, Sekizaki T (2011) Loss of capsule among *Streptococcus suis* isolates from porcine endocarditis and its biological significance. J Med Microbiol 60:1669–1676

42. Auger JP, Meekhanon N, Okura M, Osaki M, Gottschalk M, Sekizaki T, Takamatsu D (2016) *Streptococcus suis* serotype 2 capsule in vivo. Emerg Infect Dis 22:1793–1796

43. Takeuchi D, Akeda Y, Nakayama T, Kerdsin A, Sano Y, Kanda T, Hamada S, Dejsirilert S, Oishi K (2014) The contribution of suilysin to the pathogenesis of *Streptococcus suis* meningitis. J Infect Dis 209:1509–1519

44. Vecht U, Wisselink HJ, Jellema ML, Smith HE (1991) Identification of two proteins associated with virulence of *Streptococcus suis* type 2. Infect Immun 59:3156–3162

14

Frequency of Th17 cells correlates with the presence of lung lesions in pigs chronically infected with *Actinobacillus pleuropneumoniae*

Elena L. Sassu[1], Andrea Ladinig[1], Stephanie C. Talker[2], Maria Stadler[2], Christian Knecht[1], Heiko Stein[1], Janna Frömbling[3], Barbara Richter[4], Joachim Spergser[3], Monika Ehling-Schulz[3], Robert Graage[5], Isabel Hennig-Pauka[1†] and Wilhelm Gerner[2*†]

Abstract

Porcine contagious pleuropneumonia caused by *Actinobacillus pleuropneumoniae* (APP) remains one of the major causes of poor growth performance and respiratory disease in pig herds. While the role of antibodies against APP has been intensely studied, the porcine T cell response remains poorly characterized. To address this, pigs were intranasally infected with APP serotype 2 and euthanized during the acute phase [6–10 days post-infection (dpi)] or the chronic phase of APP infection (27–31 dpi). Lymphocytes isolated from blood, tonsils, lung tissue and tracheo-bronchial lymph nodes were analyzed by intracellular cytokine staining (ICS) for IL-17A, IL-10 and TNF-α production after in vitro stimulation with crude capsular extract (CCE) of the APP inoculation strain. This was combined with cell surface staining for the expression of CD4, CD8α and TCR-γδ. Clinical records, microbiological investigations and pathological findings confirmed the induction of a subclinical APP infection. ICS-assays revealed the presence of APP-CCE specific CD4$^+$CD8α^{dim} IL-17A-producing T cells in blood and lung tissue in most infected animals during the acute and chronic phase of infection and a minor fraction of these cells co-produced TNF-α. APP-CCE specific IL-17A-producing γδ T cells could not be found and APP-CCE specific IL-10-producing CD4$^+$ T cells were present in various organs but only in a few infected animals. The frequency of identified putative Th17 cells (CD4$^+$CD8α^{dim}IL-17A$^+$) in lung and blood correlated positively with lung lesion scores and APP-specific antibody titers during the chronic phase. These results suggest a potential role of Th17 cells in the immune pathogenesis of APP infection.

Introduction

Actinobacillus pleuropneumoniae (APP) is a gram negative bacterium, belonging to the *Pasteurellaceae* family that causes porcine respiratory disease worldwide. The outcome of the infection can vary from sudden death with bloody nasal discharge to an acute disease with fever and coughing that frequently results in chronic infections [1]. Vaccination and antibiotic based therapies can

help to reduce the severity of the symptoms and decrease the mortality rates, but are not effective in clearing the bacteria [2]. In fact, pigs overcoming the acute phase can become subclinically infected and persistent carriers, harboring APP in tonsils and chronic lung lesions [3]. Since 1957, when APP was first reported, most research activities were focused on the elucidation of the humoral immune response [4–6]. Thereby it also became clear that APP developed several strategies to avoid humoral host defense mechanisms. For example, in vitro experiments indicated that APP can survive in alveolar macrophages [7], has the capacity for enhanced biofilm formation in anaerobic conditions [8], and changes the polysaccharide composition of the capsule [3]; all possibly contributing

*Correspondence: Wilhelm.Gerner@vetmeduni.ac.at
†Isabel Hennig-Pauka and Wilhelm Gerner contributed equally to this work
2 Institute of Immunology, Department of Pathobiology, University of Veterinary Medicine Vienna, Vienna, Austria
Full list of author information is available at the end of the article

to an escape from humoral immunity and to the establishment of chronic infection in lung tissue and tonsils.

For a more thorough understanding of APP pathogenesis and persistence, cell-mediated immune mechanisms also need to be taken into focus. In particular, T-cell responses may equip the host with additional means to combat APP infections, but could also be involved in dysfunctional immune responses [9] or could support immune escape mechanisms [10]. Hitherto, the T-cell mediated immune response to APP has been poorly characterized in swine. Early studies indicated the potential relevance of T cells, because the intensity of a T-cell dependent delayed-type hypersensitivity reaction was associated with protection against an APP challenge infection [11]. In addition, a change in the CD4:CD8 ratio in peripheral blood following low-dose APP immunization and high-dose APP challenge has been reported, but the phenotype of involved cells was not further studied [12]. Furthermore, Faldyna et al. [13] described an increase of CD8α⁻ γδ T cells in bronchoalveolar lavage fluid (BALF) as well as B-cells in tracheobronchial lymph nodes of pigs challenged with APP suggesting a role of γδ T cells in this infection. More recently, IL-17 was shown to be induced on the transcriptional level in lungs of pigs affected by APP [14] and it has been demonstrated that CD4⁺ and γδ T cells are capable to produce IL-17 in swine [15–17]. From studies in mice and humans it is known that IL-17-producing CD4⁺ T (Th17) cells are involved in the clearance of extracellular pathogens in peripheral organs by attraction and stimulation of neutrophils [18]. There is also some evidence that Th17 cells can be involved in chronic airway inflammation [19]. Moreover, in vivo and in vitro studies with *Mannheimia haemolytica*, which like APP belongs to the *Pasteurellaceae* family and induces neutrophilic infiltration in the lung, suggested an IL-17 production by bovine γδ T cells [20]. Thus we hypothesized that IL-17 production by Th17 but also γδ T cells might be involved in the porcine immune response to APP. Since the anti-inflammatory cytokine IL-10 may support the survival of microorganisms in the host via inhibiting their cell-mediated immune response [21–23], we investigated in parallel its role in persistence of APP.

To address these issues we developed an APP infection model and an in vitro stimulation assay making use of an APP crude capsular extract (APP-CCE). Cytokine production by CD4⁺ and γδ T cells was investigated by intracellular cytokine staining (ICS) of lymphocytes isolated from different host compartments during the acute and chronic phase of APP infection. We found that the majority of pigs infected with APP harbor APP-CCE specific IL-17A⁺ CD4⁺ T cells in the lung and in the blood during the acute and the chronic phase of APP infection.

In chronically infected animals, the frequency of these cells in lung and peripheral blood was found to correlate positively with lung lesions and APP-specific antibody titers.

Materials and methods
Experimental APP infection model
Thirty 5-week-old male castrated pigs (German Landrace), routinely tested to be negative for APP, porcine reproductive and respiratory syndrome virus (PRRSV), toxigenic *Pasteurella multocida*, endo- and ectoparasites, were derived from a closed breeding herd of high health status in Mecklenburg-Western Pomerania, Germany. Animals were moved to Austria, following European guidelines on protecting the welfare of animals during transport, stated by Regulation (EC) No 1/2005. Upon arrival, animals entered a biosafety level 2 facility at the University of Veterinary Medicine Vienna, where they were kept for the entire duration of the experiment. Animals were weighed, individually marked with ear tags, and then, according to their body weight, divided into a control and an infected group of ten and twenty animals respectively. Control and infected group were housed in separate compartments. Within the infected group, animals were assigned to two subgroups of ten animals each, which were kept under identical conditions but euthanized either 6–10 days post-infection (dpi) (acute infected group) or 27–31 dpi (chronic infected group). At the time of arrival, the APP-free status of the pigs was confirmed by bacteriological examination of nasal and tonsillar swabs and by serological testing for antibodies against Apx-IV using the commercially available IDEXX APP-ApxIV Ab Test ELISA (IDEXX Laboratories, Westbrook, USA). After 2 weeks of adaptation, at day 0 an intranasal spray infection was performed. For the infection, an APP biotype 1 serotype 2 strain (Lab number C3656/0271/11) was used, isolated originally by the Institute of Microbiology, University of Veterinary Medicine, Hanover, Germany from a diseased fattening pig during an acute outbreak of porcine pleuropneumonia in northern Germany [24]. After initial isolation, bacteria were animal-passaged once and lab-passaged four times in PPLO medium supplemented with NAD. Pigs were infected with 2 mL (1 mL into each nostril) of bacterial culture containing 2×10^4 CFU/mL. The bacterial culture was vaporized directly into the nostrils of the pigs by using a mucosal atomization device (LMA MAD Nasal™, Teleflex Medical GmbH, Athlone, Ireland). Control pigs underwent the same procedure, but received 2 mL of 154 mM sterile NaCl instead of the bacterial culture. Daily clinical examinations were carried out and assembled in a clinical score, considering rectal temperature, presence of dyspnea and/or coughing and changes

in behavior (see Additional file 1 for details). Additionally, pig body weights were recorded weekly. To screen for presence of APP in the upper respiratory tract, nasal and tonsillar swabs were examined at 14 and 21 dpi. At the end of the experiment, after animals were euthanized, tonsillar tissues were taken instead of swabs. Blood samples were taken by puncture of the *V. cava cranialis* or *V. jugularis* on the same days. Sera were used for detection of APP 2 specific antibodies, while heparinized samples were obtained to isolate peripheral blood mononuclear cells (PBMCs). Euthanasia was performed on five consecutive days (two infected pigs and one control pig per day) in two different time frames: 6–10 dpi and 27–31 dpi for the acutely and the chronically infected group, respectively. Within these two periods, animals were randomly selected for euthanasia, which was performed by intracardial administration of T61® (T61®: Embutramid, Mebezoniumiodid, Tetracainhydrochlorid, 1 mL/10 kg BW, MSD, Whitehouse Station, NJ, USA) during anesthesia (Narketan®, Stresnil®). All animal procedures were approved by the institutional ethics committee, the Advisory Committee for Animal experiments (§12 of Law for Animal Experiments, Tierversuchsgesetz—TVG) and the Federal Ministry for Science and Research (reference number bmwfw GZ 68.205/0138-WF/V/3b/2015).

Gross necropsy and pathological examination

At necropsy, a general pathological examination of the carcass was performed, with focus on the respiratory tract. Organs of interest for the study were extracted in the following order: salivary gland (*Glandula mandibularis*, GM), tonsils, tracheobronchial lymph node (TBLN) and lung. After evaluation of the thoracic cavity, the lung was extracted from the chest while paying particular attention to the presence of pleural effusion or pleural adhesions. Then the severity of the pathological findings was determined using the lung lesion score (LLS) by Hannan et al. [25] and using the slaughterhouse pleurisy evaluation system (SPES) [26] for assessment of the pleura status. After clamping off the left main bronchus, the right lung was flushed with 100 mL of 154 mM sterile NaCl for collection of BALF, while tissue samples were taken from the dorsal portion of the left caudal lobe. If no lesions were detected in this particular area, an additional sample from another affected part of the lung was taken for histologic and bacteriological investigations. For histology, samples were fixed in 10% neutral buffered formalin, processed in 3-μm-thick paraffin-embedded sections and stained with haematoxylin and eosin.

Microbiological investigation

Nasal and tonsillar swabs from living animals and nasal swabs, salivary gland, tonsils, tracheobronchial lymph node, lung and BALF from euthanized animals were investigated for the presence of APP by streaking the samples on Columbia sheep blood agar (Oxoid, Vienna, Austria). *Staphylococcus aureus* was used as nurse to facilitate the isolation of APP from organs carrying a high bacterial background flora, such as tonsils and nose [1]. Subsequently, APP was transferred to PPLO agar supplemented with 10 mg/L NAD (AppliChem GmbH, Darmstadt, Germany). Plates were incubated overnight at 37 °C and 5% CO_2. Identification of the re-isolated bacteria was confirmed by serotype 2 specific PCR, using primers for the capsular biosynthesis genes *cps2AB* [27]. In addition, snap frozen tissue samples were examined directly by a conventional PCR based on detection of the apxIVA gene [28].

Determination of APP 2-specific antibody titers in serum

Sera obtained prior to infection (day 0), at the time of euthanasia and at 14 and 21 dpi were analyzed for antibodies against APP 2 using the commercial Swinecheck® APP 2 ELISA (Biovet, St-Hyacinthe, Canada) according to the manufacturer's instructions. Results were recorded as S/P ratio, obtained by the ratio between optical density (OD) of each sample (S) and the mean OD of the positive control (P): ODs/MODp.

Preparation of APP crude capsular extract for in vitro recall experiments

To stimulate lymphocytes in vitro, a crude capsular extract (CCE) from the APP serotype 2 strain C3656/0271/11, which has been used to infect the animals, was prepared following a modified protocol from Wittkowski et al. [29]. In detail, 300 mL liquid cultures of APP biotype 1, serotype 2, strain C3656, were grown to an OD_{600} of approximately 0.2 and harvested by centrifugation at 6530 *g* for 5 min. Aqueous phenol (1%, w/v) was added to the harvested bacteria (18 mL per gram of bacterial wet weight). Thereafter, the suspensions were shaken for 10 min at 37 °C and transferred to conical 25 mL flasks and the solution was gently stirred for 4 h at 4 °C. After centrifugation at 21 420 *g* for 30 min at 4 °C, the supernatant was filtrated (0.2 μm, Filtropur, Sarstedt, Nümbrecht, Germany), dialyzed against MilliQ-H_2O (2–4 L replaced every 4 h during the first day, then every 8 h) at 4 °C for 2 days, using 1 kDa MWCO membrane (Mini Dialysis Kit, GE Healthcare) and finally lyophilized overnight. To preserve the integrity of potential immunogenic proteins in the capsular extract, no further purification was performed. Lyophilized samples were dissolved in phosphate buffered saline (PBS) to reach a final concentration of 1 mg/mL. The stimulus was tested for potential toxicity in ConA-stimulated (3 μg/mL) PBMCs labelled with violet proliferation dye as described elsewhere [30]. After 4 days of cultivation, PBMCs were harvested and stained with Live/Dead® Near-IR stain kit (Invitrogen, Carlsbad, CA, USA) according to manufacturer's instructions and subjected to flow cytometry (FCM). Frequencies of dead cells and proliferating cells were determined and by a dose titration of the CCE, the optimal working concentration was found to be 4 μg/mL.

Sample collection and isolation of lymphocytes

Blood samples were collected in Lithium-Heparin tubes (Primavette®, KABE Labortechnik, Nümbrecht, Germany) prior to infection (day 0), at 14 and 21 dpi and at the time of death. PBMCs were isolated by density gradient centrifugation (Pancoll human, density 1.077 g/mL, PAN Biotech, Aidenbach, Germany) as described elsewhere [31]. Tonsils and tracheobronchial lymph nodes were subjected to a procedure for isolation of lymphocytes as previously described [30].

For isolation of lymphocytes from lung tissue, a block of tissue (approx. $4 \times 3 \times 2$ cm) from the dorsal portion of the left caudal lobe was cut into small pieces (approx. $3 \times 3 \times 3$ mm) and lymphocytes were isolated as described elsewhere [32]. Cells from the various tissues and blood were counted and suspended in cell culture medium (RPMI1640 with stable glutamine supplemented with 10% FCS, 100 IU/mL penicillin, 100 μg/mL streptomycin, all from PAN Biotech and 90 μg/mL gentamicin, from Sigma-Aldrich, Schnelldorf, Germany) for in vitro cultivation. To standardize the isolation of lymphocytes from lung tissue, we decided to sample a defined region of the lung, independently of the presence of lesions. The dorsal portion of the left caudal lobe was selected for this purpose, since the caudal lobes have been described to be a common site for APP lesions [33] but the right lung was washed for the collection of BALF.

Histopathological analysis of lung tissue

Lung samples for histopathological analysis from acutely and chronically infected animals were fixed in neutral buffered formalin and embedded in paraffin wax. Tissue slides were routinely stained with hematoxylin and eosin and examined by a pathologist blinded to the different treatment groups. The samples were located adjacent to tissue used for lymphocyte isolation. Histopathological lesions associated with porcine pleuropneumonia, such as tissue necrosis, neutrophilic, histiocytic and lymphocytic infiltration, vascular leakage (including edema, bleeding, and fibrin in tissue or air spaces) and fibroplasia were graded (0 = not present, 1 = low grade, 2 = moderate grade, 3 = high grade).

In vitro stimulation of lymphocytes

Freshly isolated cells from lung, blood, tracheobronchial lymph nodes and tonsils were stimulated in vitro with APP-CCE (4 μg/mL) for 18 h at 37 °C in 5% CO_2. Cells were cultured in round-bottomed 96-well plates, at 5×10^5 cells per well, in a volume of 200 μL. Four hours prior to harvesting the cells, Brefeldin A (BD GolgiPlug™, BD Biosciences, San Jose, CA, USA) was added at a final concentration of 1 μg/mL. In parallel, cells incubated in cell culture medium only served as a negative control. As a positive control for cytokine production, a further set of cells was cultivated in cell culture medium overnight but stimulated with phorbol 12-myristate 13-acetate (PMA; 50 ng/mL; Sigma-Aldrich) and Ionomycin (500 ng/mL; Sigma-Aldrich) during the last 4 h of incubation.

Intracellular cytokine staining and FCM analysis

For FCM staining, cells were harvested and resuspended in PBS (without Ca^{2+}/Mg^{2+}) supplemented with 3% FCS. Monoclonal antibodies (mAbs) and secondary reagents that were used for cell surface staining and subsequent intracellular cytokine staining are listed in Table 1. Staining was performed in 96-well round-bottom plates with all incubation steps lasting for 20 min at 4 °C. For discrimination of dead cells, Live/Dead® Near-IR stain kit (Invitrogen) was used. To fix and permeabilize the cells, BD Cytofix/Cytoperm and BD Perm/Wash (BD Biosciences, CA, USA) was employed according to manufacturer's instructions.

FCM samples were analyzed on a FACSCanto™ II flow cytometer (BD Biosciences) equipped with three lasers (405, 488 and 633 nm). For automatic calculation of the compensation, single-stain samples were prepared. Between 5×10^5 and 1×10^6 lymphocytes were recorded per sample. Gating of the lymphocytes, doublet discrimination and dead-cell exclusion were performed for all samples as displayed in Additional file 2. Data were processed by FACSDiva software (Version 6.1.3 BD Biosciences) and transferred to Microsoft Excel (Office 2010; Microsoft, Redmond, WA, USA) for further calculations and preparation of graphs.

Statistical analysis

Spearman's rank correlation test was used to investigate the correlation between the frequency of Th17 cells and disease parameters in individual pigs. Spearman's rank correlation coefficients (ρ) and corresponding p values were calculated in SPSS software (2011, IBM, SPSS Statistics for Windows, Version 20.0, Armonk, NY, IBM Corp.). SPSS was also applied to produce correlation graphs. For further elaboration of graphs, Inkscape

Table 1 Antibody panels

Antigen	Clone	Isotype	Fluorochrome	Labelling strategy	Source of primary Ab
Intracellular cytokine staining for IL-17A and TNF-α					
CD4	74-12-4	IgG2b	PerCP-Cy5.5	Directly conjugated	BD Biosciences
CD8α	11/295/33	IgG2a	Pe-Cy7	Secondary antibody[a]	In house
TCR-γδ	PPT16	IgG2b	BV421	Biotin–streptavidin[b]	In house
IL-17A	SCPL1362	IgG1	Alexa647	Directly conjugated	BD Biosciences
TNF-α	MAb11	IgG1	BV605	Directly conjugated	BioLegend
Intracellular cytokine staining for IL-10					
CD4	74-12-4	IgG2b	Alexa647	Secondary antibody[c]	In house
CD8α	11/295/33	IgG2a	BV421	Biotin–streptavidin[b]	In house
IL-10	945A 4C4 37B1	IgG1	PE	Secondary antibody[d]	Invitrogen

[a] Goat Anti-Mouse IgG$_{2a}$-PE-Cy7, SouthernBiotech.

[b] Brilliant Violet 421™ Streptavidin, BioLegend.

[c] Goat Anti-Mouse IgG$_{2b}$-AlexaFluor647, Invitrogen.

[d] Goat Anti-Mouse IgG$_1$-PE, SouthernBiotech.

(Version 0.91; Free and Open Source Software licensed under the GPL) was used.

Results

Establishment of an infection model for APP subclinical infection

To confirm the establishment of a subclinical APP infection in the pigs of our study, bacteriological and clinical parameters were investigated (Figure 1). APP could be isolated from the nose of the majority of infected animals both from the acute (6–10 dpi) and from the chronic period (27–31 dpi) (Figure 1A). Animals belonging to the latter group were additionally tested at 14 and 21 dpi, for weekly monitoring. The nasal swabs of some of these animals were positive during weekly monitoring but not at the time of death (indicated by a § in Figure 1A). Isolation of APP from tonsils was often impaired by overgrowth of contaminating flora, but for the majority of animals from the chronic phase (8 out of 10) APP could be identified by PCR. At the early endpoint (6–10 dpi), the location from which APP was most frequently isolated was the lung, with 7 positive samples out of 10. In contrast, at the late endpoint (27–31 dpi) only 1 out of 10 samples was positive in the lung. APP was detected in BALF and TBLN of only one animal, which died suddenly at 8 dpi (#19). APP could not be detected in salivary glands (*G. mandibularis*, GM) of any animal.

Macroscopically visible lung tissue alterations were highly variable, which is partially reflected by the lung lesion and SPES scores (Figure 1B; Additional file 3 for representative animals). On average, LLS scores from animals sacrificed during the acute phase were higher than during the chronic phase. Typical histopathological findings indicating porcine pleuropneumonia were found

in infected pigs varying from acute (hyperemia, edema, neutrophilic infiltration) to chronic (sequestration of necrotic areas by a mixed inflammatory infiltrate and fibroplasia) inflammatory tissue alterations (Additional file 4).

To evaluate the health status of the pigs, rectal temperature was measured daily together with other clinical parameters. Generally, infected animals developed clinical symptoms like dyspnea and coughing and were more lethargic than controls within the first 10 dpi. No significant differences in average daily weight gain were observed between infected (mean 724.7 g ± standard deviation of 92.6 g) and control (785.3 g ± standard deviation of 130.7 g) animals during the first 3 weeks post infection. Body temperature of infected animals started rising towards 40 °C immediately after the day of infection (day 0), with some animals reaching high temperature levels within 1–10 dpi (Figure 1C). Then, the rectal temperature stabilized between 39.5 and 40 °C for 2 weeks to finally align with the levels of control animals at the end of the study period (25–31 dpi). In parallel, the APP 2-specific humoral response was evaluated throughout the experiment (Figure 1D). Most of the infected animals produced antibodies against APP 2 after 14 days, i.e., antibodies were only detectable in animals that survived until the chronic phase of infection. No APP 2 antibodies were detectable in control animals at any time point.

Production of IL-17A and/or TNF-α by CD4$^+$ T cells in response to APP-CCE

For characterization of the T-cell mediated immune response, freshly isolated cells from lung, PBMCs, TBLN and tonsils were subjected to in vitro stimulation with

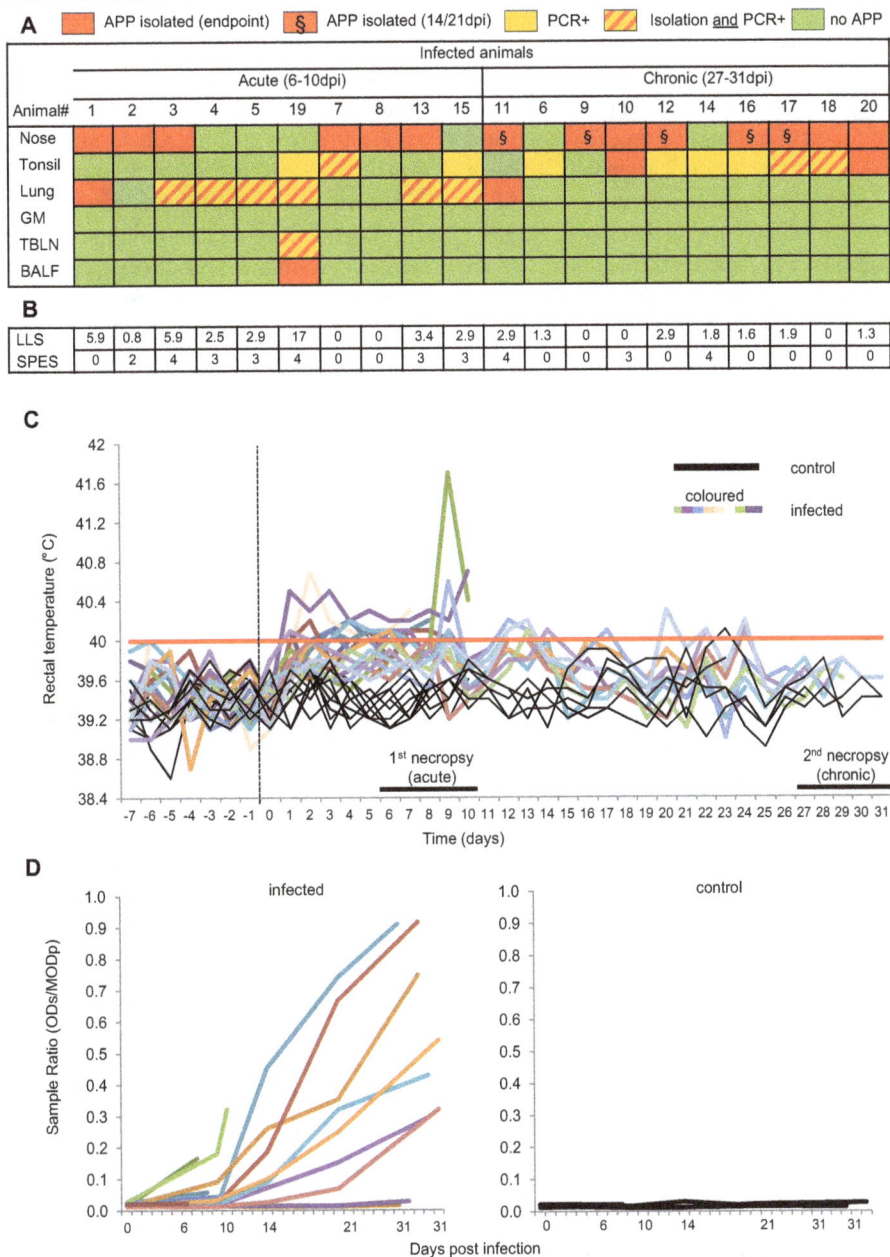

Figure 1 Microbiological investigation, lung pathology, clinical signs and antibody titers of APP-infected pigs. A The presence of APP was investigated at different host locations during necropsy (GM, *Glandula mandibularis*; TBLN, tracheobronchial lymph node; BALF, bronchoalveolar lavage fluid). Red boxes indicate APP detection by agar isolation, orange boxes indicate APP detection by PCR and orange boxes with red lines indicate positive results by both techniques. Green boxes indicate negative findings for APP. Results shown in the table refer to sampling on the day of euthanasia. The nasal swabs of animals #11, 9, 12, 16 and 17 were tested positive only on day 14 and/or 21 pi. This is indicated by red boxes with §. **B** Pathology of the lung was assessed by lung lesion score (LLS) for the lung tissue and by slaughterhouse pleurisy evaluation system (SPES) for the pleura. **C** Rectal temperatures were measured daily in both infected (colored lines) and control (black lines) animals. Body temperature of 40 °C or higher was considered as fever (red line). **D** Humoral response against APP serotype 2. Data are expressed as a ratio between optical density of the sample (ODs) and the mean of the optical density of the positive control (MODp). Colored lines in the left graph show ratios for infected animals, black lines in the right graph indicate ratios from sera of control animals.

APP-CCE of APP 2 followed by ICS for IL-17A and TNF-α. Medium- and PMA/Ionomycin-stimulated cultures served as negative and positive controls, respectively.

Total living lymphocytes were gated and analyzed for CD4 expression and IL-17A production (Additional files 2A–D). A considerable variability in frequencies of

IL-17A$^+$ CD4$^+$ T cells was found between different animals and organs following APP-CCE stimulation (Figure 2). Figure 2A shows representative data of IL-17A production and CD4 expression in lung-derived lymphocytes isolated from different animals during the acute and chronic phase. For each time point, original FCM data from one animal with a high and a low frequency of APP-CCE-responsive IL-17A$^+$ CD4$^+$ T cells is shown. In addition, respective contour plots for lymphocytes from an APP-infected but apparently non-responding animal (frequency of IL-17A$^+$ CD4$^+$ T cells was higher or at the same level for medium stimulation as compared to APP-CCE stimulation) as well as an animal from the control group are presented. Following PMA/Ionomycin stimulation IL-17A production was found in a subpopulation of CD4$^+$ T cells from all animals. Similar findings were obtained in PBMC cultures, albeit frequencies of IL-17A$^+$ CD4$^+$ T cells were somewhat lower (Additional file 5). Overall, the highest number of animals with elevated frequencies of APP-CCE reactive-IL-17A$^+$ CD4$^+$ T cells was found within lung and PBMCs (Figure 2B). During the acute phase the frequencies of IL-17A$^+$ CD4$^+$ T cells in the lung were substantially higher in five out of nine animals compared to the control animals. This was similar during the chronic phase, with two animals (#11, #12) showing even increased frequencies of IL-17A$^+$ CD4$^+$ T cells. Within PBMCs the number of responding animals was similar to the lung during the acute phase but, later in the chronic phase, the median of the frequency of IL-17A$^+$ CD4$^+$ T cells dropped down to control levels. In TBLN and tonsils, CD4$^+$ T cells of only a few infected animals responded with IL-17A production to APP-CCE stimulation, regardless of the time post infection (Figure 2B).

Expression of CD8α is correlated with activation and/or memory formation of porcine CD4$^+$ T cells [34] and following PMA/Ionomycin stimulation, IL-17A producing CD4$^+$ T cells mainly have a CD8α$^+$ phenotype [17]. We therefore analyzed CD8α expression and IL-17A production in gated CD4$^+$ T cells following APP-CCE stimulation (Figure 3; Additional file 6). In the lungs of animals belonging to the acute group, the majority of IL-17A$^+$ CD4$^+$ T cells following APP-CCE and PMA/Ionomycin stimulation were CD8α^{dim}, whereas in the chronic phase CD8α expression tended to be higher and this applied equally to APP-CCE and PMA/Ionomycin stimulated cells (Figure 3). Similar results were obtained with PBMCs albeit here an up-regulation of CD8α in IL-17A-producing CD4$^+$ T cells from the acute to the chronic phase was less obvious (Additional file 6).

Next, we analyzed co-production of IL-17A and TNF-α within APP-CCE-stimulated CD4$^+$ T cells (Figure 4; Additional file 7; for gating strategy see Additional files 2E and F), since frequent co-production of TNF-α has

been observed in PMA/Ionomycin-stimulated porcine IL-17A$^+$ CD4$^+$ T cells [17]. The majority of IL-17A-producing CD4$^+$ T cells isolated from lung tissue (Figure 4) or within PBMC (Additional file 7) did not co-produce TNF-α following APP-CCE stimulation (Figure 4A; Additional file 7A, indicated by arrowhead 1). In contrast, but in accordance with previously published data [17] following PMA/Ionomycin stimulation most IL-17A$^+$ CD4$^+$ T cells co-produced TNF-α (Figure 4A; Additional file 7A, arrowhead 2). Despite low frequencies for the majority of APP-infected animals, a tendency of higher frequencies of TNF-α$^+$ IL-17A$^+$ CD4$^+$ T cells was found within lymphocytes from APP-infected pigs compared to control animals following APP-CCE stimulation. This applied to cells isolated from lung tissue (Figure 4B) and blood (Additional file 7B).

APP-CCE stimulation induced production of IL-17A by a subset of lymphocytes that is neither TCR-γδ$^+$ nor CD4$^+$

After stimulation with APP-CCE, at least for some animals a considerable number of CD4$^-$ cells showed the ability to produce IL-17A in parallel to CD4$^+$ T cells (Figure 2A). This finding was more prominent in the lung, but it was detected also in PBMCs (Additional file 5). Since porcine γδ T cells were previously identified as potential IL-17A producers following PMA/Ionomycin stimulation [16], we hypothesized that these cells might also contribute to IL-17A production following APP-CCE stimulation. Hence, CD4$^-$ cells were further gated for expression of TCR-γδ and IL-17A (Additional files 2E and G). Interestingly, these IL-17A-producing cells induced by APP-CCE stimulation were TCR-γδ$^-$ (Figure 5; Additional file 8, arrowhead 1). However, they were also present in lymphocytes isolated from control animals (Figure 5; Additional file 8, last column), which seems to indicate that these cells did not require a preceding in vivo priming by APP. Their frequency was quite variable between individual animals but mostly exceeded the very low frequency of IL-17A-producing CD4$^-$ TCR-γδ$^-$ cells identified in medium stimulated cultures. Following PMA/Ionomycin stimulation, IL-17A-producing γδ T cells could be identified (Figure 5; Additional file 8, bottom panel, arrowhead 2), although IL-17A producing cells isolated from lung tissue showed a dim expression of TCR-γδ. Overall, this confirms the potential of porcine γδ T cells for IL-17A production but our data suggests that APP-CCE stimulation does not induce IL-17A production in this prominent porcine T-cell subset.

Inconsistent IL-10 production by CD4$^+$ T cells following APP-CCE stimulation

To investigate a potential induction of IL-10-producing lymphocytes in our APP-CCE in vitro stimulation assay

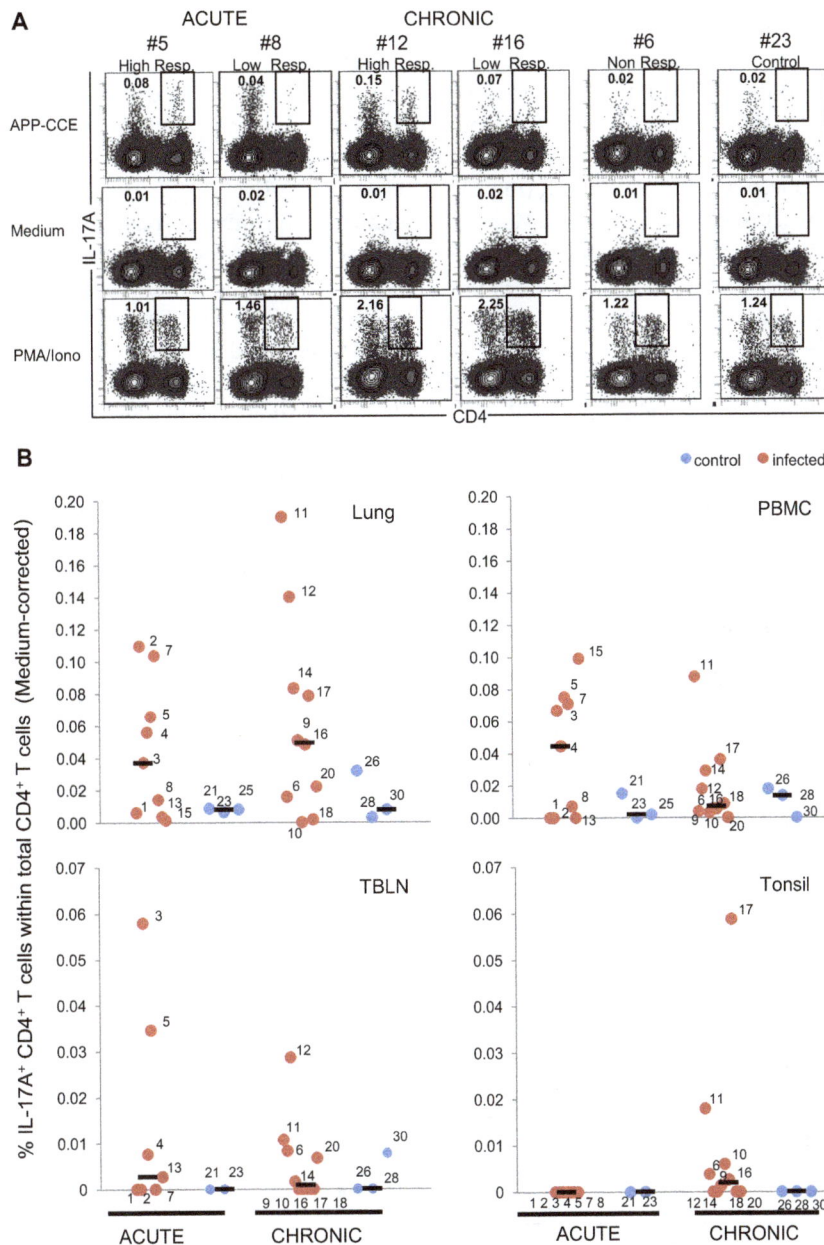

Figure 2 APP-CCE specific IL-17A-producing CD4⁺ T cells in lung, blood, tracheobronchial lymph nodes and tonsils. Cells isolated from lung, blood (PBMC), tracheobronchial lymph nodes (TBLN) and tonsils were incubated overnight with APP crude capsular extract (APP-CCE), medium or PMA/Ionomycin. Living lymphocytes were gated (not shown; see Additional file 1) and further analyzed for the expression of IL-17A and CD4. **A** For the lung, data from representative animals from different groups are displayed: #5 and #8 for the acute phase, designated as "high responder" and "low responder" respectively; #12 and #16 for the chronic phase designated as "high responder" and "low responder" respectively; #6, designated as non-responder and control #23. Approximately 1×10^6 (APP and medium) and 2×10^5 (PMA/Ionomycin) cells are shown in the contour plots. Numbers displayed within the contour plots indicate the percentages of IL-17A⁺ CD4⁺ T cells within total CD4⁺ T cells. **B** Frequency of IL-17A⁺ CD4⁺ T cells within total CD4⁺ T cells in lung, blood (PBMC), tracheobronchial lymph node (TBLN) and tonsils of all infected animals (red dots) and control animals (blue dots) during acute and chronic phase. Numbers next to colored dots indicate numbers of individual animals. Median percent values are indicated by black bars. Medium-corrected percent values are presented (% of IL-17A⁺ CD4⁺ T cells within total CD4⁺ T cells for APP-CCE stimulation minus % of IL-17A⁺ CD4⁺ T cells within total CD4⁺ T cells for medium incubation).

the production of IL-10 was analyzed in parallel samples to that of IL-17A/TNF-α in combination with cell surface staining for CD4 and CD8α expression. Overall, with the exception of cells isolated from the APP-infected pig #17, frequencies of IL-10⁺ CD4⁺ T cells were low and inconsistently distributed between individual animals during the acute and the chronic phase as well as different organs (Figure 6). However, in cells of some animals, the frequency of IL-10$^+$ CD4$^+$ T cells was at least two-fold higher following APP-CCE stimulation compared to medium and was also higher compared to that from control animals. This applied to animals #3, 5 and 7 in the lung during the acute phase and animal #18 during the chronic phase (see also Figure 6A for original FCM data). Similarly, within PBMCs, animals #7, 4, 5, 11 and 15 appeared to have APP-CCE-reactive IL-10$^+$ CD4$^+$ T cells above background levels (see also Additional file 9 for original FCM data). Isolated during the chronic phase, CD4$^+$ T cells from animal #17 showed an exceptionally high frequency of IL-10 producing cells after APP-CCE stimulation, both in lung and in tonsils (Figures 6A and B). The reasons for this are unknown. CD4$^-$ IL-10-producing cells were identified (Figure 6A; Additional file 9 and data not shown) but similar frequencies were found for APP-CCE- and medium-stimulated cultures.

Frequency of IL-17A$^+$ CD4$^+$ T cells correlates positively with disease parameters during the chronic phase of infection

We next investigated whether the variable frequency of APP-CCE-reactive IL-17A$^+$ CD4$^+$ T cells between different animals and organs correlated with parameters of APP pathogenesis and also APP-specific antibody titers. In chronically infected animals, the frequency of APP-CCE-reactive IL-17A$^+$ CD4$^+$ T cells isolated from the

lung showed a positive correlation with LLS (Spearman's rho = 0.858; p = 0.001) and with APP 2 antibody titers (Spearman's rho = 0.632, p = 0.05). For IL-17A$^+$CD4$^+$ T cells within PBMCs of the same group of animals also a positive correlation with LLS and antibody titers was found (Spearman's rho of 0.679; p = 0.031 and 0.742, p = 0.014 respectively) (Figure 7). In contrast, for acutely infected animals no positive correlation of IL-17A$^+$ CD4$^+$ T cells isolated from lung or blood with the LLS was found (Additional file 10). Additionally, the frequencies of APP-CCE-reactive IL-17A$^+$ CD4$^+$ T cells isolated from the lung and blood were tested for correlation with histological scores of the lung tissue adjacent to tissue used for isolation of lymphocytes (Additional file 11). A total histological score for each sample was calculated by summing up all analyzed parameters (see Additional file 4) and was used to calculate the correlation. No significant correlation was found, which may indicate that APP-CCE-reactive IL-17A$^+$ CD4$^+$ T cells have a general capacity for lung homing.

Discussion

The main focus of the study was to characterize the cytokine response of T cells isolated from pigs undergoing either an acute or a subclinical APP infection. To address this question, we first aimed to establish an infection model that evokes typical but not lethal APP disease symptoms and induces a status of subclinical infection. Most of the experimental infections described in the literature so far focused on studying the acute phase of

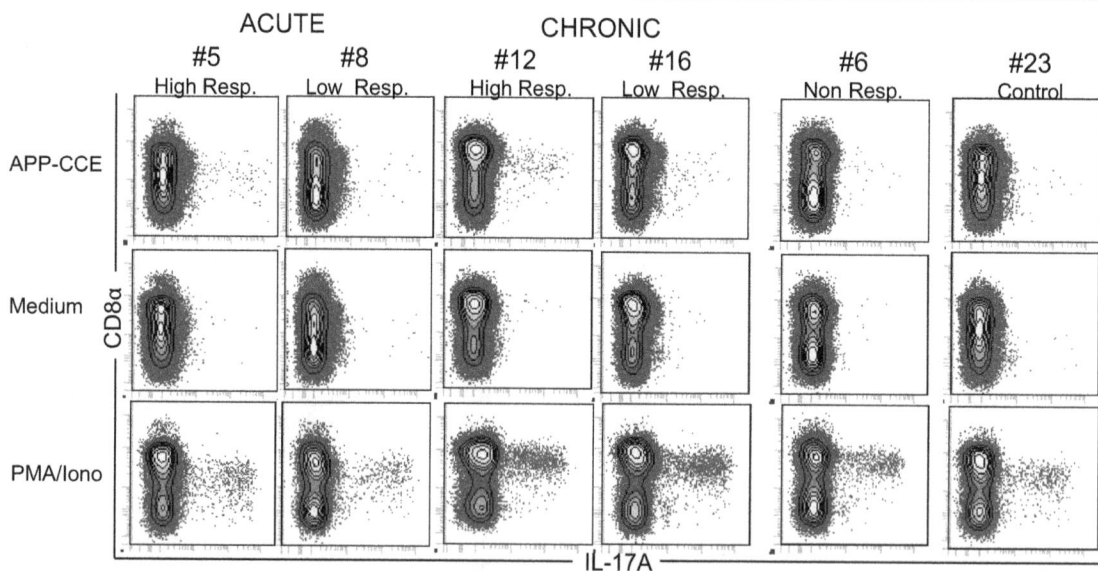

Figure 3 Expression of CD8α by IL-17A$^+$ CD4$^+$ T cells in the lung. Cells isolated from lung tissue were incubated overnight with APP crude capsular extract (APP-CCE), medium or PMA/Ionomycin and subsequently analyzed for CD4, CD8α and IL-17A expression by FCM. Living CD4$^+$ T cells were gated (not shown; see Additional file 1) and subsequently investigated for expression of CD8α and IL-17A. Data from the same animals as in Figure 2 are shown. Approximately 1 × 10^5 (APP and medium) and 5 × 10^4 (PMA/Ionomycin) CD4$^+$ T cells are shown in the contour plots.

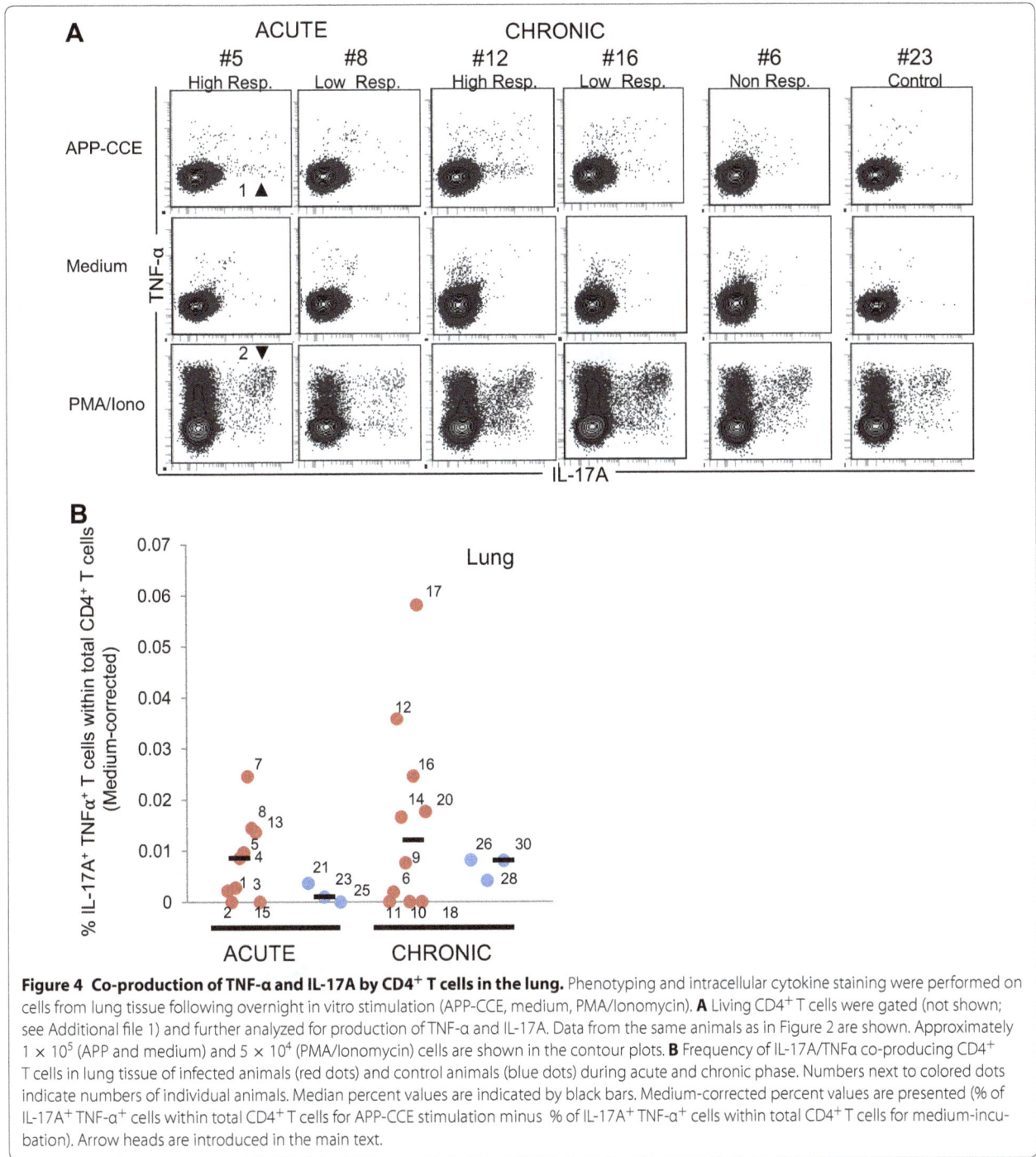

Figure 4 Co-production of TNF-α and IL-17A by CD4⁺ T cells in the lung. Phenotyping and intracellular cytokine staining were performed on cells from lung tissue following overnight in vitro stimulation (APP-CCE, medium, PMA/Ionomycin). **A** Living CD4⁺ T cells were gated (not shown; see Additional file 1) and further analyzed for production of TNF-α and IL-17A. Data from the same animals as in Figure 2 are shown. Approximately 1×10^5 (APP and medium) and 5×10^4 (PMA/Ionomycin) cells are shown in the contour plots. **B** Frequency of IL-17A/TNFα co-producing CD4⁺ T cells in lung tissue of infected animals (red dots) and control animals (blue dots) during acute and chronic phase. Numbers next to colored dots indicate numbers of individual animals. Median percent values are indicated by black bars. Medium-corrected percent values are presented (% of IL-17A⁺ TNF-α⁺ cells within total CD4⁺ T cells for APP-CCE stimulation minus % of IL-17A⁺ TNF-α⁺ cells within total CD4⁺ T cells for medium-incubation). Arrow heads are introduced in the main text.

APP infection [35–37]. The outcome of APP infection is depending on the route of infection, the dose and the virulence of the strain [38]. Baarsch et al. [39] demonstrated that the route of infection influences the distribution of lung lesions, with the intranasal inoculation provoking mainly unilateral lesions and the endotracheal infection inducing diffuse bilateral pneumonia. To

better mimic natural infection, we decided to perform an intranasal inoculation. To avoid loss of bacterial solution by swallowing or miscalculation of the actual infection dose by aerosol administration, the inoculum was sprayed directly into the nostrils rather than deposited as a liquid. Considering that vaporizing the bacterial solution into finely atomized particles increases the chance of

APP reaching the alveoli [1], the infection dose was kept to low levels to avoid the induction of a per-acute form. The endpoints where chosen to compare acute and sub-clinical phase of infection. We hypothesized that at days 6–10 a first activation of T cells may be measurable like previously reported for acute influenza A virus infection [40]. Additionally, the median duration of APP tonsillar colonization was reported around 7–8 weeks post-infection (pi) [41] leading to the assumption that APP would still be present at days 27–31 pi causing a subclinical infection. Pathological and clinical findings confirmed the establishment of a bi-phasic course of infection. The variety of rectal temperatures obtained during the acute phase paralleled with the variety of lung lesions observed at necropsy, with patterns ranging from severe and diffuse pneumonia with dark red–purple areas (per-acute), local-ized necrotizing pneumonia accompanied by fibrinous pleurisy (acute) to firm adhesive pleurisy and organized sequestra (chronic). On the opposite, during the chronic phase animals showed more uniform lesions and their body temperatures dropped down to physiological levels. These results indicate that our infection model success-fully induced an acute infection that resolved into a sub-clinical one. Furthermore, this dichotomy could also be found by analyzing the presence of APP at different host compartments. During the acute phase, APP was mostly detected in the lung (7 out of 10), and hardly in the tonsils (3 out of 10). During the chronic phase, only one animal

was positive in the lung, whereas in the tonsils 8 out of 10 tested positive. This might indicate a shift in the tropism of the bacteria from the lower to the upper respiratory tract and might be interpreted as an attempt of the bacte-ria to escape from the local immune response in the lung.

In frame of this study, we developed an in vitro stimula-tion assay using a crude capsular extract of APP. This assay was used to investigate the production of IL-17A, TNF-α and IL-10 in lymphocytes isolated from lung, peripheral blood, tracheobronchial lymph node and tonsil. Our data suggest that IL-17A-producing CD4$^+$ T cells are induced in the lung tissue and blood of most APP-infected pigs. IL-17 is a pro-inflammatory cytokine, known to play a role in pul-monary infection and neutrophil recruitment [42, 43]. Its role in veterinary animal species [44] and its up-regulation in the surroundings of APP colonies in affected lung lesions on mRNA level have been previously described [14]. Thus it is tempting to speculate that the APP-CCE-reactive IL-17A producing CD4$^+$ T cells identified in this study repre-sent APP-specific Th17 cells. The specificity of these cells is corroborated by two findings. First, similar to PMA/Iono-mycin-induced IL-17A$^+$ CD4$^+$ T cells, these putative APP-specific Th17 cells expressed low or intermediate levels of CD8α. Its expression in porcine CD4$^+$ T cells is related to activation and/or memory formation [34, 45]. Therefore, this CD8α expression can be interpreted as an indication that APP-CCE-reactive IL-17A-producing CD4$^+$ T cells performed an in vitro recall response. Secondly, APP-CCE

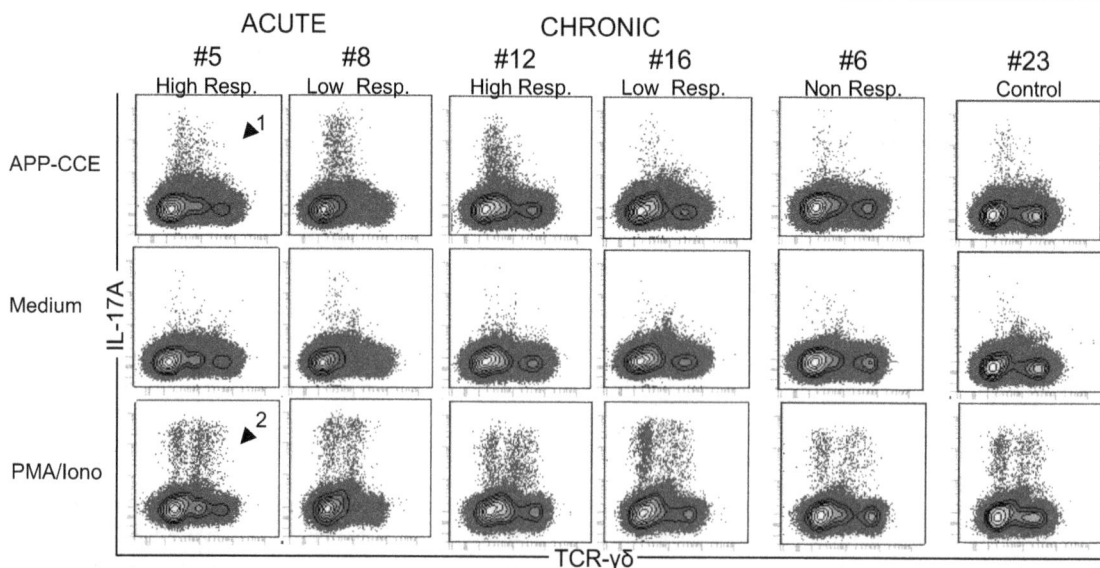

Figure 5 Production of IL-17A by non-CD4$^+$ cells and γδ T cells in the lung. Cells isolated from lung tissue were incubated overnight with APP-CCE, medium or PMA/Ionomycin and subsequently analyzed for CD4, TCR-γδ and IL-17A expression by FCM. Living lymphocytes excluding CD4$^+$ T cells (not shown; see Additional file 1) were gated and further analyzed for expression of IL-17A and TCR-γδ. Data from the same animals as in Figure 2 are shown. Approximately 1 × 10^6 (APP and medium) and 2 × 10^5 (PMA/Ionomycin) cells are shown in the contour plots. Arrow heads are introduced in the main text.

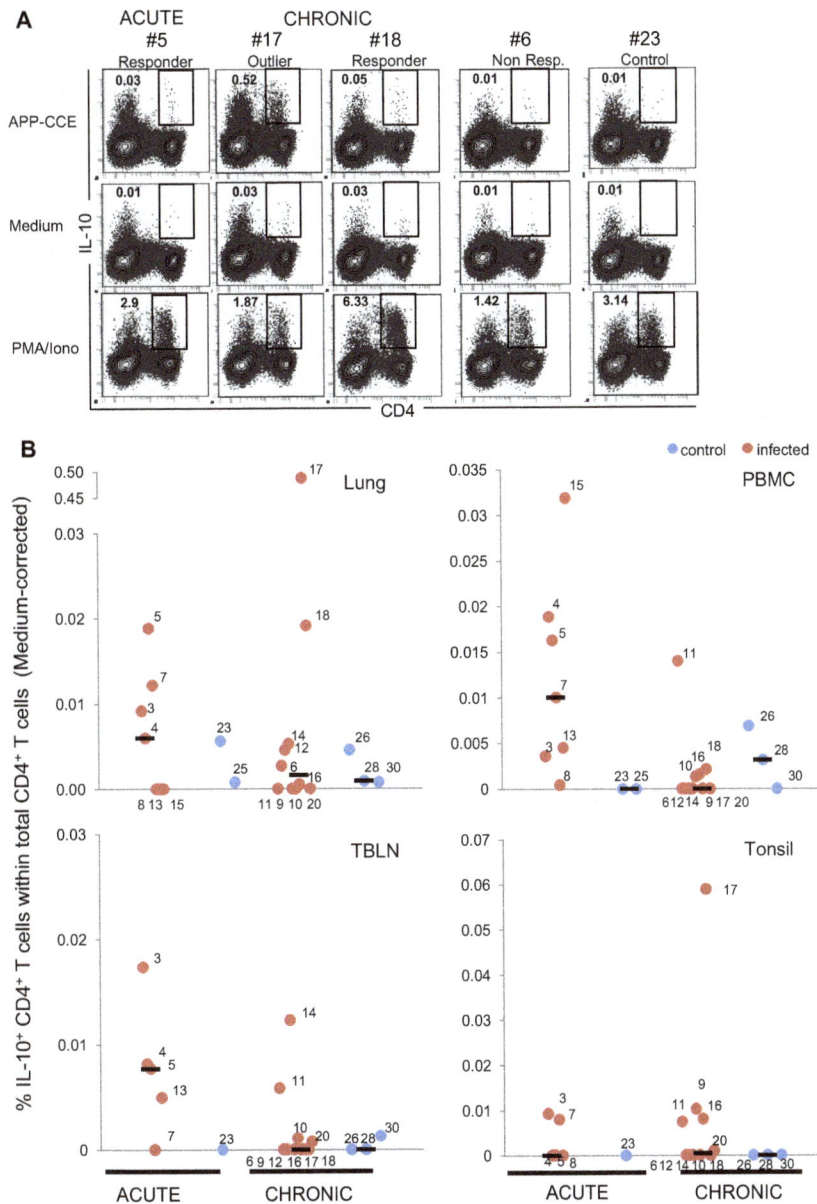

Figure 6 APP-CCE specific IL-10-producing CD4+ T cells in lung, peripheral blood, tracheobronchial lymph nodes and tonsils. Cells isolated from lung, blood (PBMC), tracheobronchial lymph nodes (TBLN) and tonsils were incubated overnight with APP-CCE, medium or PMA/Ionomycin and subsequently analyzed by FCM. Living cells were gated (not shown; see Additional file 1) and further analyzed for expression of IL-10 and CD4. **A** For the lung, data from representative animals from different groups are displayed: #5 for the acute phase, designated as "responder"; #17 and #18 for the chronic phase, designated as "outlier" and "responder", respectively; #6, designated as "non-responder" and control pig #23. Approximately 5 × 10^5 (APP and medium) and 1.5 × 10^5 (PMA/Ionomycin) cells are shown in the contour plots. Numbers displayed within the contour plots indicate the percentage of IL-10+ CD4+ T cells within total CD4+ T cells. **B** Frequency of IL-10+ CD4+ T cells in lung, PBMC, TBLN and tonsils of infected animals (red dots) and control animals (blue dots) during acute and chronic phase. Numbers next to colored dots indicate numbers of individual animals. Median percent values are indicated by black bars. Medium-corrected percent values are presented (% of IL-10+ CD4+ T cells within total CD4+ T cells for APP-CCE stimulation minus % of IL-10+ CD4+ T cells within total CD4+ T cells for medium incubation).

reactive IL-17A producing CD4+ T cells were nearly completely absent in lymphocytes isolated from control pigs, indicating that APP-naive CD4+ T cells did not respond to in vitro stimulation with APP-CCE.

Human [46] and porcine [17] CD4+ T cells have the capacity to co-produce IL-17A and TNF-α following PMA/Ionomycin stimulation. Furthermore, a synergistic effect between IL-17 and TNF-α has been reported, enhancing neutrophil migration [47]. Also, TNF-α is known to play a major role in the immune-pathogenesis of APP infection [35, 48]. Following APP-CCE stimulation, we found that the majority of CD4$^+$ T cells that produced IL-17A did not co-produce TNF-α. This suggests that CD4$^+$ T cells are not a main source of TNF-α during APP infection.

Interestingly, a small subset of CD4$^-$ TCR-γδ$^-$ cells showed production of IL-17A upon APP-CCE stimulation but was also identified in control animals. Innate sources of IL-17 are described [49] such us iNKT cells [50], NK cells [51] and innate lymphoid cells type 3 (ILC3) [52]. To affirm that the population revealed in our study is actually belonging to one of the subsets mentioned above, further investigations would be needed.

For several persistent pathogens like *Mycobacterium tuberculosis* [21], *Leishmania* spp. [23] and *Toxoplasma gondii* [22], IL-10 has been reported to impair their clearance by influencing the delicate balance between suppression and activation of host immune responses. In this study we therefore evaluated the production of IL-10 by CD4$^+$ T cells in different organs but a specific induction upon APP-CCE stimulation was found only in few animals and frequencies of IL-10$^+$ CD4$^+$ T cells were rather low. In a previous study, IL-10 mRNA was predominantly found within lung lesions of APP-infected pigs but was only minimal in non-affected areas. [53]. Of note, lung tissue samples in our study were derived from a defined anatomic area (dorsal portion of the left caudal lobe) and only in a single animal (#11) sequestra were included in that area. The frequency of IL-10-producing CD4$^+$ T cells derived from this animal was high in both APP-CCE-(0.17%) and medium-(0.17%) stimulated cultures, resulting in a medium-corrected value of zero (Figure 6B, lung). Thus, we cannot exclude a potential role of IL-10 in the immune

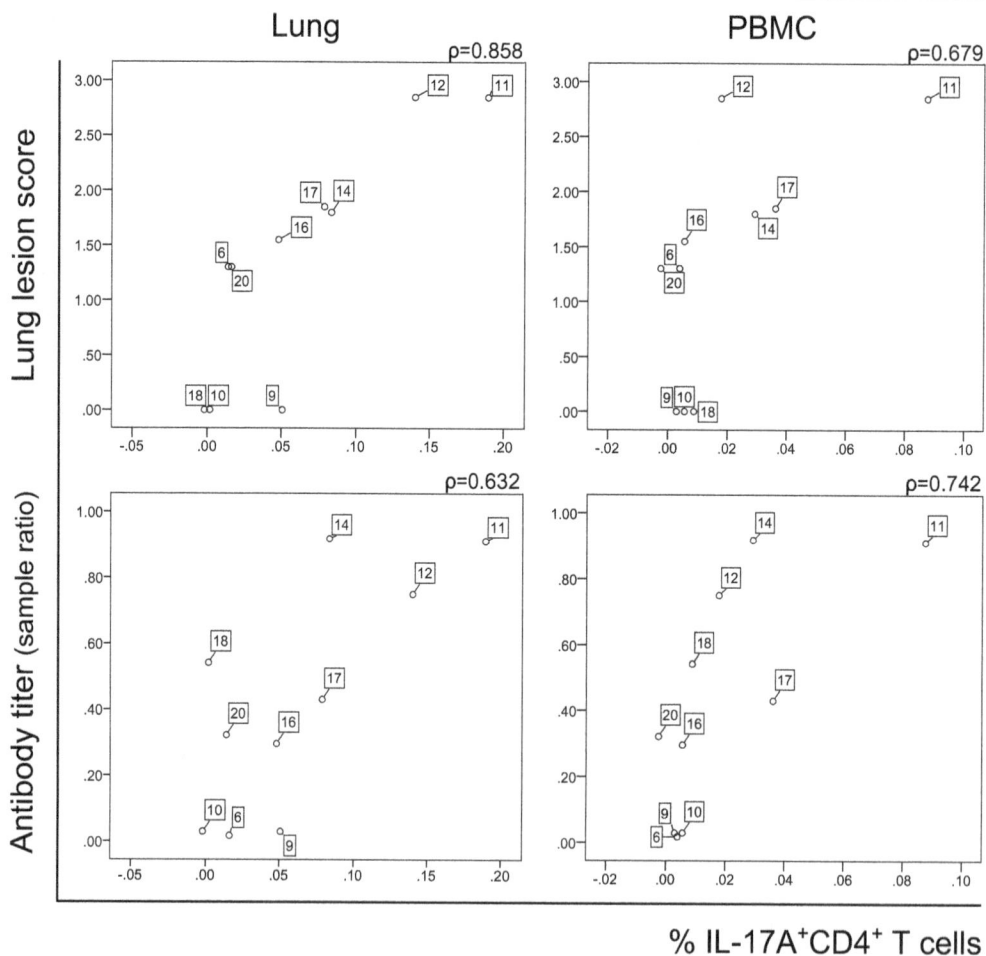

Figure 7 Correlation of the frequency of IL-17A$^+$ CD4$^+$ T cells with lung lesion score and antibody titers during the chronic phase.
Scatterplots show correlation of the frequency of IL-17A$^+$ CD4$^+$ T cells isolated from lung and blood with lung lesion score (top panel) and antibody titer (bottom panel) in chronically infected animals. Antibody titer is expressed as a ratio between optical density of the sample (ODs) and the mean of the optical density of the positive control (MODp). Spearman's Rank Correlation coefficients (ρ) are displayed above each scatterplot.

pathogenesis of APP infection. Further studies on affected lung lesions should be carried out in future studies to decipher the exact role of IL-10 in APP infections.

Finally, we observed that the frequency of Th17 cells in lung and PBMCs from chronically infected animals correlated positively with the lung lesion score and APP-specific antibody titers. Such a correlation was not found in the animals during the acute infection phase. This could be related to the enormous variety of lung lesions (diffuse/local necrotic and hemorrhagic areas, fibrosis, formation of sequestra, absence of lesions) observed at the necropsy during the acute phase, as described above. Moreover, no positive correlation between Th17 cells and the histological score of lung tissue samples from which lymphocytes had been isolated was found in the chronic phase of infection. Together with the positive correlation between frequency of Th17 cells in lung tissue as well as blood and the lung lesion score, this may indicate that these APP-specific Th17 cells have a general capacity for lung homing and also recirculate via the bloodstream. This would correspond with functional attributes ascribed to effector memory T cells [54]. However, the precise functional role of these Th17 cells in APP pathology and persistence remains speculative. It is well established that cytokine production by Th17 cells can have protective but also pathologic roles in lung immunity [19]. An excessive recruitment of neutrophils due to IL-17 production by $CD4^+$ T cells could lead to progressive inflammation, which might explain the positive correlation between lung lesion and IL-17 production. Additionally, APP chronic lung lesions are usually characterized by fibroplasia [1] and IL-17 was shown to be involved in the occurrence and the development of pulmonary fibrosis in rats [55]. Nevertheless, our in vitro stimulation system does not allow a distinction between actively IL-17A-producing $CD4^+$ T cells in vivo (at the time of isolation) and the re-stimulation of quiescent APP-specific Th17 memory cells upon a second exposure to the antigen. Therefore, the precise role of the putative APP-specific Th17 cells in APP immunity, identified in our study, remains to be elucidated.

In conclusion, our results support previous findings that T cells are involved in the immune response to APP infection. We could show for the first time that APP-specific T cells with functional attributes of Th17 cells are induced in most APP-infected animals, which during the chronic phase of infection seem to positively correlate with lung lesion formation. Thus, our findings highlight the relevance of detailed immunological studies addressing T-cell differentiation for a better understanding of host-pathogen interactions in APP. Moreover, our infection model provides a solid basis for such studies in a controlled setting. This will contribute to a better understanding of APP pathogenesis and persistence.

Additional files

Additional file 1. Clinical score protocol. Clinical examinations were performed daily throughout the experiment. Alterations in behavior, gait, presence of respiratory symptoms (cough and dyspnea), and body temperature were assessed and scored on a scale from 0 to 4 based on the listed symptoms or traits.

Additional file 2. FCM gating hierarchy. Representative example of the FCM gating strategy used in this study. Data is derived from lung of animal #12 (APP-infected). (**A**) Lymphocytes were gated according to their light scatter properties. (**B**) A FSC-W/H gate coupled with a SSC-W/H gate was applied in order to exclude potential doublet cells. (**C**) Near-IR stain was used for Live/Dead discrimination. Only Near-IR negative cells (live cells) were included in the following analyses. (**D**) Co-expression of CD4 and IL-17A for identification of IL-17A$^+$ CD4$^+$ T cells. (**E**) Cells were further distinguished in either CD4$^+$ or CD4$^-$ T cells. (**F**) Within the CD4$^+$ subpopulation, the production of IL-17A and TNF-α was investigated. (**G**) Within the CD4$^-$ subpopulation, the expression of IL-17A and TCR-γδ was investigated.

Additional file 3. Pathological findings in the lung of acutely and chronically infected animals. Lungs from representative animals, one for the acute and one for the chronic phase, are shown. (**A**) Bilateral diffuse hemorrhagic pneumonia and fibrinous pleurisy in an acutely infected animal (#3). (**B**) Necrotic foci surrounded by scar tissue (sequestra) and adhesive pleurisy with evidence of firm adhesions between visceral and parietal pleura in a chronically infected animal (#11).

Additional file 4. Histological evaluation of lung tissue from infected animals. Lung tissue of the dorsal portion of left caudal lung lobe (adjacent to samples used for lymphocyte isolation) was taken from acutely and chronically infected animals. This tissue was paraffin embedded, stained with hematoxylin and eosin, and examined for presence and quantity of parameters A–H (see legend). The quantity and presence of each parameter were assessed by using a score from 0 to 3 (0 = not present, 1 = low grade, 2 = moderate grade, 3 = high grade). No sample in this study presented lesions of grade 3; therefore this grade is not shown in the legend.

Additional file 5. APP-specific induction of IL-17A$^+$ CD4$^+$ T cells in peripheral blood. PBMCs were incubated overnight with APP crude capsular extract (APP-CCE), medium or PMA/Ionomycin. Living lymphocytes were gated (not shown; see Additional file 1) and further analyzed for the expression of IL-17A and CD4. Data from representative animals from different groups are displayed: #5 and #4 for the acute phase, designated as "high responder" and "low responder" respectively; #11 and #17 for the chronic phase designated as "high responder" and "low responder" respectively; #6, designated as non-responder and control pig #23. Approximately 7×10^5 (APP and medium) and 2×10^5 (PMA/Ionomycin) cells are shown in the contour plots respectively. Numbers displayed within the contour plots indicate the percentage of IL-17A$^+$CD4$^+$ T cells within total CD4$^+$ T cells.

Additional file 6. Expression of CD8α by IL-17A$^+$ CD4$^+$ T cells in peripheral blood. PBMCs were incubated overnight with APP crude capsular extract (APP-CCE), medium or PMA/Ionomycin. Living lymphocytes were gated (not shown; see Additional file 1) and further analyzed for the expression of CD8α and IL-17A. Data from the same animals as in Additional file 2 is shown. Approximately 3×10^5 (APP and medium) and 5×10^4 (PMA/Ionomycin) cells are shown in the contour plots.

Additional file 7. Co-production of TNF-α and IL-17A by CD4$^+$ T cells in peripheral blood. Phenotyping and intracellular cytokine staining were performed on PBMC following overnight in vitro stimulation (APP-CCE, medium, PMA/Ionomycin). (**A**) Living CD4$^+$ T cells were gated (not shown; see Additional file 1) and further analyzed for production of TNF-α and IL-17A. Data from the same animals as in Additional file 2 is shown. Approximately 3×10^5 (APP and medium) and 5×10^4 (PMA/Ionomycin) cells are shown in the contour plots. (**B**) Frequency of IL-17A/TNF-α co-producing CD4$^+$ T cells in PBMC of infected animals (red dots) and control animals (blue dots) during acute and chronic phase. Numbers next to colored dots indicate numbers of individual animals. Median percent values are indicated by black bars. Medium-corrected percentage values are presented (% of IL-17A$^+$ TNF-α$^+$ cells within total CD4$^+$ T cells for APP-CCE stimulation minus % of IL-17A$^+$ TNF-α$^+$ cells within total CD4$^+$ T cells for medium incubation). Arrow heads are introduced in the main text.

Additional file 8. Production of IL-17A by non-CD4$^+$ cells and γδ T cells in the peripheral blood. PBMC were incubated overnight with APP-CCE, medium or PMA/Ionomycin and subsequently analyzed for CD4, TCR-γδ and IL-17A expression by FCM. Living lymphocytes excluding CD4$^+$ T cells (not shown; see Additional file 1) were gated and further analyzed for expression of IL-17A and TCR-γδ. Data from the same animals as in Additional file 2 are shown. Approximately 7 × 10^5 (APP and medium) and 2 × 10^5 (PMA/Ionomycin) cells are shown in the contour plots. Arrow heads are introduced in the main text.

Additional file 9. APP-CCE-specific IL-10-producing CD4$^+$ T cells in peripheral blood. PBMC were incubated overnight with APP-CCE, medium or PMA/Ionomycin and subsequently analyzed by FCM. Living cells were gated (not shown; see Additional file 1) and further analyzed for expression of IL-10 and CD4. Data from representative animals from different groups are displayed: #15 for the acute phase and #11 for the chronic phase, both designated as "responders"; #6, designated as "non-responder" and control pig #23. Approximately 8 × 10^5 (APP and medium) and 1.5 × 10^5 (PMA/Ionomycin) cells are shown in the contour plots. Numbers displayed within the contour plots indicate the percentage of IL-10$^+$ CD4$^+$ T cells within total CD4$^+$ T cells.

Additional file 10. Correlation of the frequency of IL-17A$^+$ CD4$^+$ T cells with lung lesion score during the acute phase. Scatterplots show correlation of the frequency of IL-17A$^+$ CD4$^+$ T cells isolated from lung and blood with lung lesion score in acutely infected animals. Spearman's Rank Correlation Coefficients (ρ) are displayed above each scatterplot.

Additional file 11. Correlation of the frequency of IL-17A$^+$ CD4$^+$ T cells with histological score of lung tissue during the chronic phase. Scatterplots show correlation of the frequency of IL-17A$^+$ CD4$^+$ T cells isolated from lung and blood during the chronic phase with the histological score of the lung tissue sampled adjacent to tissue used for lymphocyte isolation. Histological scores for each sample were calculated by summing up the grading of all parameters shown in Additional file 4. Spearman's Rank Correlation Coefficients (ρ) are displayed above each scatterplot.

Competing interests
The authors declare that they have no competing interests.

Authors' contributions
ES, WG, AL, IHP: conceived and designed the experiments; JF and JS: prepared the inoculum and carried out microbiological analysis; MS: helped to set up the in vitro assay, isolated the lymphocytes from the organs and applied the stimulus; ES and HS: performed the infection, clinical examination and collected samples; CK, HS, AL, RG: performed the necropsies and harvested samples; BR: performed histopathological analyses; ES: produced the stimulus. ES and ST performed the intracellular cytokine staining and FCM measurements; ST: established the protocol for the intracellular cytokine staining; ES and WG: analyzed and interpreted the results; AL, IHP and MES: contributed to the organization of the experiments and edited the manuscript; ES and WG: wrote the manuscript. All authors read and approved the final manuscript.

Acknowledgements
The authors thank Michaela Koch and Lisa Reiter for their excellent work in the lab and Hanna Koinig for her precious help with the organization of the animal experiment. Elena L. Sassu, Stephanie C. Talker and Janna Frömbling were supported by the Graduate School for Pig and Poultry Medicine of the University of Veterinary Medicine Vienna.

Author details
[1] University Clinic for Swine, Department of Farm Animals and Veterinary Public Health, University of Veterinary Medicine, Vienna, Austria. [2] Institute of Immunology, Department of Pathobiology, University of Veterinary Medicine Vienna, Vienna, Austria. [3] Functional Microbiology, Institute of Microbiology, Department of Pathobiology, University of Veterinary Medicine Vienna, Vienna, Austria. [4] Institute of Pathology and Forensic Veterinary Medicine, Department of Pathobiology, University of Veterinary Medicine Vienna, Vienna, Austria. [5] Division of Swine Medicine, Department of Farm Animals, University of Zurich, Vetsuisse Faculty, Zurich, Switzerland.

References
1. Gottschalk M (2012) Actinobacillosis. In: Zimmerman JJ, Karriker LA, Ramirez A, Schwartz KJ, Stevenson GW (eds) Diseases of Swine. Wiley, New York
2. Angen O, Andreasen M, Nielsen EO, Stockmarr A, Baekbo P (2008) Effect of tulathromycin on the carrier status of Actinobacillus pleuropneumoniae serotype 2 in the tonsils of pigs. Vet Rec 163:445–447
3. Chiers K, De Waele T, Pasmans F, Ducatelle R, Haesebrouck F (2010) Virulence factors of Actinobacillus pleuropneumoniae involved in colonization, persistence and induction of lesions in its porcine host. Vet Res 41:65
4. Devenish J, Rosendal S, Bosse JT (1990) Humoral antibody response and protective immunity in swine following immunization with the 104-kilodalton hemolysin of Actinobacillus pleuropneumoniae. Infect Immun 58:3829–3832
5. Krejci J, Nechvatalova K, Kudlackova H, Faldyna M, Kucerova Z, Toman M (2005) Systemic and local antibody responses after experimental infection with Actinobacillus pleuropneumoniae in piglets with passive or active immunity. J Vet Med B Infect Dis Vet Public Health 52:190–196
6. Costa G, Oliveira S, Torrison J, Dee S (2011) Evaluation of Actinobacillus pleuropneumoniae diagnostic tests using samples derived from experimentally infected pigs. Vet Microbiol 148:246–251
7. Cruijsen T, van Leengoed LA, Kamp EM, Bartelse A, Korevaar A, Verheijden JH (1995) Susceptibility to Actinobacillus pleuropneumoniae infection in pigs from an endemically infected herd is related to the presence of toxin-neutralizing antibodies. Vet Microbiol 47:219–228
8. Li L, Zhu J, Yang K, Xu Z, Liu Z, Zhou R (2014) Changes in gene expression of Actinobacillus pleuropneumoniae in response to anaerobic stress reveal induction of central metabolism and biofilm formation. J Microbiol 52:473–481
9. Wherry EJ, Kurachi M (2015) Molecular and cellular insights into T cell exhaustion. Nat Rev Immunol 15:486–499
10. Boer MC, Joosten SA, Ottenhoff TH (2015) Regulatory T-cells at the interface between human host and pathogens in infectious diseases and vaccination. Front Immunol 6:217
11. Furesz SE, Mallard BA, Bosse JT, Rosendal S, Wilkie BN, MacInnes JI (1997) Antibody- and cell-mediated immune responses of Actinobacillus pleuropneumoniae-infected and bacterin-vaccinated pigs. Infect Immun 65:358–365
12. Appleyard GD, Furesz SE, Wilkie BN (2002) Blood lymphocyte subsets in pigs vaccinated and challenged with Actinobacillus pleuropneumoniae. Vet Immunol Immunopathol 86:221–228
13. Faldyna M, Nechvatalova K, Sinkora J, Knotigova P, Leva L, Krejci J, Toman M (2005) Experimental Actinobacillus pleuropneumoniae infection in piglets with different types and levels of specific protection: immunophenotypic analysis of lymphocyte subsets in the circulation and respiratory mucosal lymphoid tissue. Vet Immunol Immunopathol 107:143–152
14. Brogaard L, Klitgaard K, Heegaard PM, Hansen MS, Jensen TK, Skovgaard K (2015) Concurrent host-pathogen gene expression in the lungs of pigs challenged with Actinobacillus pleuropneumoniae. BMC Genomics 16:417
15. Stepanova H, Mensikova M, Chlebova K, Faldyna M (2012) CD4$^+$ and γδTCR$^+$ T lymphocytes are sources of interleukin-17 in swine. Cytokine 58:152–157
16. Sedlak C, Patzl M, Saalmüller A, Gerner W (2014) CD2 and CD8α define porcine γδ T cells with distinct cytokine production profiles. Dev Comp Immunol 45:97–106

17. Gerner W, Talker SC, Koinig HC, Sedlak C, Mair KH, Saalmüller A (2015) Phenotypic and functional differentiation of porcine αβ T cells: current knowledge and available tools. Mol Immunol 66:3–13

18. McGeachy MJ (2013) Th17 memory cells: live long and proliferate. J Leukoc Biol 94:921–926

19. Way EE, Chen K, Kolls JK (2013) Dysregulation in lung immunity—the protective and pathologic Th17 response in infection. Eur J Immunol 43:3116–3124

20. McGill JL, Rusk RA, Guerra-Maupome M, Briggs RE, Sacco RE (2016) Bovine gamma delta T cells contribute to exacerbated IL-17 production in response to co-infection with bovine RSV and Mannheimia haemolytica. PLoS One 11:e0151083

21. Redford PS, Murray PJ, O'Garra A (2011) The role of IL-10 in immune regulation during M. tuberculosis infection. Mucosal Immunol 4:261–270

22. Neyer LE, Grunig G, Fort M, Remington JS, Rennick D, Hunter CA (1997) Role of interleukin-10 in regulation of T-cell-dependent and T-cell-independent mechanisms of resistance to Toxoplasma gondii. Infect Immun 65:1675–1682

23. Belkaid Y, Hoffmann KF, Mendez S, Kamhawi S, Udey MC, Wynn TA, Sacks DL (2001) The role of interleukin (IL)-10 in the persistence of Leishmania major in the skin after healing and the therapeutic potential of anti-IL-10 receptor antibody for sterile cure. J Exp Med 194:1497–1506

24. Hennig-Pauka I, Baltes N, Jacobsen I, Stratmann-Selke J, Gerlach GF, Selbitz HJ, Waldmann KH (2008) Study of the virulence of Actinobacillus pleuropneumoniae in finishing pigs as a basis for vaccination development. Berl Munch Tierarztl Wochenschr 121:189–197 (in German)

25. Hannan PC, Bhogal BS, Fish JP (1982) Tylosin tartrate and tiamutilin effects on experimental piglet pneumonia induced with pneumonic pig lung homogenate containing mycoplasmas, bacteria and viruses. Res Vet Sci 33:76–88

26. Merialdi G, Dottori M, Bonilauri P, Luppi A, Gozio S, Pozzi P, Spaggiari B, Martelli P (2012) Survey of pleuritis and pulmonary lesions in pigs at abattoir with a focus on the extent of the condition and herd risk factors. Vet J 193:234–239

27. Hussy D, Schlatter Y, Miserez R, Inzana T, Frey J (2004) PCR-based identification of serotype 2 isolates of Actinobacillus pleuropneumoniae biovars I and II. Vet Microbiol 99:307–310

28. Schaller A, Djordjevic SP, Eamens GJ, Forbes WA, Kuhn R, Kuhnert P, Gottschalk M, Nicolet J, Frey J (2001) Identification and detection of Actinobacillus pleuropneumoniae by PCR based on the gene apxIVA. Vet Microbiol 79:47–62

29. Wittkowski M, Mittelstadt J, Brandau S, Reiling N, Lindner B, Torrelles J, Brennan PJ, Holst O (2007) Capsular arabinomannans from Mycobacterium avium with morphotype-specific structural differences but identical biological activity. J Biol Chem 282:19103–19112

30. Reutner K, Leitner J, Essler SE, Witter K, Patzl M, Steinberger P, Saalmüller A, Gerner W (2012) Porcine CD27: identification, expression and functional aspects in lymphocyte subsets in swine. Dev Comp Immunol 38:321–331

31. Saalmüller A, Reddehase MJ, Buhring HJ, Jonjic S, Koszinowski UH (1987) Simultaneous expression of CD4 and CD8 antigens by a substantial proportion of resting porcine T lymphocytes. Eur J Immunol 17:1297–1301

32. Rodriguez-Gomez IM, Talker SC, Kaser T, Stadler M, Hammer SE, Saalmüller A, Gerner W (2016) Expression of T-bet, Eomesodermin and GATA-3 in porcine αβ T cells. Dev Comp Immunol 60:115–126

33. Frank RK, Chengappa MM, Oberst RD, Hennessy KJ, Henry SC, Fenwick B (1992) Pleuropneumonia caused by Actinobacillus pleuropneumoniae biotype 2 in growing and finishing pigs. J Vet Diagn Investig 4:270–278

34. Saalmüller A, Werner T, Fachinger V (2002) T-helper cells from naive to committed. Vet Immunol Immunopathol 87:137–145

35. Baarsch MJ, Scamurra RW, Burger K, Foss DL, Maheswaran SK, Murtaugh MP (1995) Inflammatory cytokine expression in swine experimentally infected with Actinobacillus pleuropneumoniae. Infect Immun 63:3587–3594

36. Heegaard PM, Klausen J, Nielsen JP, Gonzalez-Ramon N, Pineiro M, Lampreave F, Alava MA (1998) The porcine acute phase response to infection with Actinobacillus pleuropneumoniae. Haptoglobin, C-reactive protein, major acute phase protein and serum amyloid A protein are sensitive

37. indicators of infection. Comp Biochem Physiol B Biochem Mol Biol 119:365–373

38. Skovgaard K, Mortensen S, Boye M, Poulsen KT, Campbell FM, Eckersall PD, Heegaard PM (2009) Rapid and widely disseminated acute phase protein response after experimental bacterial infection of pigs. Vet Res 40:23

39. Rosendal S, Mittal KR (1985) Serological cross-reactivity between a porcine Actinobacillus strain and Haemophilus pleuropneumoniae. Can J Comp Med 49:164–170

40. Baarsch MJ, Foss DL, Murtaugh MP (2000) Pathophysiologic correlates of acute porcine pleuropneumonia. Am J Vet Res 61:684–690

41. Talker SC, Stadler M, Koinig HC, Mair KH, Rodriguez-Gomez IM, Graage R, Zell R, Durrwald R, Starick E, Harder T, Weissenbock H, Lamp B, Hammer SE, Ladinig A, Saalmüller A, Gerner W (2016) Influenza A virus infection in pigs attracts multifunctional and cross-reactive T cells to the lung. J Virol 90:9364–9382

42. Vigre H, Angen O, Barfod K, Lavritsen DT, Sorensen V (2002) Transmission of Actinobacillus pleuropneumoniae in pigs under field-like conditions: emphasis on tonsillar colonisation and passively acquired colostral antibodies. Vet Microbiol 89:151–159

43. Tabarkiewicz J, Pogoda K, Karczmarczyk A, Pozarowski P, Giannopoulos K (2015) The role of IL-17 and Th17 lymphocytes in autoimmune diseases. Arch Immunol Ther Exp 63:435–449

44. Rathore JS, Wang Y (2016) Protective role of Th17 cells in pulmonary infection. Vaccine 34:1504–1514

45. Mensikova M, Stepanova H, Faldyna M (2013) Interleukin-17 in veterinary animal species and its role in various diseases: a review. Cytokine 64:11–17

46. Zuckermann FA, Husmann RJ (1996) Functional and phenotypic analysis of porcine peripheral blood CD4/CD8 double-positive T cells. Immunology 87:500–512

47. Kim CJ, McKinnon LR, Kovacs C, Kandel G, Huibner S, Chege D, Shahabi K, Benko E, Loutfy M, Ostrowski M, Kaul R (2013) Mucosal Th17 cell function is altered during HIV infection and is an independent predictor of systemic immune activation. J Immunol 191:2164–2173

48. Griffin GK, Newton G, Tarrio ML, Bu DX, Maganto-Garcia E, Azcutia V, Alcaide P, Grabie N, Luscinskas FW, Croce KJ, Lichtman AH (2012) IL-17 and TNF-alpha sustain neutrophil recruitment during inflammation through synergistic effects on endothelial activation. J Immunol 188:6287–6299

49. Choi C, Kwon D, Min K, Chae C (1999) In-situ hybridization for the detection of inflammatory cytokines (IL-1, TNF-α and IL-6) in pigs naturally infected with Actinobacillus pleuropneumoniae. J Comp Pathol 121:349–356

50. Cua DJ, Tato CM (2010) Innate IL-17-producing cells: the sentinels of the immune system. Nat Rev Immunol 10:479–489

51. Michel ML, Keller AC, Paget C, Fujio M, Trottein F, Savage PB, Wong CH, Schneider E, Dy M, Leite-de-Moraes MC (2007) Identification of an IL-17-producing NK1.1(neg) iNKT cell population involved in airway neutrophilia. J Exp Med 204:995–1001

52. Passos ST, Silver JS, O'Hara AC, Sehy D, Stumhofer JS, Hunter CA (2010) IL-6 promotes NK cell production of IL-17 during toxoplasmosis. J Immunol 184:1776–1783

53. Spits H, Artis D, Colonna M, Diefenbach A, Di Santo JP, Eberl G, Koyasu S, Locksley RM, McKenzie AN, Mebius RE, Powrie F, Vivier E (2013) Innate lymphoid cells—a proposal for uniform nomenclature. Nat Rev Immunol 13:145–149

54. Cho WS, Jung K, Kim J, Ha Y, Chae C (2005) Expression of mRNA encoding interleukin (IL)-10, IL-12p35 and IL-12p40 in lungs from pigs experimentally infected with Actinobacillus pleuropneumoniae. Vet Res Commun 29:111–122

55. Masopust D, Picker LJ (2012) Hidden memories: frontline memory T cells and early pathogen interception. J Immunol 188:5811–5817

56. Ding W, Zhang XY, Pan M, Zhao B, Chen C, Niu ZH, Huang CL, Li YY, Fan XM, Ma YM, Zhang M, Zhang WJ (2015) Interleukin-17A promotes the formation of inflammation in the lung tissues of rats with pulmonary fibrosis. Exp Ther Med 10:491–497

15

Correlating bacterial shedding with fecal corticosterone levels and serological responses from layer hens experimentally infected with *Salmonella* Typhimurium

Pardeep Sharma, Vivek V. Pande, Talia S. Moyle, Andrea R. McWhorter and Kapil K. Chousalkar[*]

Abstract

Salmonella Enteriditis and *Salmonella* Typhimurium are commonly isolated during egg-related outbreaks of salmonellosis and represent a significant international public health issue. In Australia, *Salmonella* Typhimurium is the most common serovar identified in egg product related foodborne outbreaks. While a number of studies have investigated *Salmonella* shedding and host responses to infection, they have been conducted over a short time period. The present study sought to characterise bacterial shedding and host responses to infection in hens infected with only *Salmonella* Typhimurium or co-infected with both *Salmonella* Typhimurium and *Salmonella* Mbandaka over a 16 week period. *Salmonella* shedding was quantified using the most probable number and qPCR methods and was highly variable over the course of the experiment. On day 1, fecal corticosterone metabolites in birds infected with *Salmonella* Typhimurium (674.2 ± 109.3 pg/mg) were significantly higher than control (238.0 ± 12.62 pg/mg) or co-infected (175.4 ± 8.58 pg/mg) birds. The onset of lay occurred between weeks 6–8 post-infection (pi) and Fecal corticosterone metabolite (FCM) concentrations increased in both control and co-infected birds. Antibody responses to infection were monitored in both serum and yolk samples. *Salmonella* Typhimurium specific antibody was lower in co-infected animals than monoinfected animals. Bacterial loads in internal organs were characterised to determine persistence. Spleen, liver and caecal tonsils were positive for bacteria in both groups, indicating that *Salmonella* was not cleared from the birds and internal organ colonization could serve as a reservoir for continued bacterial shedding.

Introduction

Commercial poultry are often persistently infected with non-typhoidal serovars of *Salmonella enterica*. Eggs and raw egg based food products are often identified as the source of *Salmonella* during outbreaks of human gastrointestinal disease [1]. Thus, the zoonotic potential of *Salmonella* represents a significant global public health concern. In North America and Europe, the most common serovar isolated during egg-related outbreaks is *Salmonella* Enteritidis followed by *Salmonella* Typhimurium [2]. Strains of *Salmonella* Typhimurium, however,

are most frequently identified during Australian outbreaks of egg-related cases of salmonellosis [1].

Over the past several years, the incidence of human cases of salmonellosis in Australia has been increasing. In 2011, the total number of food related disease outbreaks had increased to over 150 and 38.4% were attributed to *Salmonella* [1]. Over the same period, the number of cases linked directly with eggs increased from 20.8 to 44.8% [1]. Despite improvements of on-farm control strategies, *Salmonella* Typhimurium remains a significant problem within the Australian layer industry [3].

Due to the public health importance of contaminated eggs, understanding the dynamics of *Salmonella* Typhimurium shedding patterns and associated host responses to infection is of critical importance. Previous experimental infection trials have examined

*Correspondence: Kapil.chousalkar@adelaide.edu.au
School of Animal and Veterinary Sciences, The University of Adelaide, Roseworthy, SA 5173, Australia

egg contamination and internal organ colonization of layer hens. These studies, however, have infected birds at different ages, using a variety of inoculation methods [4–7] limiting the degree to which the data can be directly compared. Moreover, the data obtained from these investigations was collected for 3–4 weeks pi. The productive lifetime of a layer hen, however, can extend beyond 50 weeks of age and few studies have investigated extended bacterial shedding dynamics, egg contamination and host responses to infection.During productive lifespan, layer hens may also experience many physiological and environmental stressors, such as overcrowding, extreme temperature variation and the onset of lay that may lead to increased fecal shedding of *Salmonella* [8–11]. Stress has also been linked with impaired immunity [8, 9, 12, 13] which may increase intestinal colonization by enteric pathogens such as *Salmonella* [14]. The host immune response to *Salmonella* infection may also contribute to increased corticosterone levels however, relationship between persistent *Salmonella* colonisation and stress in birds is unclear.

In the Australian egg industry, *Salmonella* Typhimurium is frequently isolated from eggshell surfaces but it is not the only serovar isolated from egg farms [15, 16]. The poultry farm environment is often contaminated with multiple serovars [15–17]. Field epidemiological investigations suggested that *Salmonella* Mbandaka was commonly isolated along with *Salmonella* Typhimurium in layer flocks without any clinical signs in chickens [16, 18]. *Salmonella* Mbandaka has not been associated with any egg related outbreaks in Australia [19], although this serovar has been associated with egg product related *Salmonella* outbreaks in the US [20].

Competition between co-infecting strains may affect the dynamics of one or more serovars. Layer hens environmentally infected with *Salmonella* Kentucky, for example, mitigated *Salmonella* Enteritidis colonisation of internal organs [21]. In addition, coinfection of layer hens with *Salmonella* Enteritidis, *Salmonella* Gallinarum and *Salmonella* Isangi has recently been shown to enhance disease in infected birds [22]. To date, there have been limited studies investigating how co-infection affects the dynamics of *Salmonella* Typhimurium shedding as well as host responses to infection.

Our hypothesis was that *Salmonella* Mbandaka can affect the shedding of *Salmonella* Typhimurium and internal organ colonization. We have conducted a 16 week infection trial, using layer hens reared free from exogenous *Salmonella*. Results from a companion study demonstrated that over the 16 week infection period, bacterial shedding was variable and that vertical transmission of *Salmonella* Typhimurium DT9 into egg internal did not occur [23]. The aims of the present study

were to correlate fecal shedding and egg contamination patterns with host responses to infection (single and mixed) including fecal corticosterone levels as a marker of the host stress response as well as levels of *Salmonella* Typhimurium specific antibodies in the serum and yolk. A final aim of this study was to characterise persistence of *Salmonella* infection in peripheral organs.

Materials and methods

Birds

Fertile eggs were obtained from a commercial brown layer flock hatchery. Eggs were fumigated using formaldehyde and incubated for 21 days. A total of 32 pullets were hatched and raised in floor pens in positive pressure rooms within an animal housing facility located on the Roseworthy Campus of the University of Adelaide. The rooms within this facility, all animal cages, trays, and feeders had previously been cleaned and decontaminated using FoamCleanS and SaniGuard (Chemtall, Australia). At 10 weeks of age, birds were divided into three treatment groups: control ($n = 4$), *Salmonella* Typhimurium ($n = 14$) and *Salmonella* Typhimurium + *Salmonella* Mbandaka ($n = 14$) and housed individually in cages in separate rooms. Fumigated feed and sanitised water (Aquatabs, Ireland) were provided ad libitum to all birds. Feed, water and fecal samples were screened for *Salmonella* fortnightly by culture method as described previously [16]. This experiment was performed according to the Australian Code for the Care and Use of Animals for Scientific Purposes and was approved by the University of Adelaide Animal Ethics Committee (approval number: S-2014-008).

Bacterial isolates

Single isolates of *Salmonella* Typhimurium definitive type 9 (DT9) and *Salmonella* Mbandaka were used in this study. These *Salmonella* had been previously isolated from samples collected from layer hen farms during a previous epidemiology study [16] and serotyped at the *Salmonella* Reference Laboratory, Institute of Veterinary Medical Science (IMVS), Adelaide, South Australia.

Challenge experiment

At 14 weeks of age, just prior to lay, hens were orally inoculated with 1×10^9 colony forming units (CFU) of either *Salmonella* Typhimurium DT9 or a combination containing equal amounts of both *Salmonella* Typhimurium DT9 and *Salmonella* Mbandaka (5.0×10^8 CFU of each serovar) suspended in Luria–Bertani (LB) broth (Oxoid, Australia). Serial tenfold dilutions of the inoculum were prepared and plated onto nutrient agar to confirm the total number of bacteria. Control birds received a sham inoculum containing only sterile LB broth. Clinical signs of infection were recorded throughout the experiment. At 30 weeks of age, [16 weeks post-infection (pi)] all birds were euthanized with Lethabarb (Virbac, Australia). Bone marrow, spleen, liver and caecal tonsils were collected from each bird for bacteriological examination.

Enumeration of *Salmonella* in fecal samples

A total of 320 fecal samples from individual hens were collected aseptically using sterile plastic bags on day 1 post-infection (pi) followed by 1, 2, 4, 6, 8, 10, 12, 14 and 16 weeks pi. *Salmonella* enumeration using the three tube most probably number (MPN) method was performed on all faecal samples as described previously [24]. *Salmonella* suspected samples were streaked onto xylose lysine deoxycholate (XLD) agar plates (Oxoid, Australia) and *Salmonella* Brilliance agar plates (Oxoid, Australia) for confirmation of *Salmonella* spp.

Bacterial DNA extractions from fecal samples, egg shell wash and internal organs

DNA was extracted from fecal samples using the Isolate Fecal DNA Kit (Bioline, Australia) following manufacturer instruction. DNA extraction from eggshell washes (enriched in RVS broth) collected from both infection groups was performed using Chelex® (Bio-Rad, Sydney, NSW, Australia) [25] The Wizard genomic DNA purification kit (Promega, Australia) was used to extract DNA from the tissue samples as per manufacturer instructions.

Standard curve and qPCR for fecal samples for *Salmonella* Typhimurium and *Salmonella* Mbandaka

The PCR detection of *Salmonella* was performed using the Quantifast® SYBER® Green qPCR kit (Qiagen, Australia) in a total reaction volume of 10 μL containing 2 μL sample (5 ng/μL), 5 μL of 2× Quantifast SYBER Green Master Mix and 1 μM of reverse and forward primers. *Salmonella* Typhimurium serovar specific primers *TSR*3 were used to detect *Salmonella* Typhimurium DT9. Further, to differentiate *Salmonella* Mbandaka from *Salmonella* Typhimurium DT9 in the co-infection group, primers for class 1 integron were used to specifically detect *Salmonella* Mbandaka [26]. The qPCR conditions were 5 min of denaturation at 95 °C, followed by 40 cycles of denaturation at 95 °C for 10 s and 60 °C for 30 s each. Rotor-gene 1.7.75 (Corbett Research, Qiagen, Australia) software version was used for the data analysis. A standard curve was generated to establish the limit of detection and quantification of positive samples, by determining a serial tenfold dilution of spiked fecal samples with known concentrations of *Salmonella* Typhimurium or *Salmonella* Typhimurium + *Salmonella* Mbandaka.

Fecal corticosterone analysis

Fecal samples collected at day 1 (pi) followed by 1, 2, 4, 6, 8, 10, 12, 14 and 16 weeks pi were thawed, mixed, and dried at 103 °C overnight. After cooling to room temperature, samples were ground to a fine powder. Corticosterone metabolites were extracted using methods recommended by the DetectX Corticosterone EIA kit manufacturer (Arbor Assays, Ann Arbor, USA). The concentration of fecal corticosterone metabolites (FCM) was measured by DetectX Corticosterone EIA kit as per manufacturer instruction.

Survey of egg shell and egg internal contents for *Salmonella* contamination

Eggs laid daily during 6, 8, 10, 12 and 14 weeks pi were collected and processed for *Salmonella* detection from both the eggshell and internal contents (Total eggs: 892; Control = 118, *Salmonella* Typhimurium only = 365, *Salmonella* Typhimurium + *Salmonella* Mbandaka co-infection = 409) using previously described methods [16]. Eggshell wash enriched in Rappaport–Vassiliadis broth (RVS; Oxoid, Australia) was stored in 80% glycerol at −80 °C to differentiate between *Salmonella* Typhimurium DT9 and *Salmonella* Mbandaka by standard PCR.

PCR for egg shell wash and internal organ samples for *Salmonella* Typhimurium and *Salmonella* Mbandaka

Salmonella positive eggshell wash and internal organ samples from both infection groups were screened for the amplification of *invA* and *TSR*3 gene for detection of *Salmonella* Typhimurium by multiplex PCR [26]. *TSR*3 gene was not amplified in *Salmonella* Mbandaka isolates [26]. Samples from both groups were also tested for the presence of *Salmonella* Mbandaka.

Bacteriology of internal organs

Bone marrow, spleen, liver and caecal tonsils were collected at week 16 pi and processed for bacteriology. Briefly, 0.1–0.2 grams of tissue sample were homogenised and serial tenfold dilutions were prepared in phosphate buffer saline (PBS). One hundred micro litre of each dilution was spread onto XLD agar plates and incubated overnight at 37 °C. After 24 h, the bacterial colonies were enumerated and the number of *Salmonella* in tissues was expressed as mean $\log_{10}$ CFU/g of tissue.

Serum and egg yolk sample collection and serologic examination by ELISA

On day 0 and at 1, 2, 4, 6, 8, 10, 12, and 14 weeks pi, 2 mL blood samples were collected from each bird and placed into serum clot activator tubes (Vacuette® tube, Greiner Bio-One, Australia). A total of 145 (Control; $n = 20$,

Salmonella Typhimurium only; $n = 57$, Co-infection group; $n = 68$) egg samples collected at weeks 6, 8, 10, 12 and 14 pi were processed for the antibody extraction from the yolk samples. Egg yolk antibodies were extracted as described previously [27]. Dilutions of chloroform-extract egg yolk antibody were prepared from the pools of known positive and known negative eggs from control birds. Samples were tested in duplicate for the following dilutions; 1:10, 1:50, 1:100, 1:500 and 1:1000. From the curve produced, the linear part was expanded. Readings of known positive and negative samples individually at the selected dilution produced a cut-off value for the test. Threshold value were determined by plotting sensitivity and specificity against the cut off value using two graph receiver operating characteristics (TG-ROC) analysis as described [28]. A dilution factor of 1:100 was selected because it was on the linear part of the standard curve.

Antibody detection from both serum and egg yolk samples was tested using the Chicken *Salmonella* Typhimurium Antibody Kit LPS Group B (BioChek, Holland) and antibody titres were calculated according to manufacturer instruction.

Statistical analysis

The data for average $\log_{10}$ CFU/qPCR, corticosterone level, and serum and egg yolk was analyzed using a two way analysis of variance (ANOVA) followed by a Tukey's multiple comparison of the mean. Significance between bacterial titres in organs was tested using a Mann–Whitney test. The correlation between MPN/g fecal count and *Salmonella* positive eggshell wash, average $\log_{10}$ CFU/qPCR and corticosterone concentration was determined by Pearson correlation test (r^2 value). All data was analysed using either by GraphPad Prism version 6 software or IBM®SPSS Statistics® version 21. p values <0.05 were considered statistically significant. A D'Agostino-Pearson omnibus normality test was conducted for all data. Serum and egg yolk antibody titres were normally distributed. MPN data were not normally distributed. MPN data was analysed by a Kruskal–Wallis with a Dunn's comparison of the means.

Results
Shedding and viable bacterial counts of *Salmonella* in fecal samples

Bacterial shedding varied significantly over time ($p < 0.01$) in both experimental treatment groups (Figure 1). The greatest number of viable bacteria observed in birds infected with only *Salmonella* Typhimurium occurred during week 1 pi, with a mean MPN/g of 48.53 ± 16.55. Samples collected from the *Salmonella* Typhimurium infection group in week 10 exhibited the

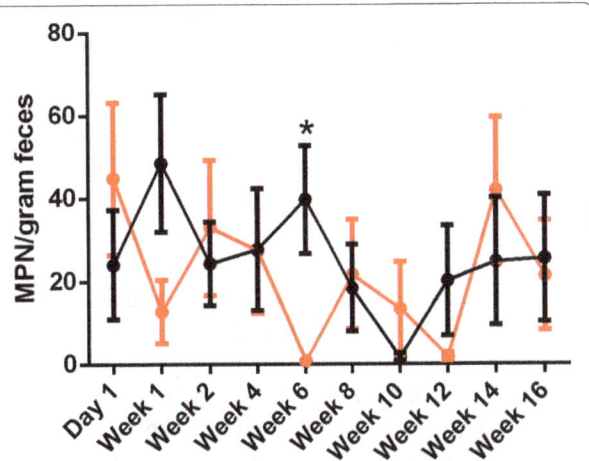

Figure 1　Enumeration of *Salmonella* in feces using most probable number (MPN) method. Fecal samples were collected from birds orally infected with 1×10^9 CFU of *Salmonella* Typhimurium (Black line) or a combination of both *Salmonella* Typhimurium + *Salmonella* Mbandaka (5×10^8 CFU of each serovar) (Red line) on day 1 and weeks 1, 2, 4, 6, 8, 10, 12, 14 and 16 pi. Data is presented as mean MPN/gram feces ± standard error of the mean. Bacterial shedding in both infection groups varied significantly over the course of the experiment ($p < 0.01$). At week 6 pi, bacterial shedding was significantly higher in birds infected with only *Salmonella* Typhimurium group (*$p < 0.05$).

lowest mean MPN/g, 1.535 ± 1.05. For birds infected with both *Salmonella* Typhimurium and *Salmonella* Mbandaka, the greatest number of viable *Salmonella* was detected on day 1 pi with a mean MPN/g of 44.80 ± 18.30. The lowest mean MPN/g, 0.78 ± 0.27, was observed in the multi-serovar infection group at week 6 pi.

Over the entire experiment, no significant effect of time or treatment was detected between single and multi-serovar treatment groups ($p > 0.05$). At week 6 pi, however, birds infected with only *Salmonella* Typhimurium exhibited a significantly greater mean MPN/g than birds infected with both *Salmonella* Typhimurium and *Salmonella* Mbandaka ($p < 0.05$). This difference correlated with the onset of lay. No *Salmonella* was detected in uninfected birds over the course of the experiment.

Quantification of *Salmonella* in fecal samples using a serovar specific qPCR

A quantitative PCR was developed to detect total *Salmonella* Typhimurium in single infection fecal samples and differentiate between *Salmonella* Typhimurium and *Salmonella* Mbandaka co-infection samples. A standard curve was generated by spiking uninfected, control feces spiked with known quantities of *Salmonella* Typhimurium. A cut-off Ct of 32 was used to exclude the detection of false positives and corresponded to 100 CFU of

Salmonella. For fecal samples spiked with both *Salmonella* Typhimurium and *Salmonella* Mbandaka, a cut-off Ct of 33 was used to exclude the detection of false positives. A Ct of 33 represented 1000 CFU of *Salmonella*. Data are presented as mean $\log_{10}$ CFU/gram feces ± standard error of the mean.

The number of *Salmonella* detected by qPCR varied significantly in both treatment groups over the course of the experiment (Figure 2). The greatest amount of *Salmonella* detected in all groups was observed at week 1 pi (Figure 2) with *Salmonella* Mbandaka in the co-infection group exhibiting the highest mean $\log_{10}$ CFU/gram feces (8.13 ± 0.65). Interestingly, *Salmonella* Mbandaka had the highest mean $\log_{10}$ CFU/gram feces between weeks 1 through 14 pi, though this difference was not significant than *Salmonella* Typhimurium. After week 1, *Salmonella* detection was relatively stable and consistent and did not vary significantly. No significant correlation was observed between MPN counts and qPCR results.

Fecal corticosterone metabolites in dried fecal extracts

Measuring fecal corticosterone metabolites (FCM) is a non-invasive method enabling the measurement of one stress parameter [29, 30]. It has been previously shown that during point of lay, birds experience increased physiological stress and are thought to be immunocompromised [31]. Infection, however, has also been shown to affect plasma corticosterone levels [12]. Therefore, it was hypothesized that corticosterone should increase in all chickens around the onset of lay, and infection may lead to further increase in level of corticosterone.

Fecal samples collected for enumeration of bacteria were also processed for FCM. A significant effect of time ($p < 0.05$) and treatment ($p < 0.001$) were observed between FCM concentrations (Figure 3). At day 1 pi, the FCM in birds infected with *Salmonella* Typhimurium (674.2 ± 109.3 pg/mg) was significantly higher than the FCM observed for control birds (238.0 ± 12.62 pg/mg) or birds infected with a mixed inoculum of both *Salmonella* Typhimurium and *Salmonella* Mbandaka (175.4 ± 8.58 pg/mg) ($p < 0.001$).

At week 6 pi, the mean FCM (625.2 ± 113.2 pg/mg) increased in birds co-infected with both *Salmonella* Typhimurium and *Salmonella* Mbandaka. At this time point, no significant difference between the two infection groups was detected. The mean FCM in control birds (268.7 ± 24.19 pg/mg), however, was significantly less than both treatment groups ($p < 0.01$). At weeks 8, 12, 14 and 16 pi, the mean FCM obtained for all groups varied but did not differ significantly (Figure 3).

No significant correlation was detected between the mean FCM concentration and MPN counts in singly or co-infected birds ($r^2 = -0.036$, $p = 0.699$). A significant but weak positive correlation ($r^2 = 0.26$, $p = 0.02$) was observed between the mean log copy number/gram and FCM concentration in birds infected with *Salmonella* Typhimurium only.

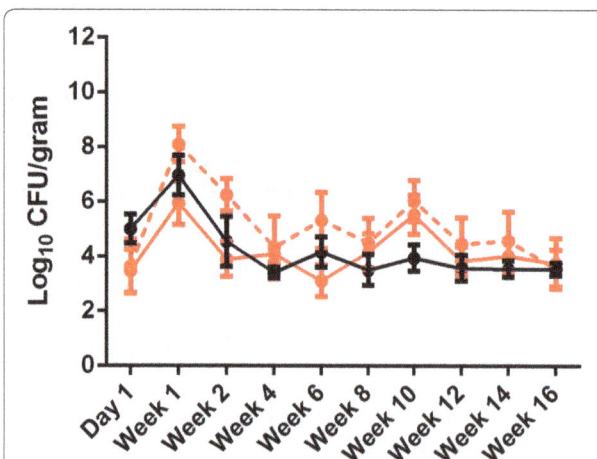

Figure 2 Quantification and differentiation of *Salmonella* by qPCR. Bacterial loads of fecal samples collected from birds infected with *Salmonella* Typhimurium only (black line) or co-infected with *Salmonella* Typhimurium (red line) and *Salmonella* Mbandaka (red hashed line) were quantified using a serovar specific qPCR. *Salmonella* Typhimurium was detected using a primers designed to the *TSR3* gene while *Salmonella* Mbandaka was detected using the *dhrfV* gene. Data are presented as mean $\log_{10}$ CFU/gram feces ± SEM. The amount of bacteria varied significantly over time ($p < 0.01$).

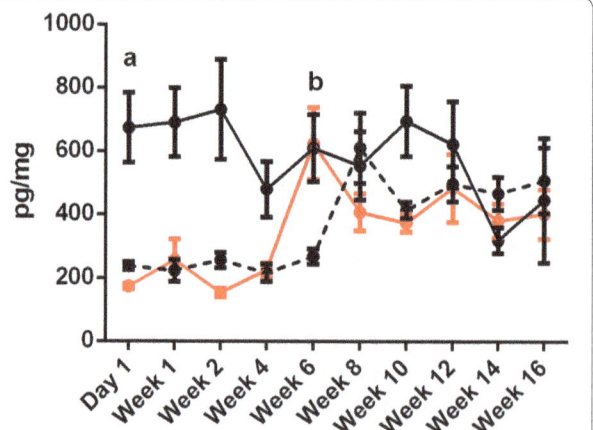

Figure 3 Measurement of fecal corticosterone metabolites (FCM). FCM concentrations were measured at day 1 and weeks 1, 2, 4, 6, 8, 10, 12, 14, and 16 pi. Data is presented as mean pg/mg feces ± SEM. A significant effect of time ($p < 0.05$) and treatment ($p < 0.001$) was detected for FCM concentrations. At day 1 pi, the mean FCM in birds infected with *Salmonella* Typhimurium (black line) was significantly higher than either control (black hashed line) or co-infected birds (red line) (a; $p < 0.001$). At week 6 pi, the mean FCM in co-infected birds increased. At this time point, both infection groups were exhibited significantly higher FCM concentrations than control birds (b; $p < 0.01$).

Detection of *Salmonella* from eggshell wash and internal contents

Eggs were collected at weeks 6, 8, 10, 12, and 14 pi and tested for the presence of *Salmonella* on the shell surface and within the internal contents. *Salmonella* was isolated throughout the experiment from the eggshell wash of experimentally infected hens. In birds infected with only *Salmonella* Typhimurium, the percentage of eggshell contamination ranged from 9.52 to 21.74%. Birds infected with both *Salmonella* Typhimurium and *Salmonella* Mbandaka exhibited a similar level of eggshell contamination, 10.89–33.33% (Table 1). By culture methods, the percentage of eggshell contamination was highest in both the groups at week 6 pi (onset of lay). No significant difference in eggshell contamination frequency was detected between *Salmonella* infection treatment groups. PCR results of egg shell samples indicated that the recovery rate of *Salmonella* Typhimurium (11.74%) was higher than *Salmonella* Mbandaka (6.60%) in co-infection group (Table 1).

No linear correlation was observed between the *Salmonella* MPN count in feces and eggshell contamination of infected birds ($r^2 = 0.001$, $p = 0.99$). *Salmonella* was not detected in egg internal contents of either infection treatment group at any point during this experiment. Eggshells and internal contents from control hens were also negative for *Salmonella*.

Salmonella Typhimurium antibody titres in serum and egg yolk samples

The titres of *Salmonella* Typhimurium specific serum and yolk antibodies were measured over the course of the experiment (Figures 4A and B). The lowest mean antibody titre (antilog) in birds infected with only *Salmonella* Typhimurium was observed at week 1 pi (1286 ± 168.1) and peaked at week 6 pi (2678 ± 179.5). After week 6 pi,

antibody titres remained constant during the remainder of the experiment. A similar pattern was observed for *Salmonella* Typhimurium antibodies measured from the co-infection group. In birds infected with both *Salmonella* Typhimurium and *Salmonella* Mbandaka, the mean titre was lowest at week 1 pi (997.7 ± 170.5) and highest at week 6 pi (1949 ± 239.1). Mean antibody titres of birds infected with *Salmonella* Typhimurium only were significantly higher than those obtained for the co-infection group at weeks 6, 8, 10, 12, and 14 pi ($p < 0.01$). Control birds were negative for *Salmonella* Typhimurium antibodies over the course of the experiment.

Eggs collected from both infection groups tested positive for *Salmonella* yolk antibodies (Figure 4B). A significant effect of treatment was detected between the experimental groups ($p \leq 0.01$).

Persistence of *Salmonella* in internal organs

At 30 weeks of age (week 16 pi), the experiment was terminated and birds were euthanized. Spleen, liver, bone marrow and caecal tonsils from all hens were collected and processed for *Salmonella* to characterise the persistence of the bacteria in these organs. All samples collected from control hens were negative for *Salmonella*. Bacteria were detected in all tissues except for the bone marrow samples. The total number of positive samples was greatest in the spleen, followed by the liver and caecal tonsils (Figure 5). The mean splenic bacterial load observed in birds infected with only *Salmonella* Typhimurium (757.4 ± 301.1 CFU/g tissue) was significantly greater than the mean titre observed for birds inoculated with both *Salmonella* Typhimurium and *Salmonella* Mbandaka (236.0 ± 54.51 CFU/g tissue) ($p < 0.01$).

Birds infected with both *Salmonella* Typhimurium and *Salmonella* Mbandaka exhibited the highest number of individuals positive for *Salmonella* in the liver

Table 1 Percentage of isolation of *Salmonella* and *Salmonella* Typhimurium by culture and PCR method respectively from eggshell samples of orally infected birds at different weeks of pi

Weeks pi	*Salmonella* Typhimurium only group		Co-infection group		
	Salmonella detection by culture method	*Salmonella* Typhimurium detection by PCR	*Salmonella* detection by culture method	*Salmonella* Typhimurium detection by PCR	*Salmonella* Mbandaka detection by PCR
Week 6	21.74[c] (5/23)[a]	17.39 (4/23)	33.33 (8/24)	8.33 (2/24)[b]	8.33 (2/24)[b]
Week 8	9.52 (8/84)	8.33 (7/84)	10.89 (11/101)	8.91 (9/101)	0.00 (0/101)
Week 10	15.85 (13/82)	15.85 (13/82)	15.22 (14/92)	10.87 (10/92)	5.43 (5/92)
Week 12	13.48 (12/89)	12.36 (11/89)	22.92 (22/96)	14.58 (14/96)	13.54 (13/96)
Week 14	11.49 (10/87)	10.34 (9/87)	21.88 (21/96)	13.54 (13/96)	7.29 (7/96)
Total	13.15 (48/365)	12.05 (44/365)	13.20 (54/409)	11.74 (48/409)	6.60 (27/409)

[a] Number of positive eggs/total number of eggs tested.

[b] Results confirmed by PCR.

[c] Values in %.

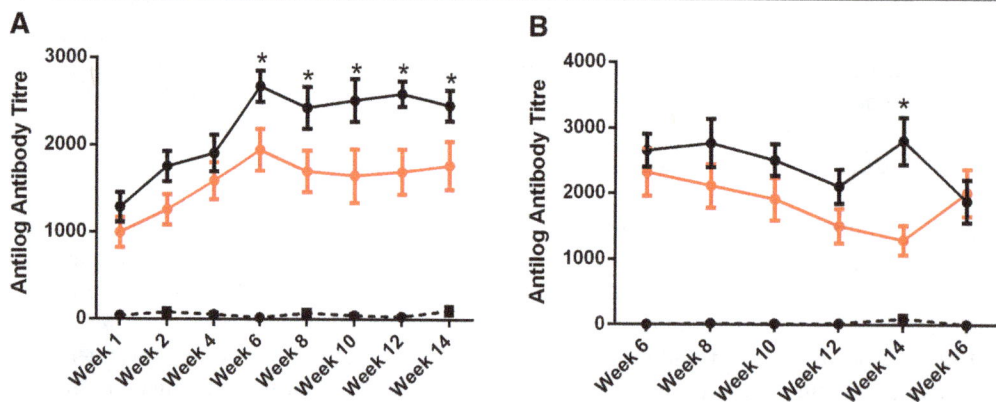

Figure 4 Quantification of *Salmonella* Typhimurium specific antibodies in serum and yolk. *Salmonella* Typhimurium specific antibody titers (antilog antibody titres ± SEM) were characterised over the course of the experiment in both serum (**A**) and yolk (**B**) in control birds (black hashed line) as well as hens infected with only *Salmonella* Typhimurium (black line) or a combination of both *Salmonella* Typhimurium and *Salmonella* Mbandaka (red line). In the serum, the amount of *Salmonella* Typhimurium antibody was significantly higher in singly infected birds compare with co-infected birds from week 6 pi till the end of the experiment (*$p < 0.01$). Mean antibody titres detected in yolk samples collected from *Salmonella* Typhimurium infected birds were only significantly different from co-infected birds at week 14 pi (*$p < 0.01$).

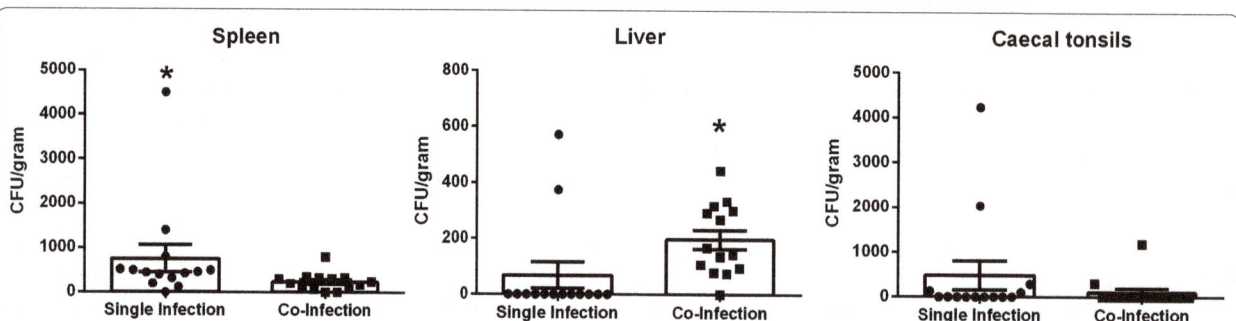

Figure 5 Bacterial persistence in spleen, liver and caecal tonsils. The total amount of viable bacteria was quantified from internal organs at week 16 pi. Data is presented as mean CFU/gram tissue ± standard error of the mean. Individual data points have also been included to highlight the variation within each group. In splenic samples, bacterial loads in birds infected with only *Salmonella* Typhimurium were significantly higher than the titre observed in the co-infection group (*$p < 0.01$). Only 2/14 liver samples from the *Salmonella* Typhimurium treatment group were positive for bacteria, while 13/14 positive samples were detected for co-infected birds. The mean for the liver was significantly higher in the co-infection group (*$p < 0.01$). No significant difference was detected in bacterial loads from the caecal tonsils.

(92.9%) (Figure 5). The mean bacterial titre for the co-infection group was 197.1 ± 34.17 CFU/g tissue and was significantly higher than the mean titre observed for birds infected with *Salmonella* Typhimurium, 68.46 ± 46.97 CFU/g tissue (Mann–Whitney, $p < 0.01$). The lowest overall level of *Salmonella* colonisation was observed in the caecal tonsils with 35.7% positive individuals in the single infection group and 14.3% positive birds in the multi-serovar group (Figure 5). Bacterial titres in caecal tonsils collected from birds infected with only *Salmonella* Typhimurium ranged from 0 to 4.2×10^3 CFU/g tissue with a mean titre of 485.7 ± 321.9 CFU/g tissue. Birds infected with both *Salmonella* Typhimurium and *Salmonella* Mbandaka ranged from 0 to 1.2×10^3 CFU/g

tissue with a mean of 107.1 ± 85.79 CFU/g tissue. No significant difference was detected between the two infection treatment groups.

The culture positive internal organs were further tested by PCR to differentiate *Salmonella* Typhimurium and *Salmonella* Mbandaka in the co-infection group (Table 2). In splenic samples, 1 of 14 was positive for *Salmonella* Typhimurium while 4/14 samples were positive for *Salmonella* Mbandaka. Three of 14 liver samples from the co-infection group were positive for *Salmonella* Mbandaka, however, no *Salmonella* Typhimurium was detected. In the caecal tonsils, 1/14 samples were positive for *Salmonella* Typhimurium and 1/14 tested positive for *Salmonella* Mbandaka.

Table 2 Recovery and enumeration of _Salmonella_ from internal organs

| Organ | _Salmonella_ Typhimurium only group | | | Co-infection group | | | |
	Salmonella detection by culture method	Mean log$_{10}$ CFU/g and SEM	_Salmonella_ Typhimurium detection by PCR	_Salmonella_ detection by culture method	Mean log$_{10}$ CFU/g and SEM	_Salmonella_ Typhimurium detection by PCR	_Salmonella_ Mbandaka detection by PCR
Spleen	13/14 (92.85%)	2.52 ± 0.22 (n = 13)	3/14 (21.43%)	12/14 (85.71%)	2.01 ± 0.24 (n = 12)	1/14 (7.14%)	4/14 (28.57%)
Liver	2/14 (14.29%)	0.38 ± 0.26 (n = 2)	2/14 (14.29%)	13/14 (92.85%)	2.10 ± 0.17 (n = 13)	0/14 (0.00%)	3/14 (21.43%)
Caecal tonsils	5/14 (35.71%)	0.97 ± 0.38 (n = 5)	2/14 (14.29%)	2/14 (14.29%)	0.40 ± 0.27 (n = 2)	1/14 (7.14%)	1/14 (7.14%)

Discussion

This study indicated that layers infected with *Salmonella* Typhimurium DT9 became persistently infected causing intermittent bacterial shedding in faeces. At week 6 pi, the MPN count in *Salmonella* Typhimurium infected group was significantly higher than multi-serovar infection group. Week 6 corresponded to the onset of lay in experimental birds and it was postulated that this increase could be related to physiological stress induced by onset of lay [16].

FCM levels in the *Salmonella* Typhimurium group were higher than either the control or multi-serovar treatment groups from day 1 until week 6 pi. Bacterial lipopolysaccharide (LPS) can induce inflammation within a host and has been associated with increased serum and corticosterone [12]. The LPS of *Salmonella enterica* is variable, serovar dependent and contributes to different degrees of virulence. This may account for lower mean FCM concentrations in the multi-serovar group. Increase in FCM in all treatment groups between 6-8 weeks could be attributed to the onset of lay, and infection may lead to further increase in level of FCM. However, it important to note that no positive correlation was observed between bacterial shedding and FCM levels in this study.

During this study, higher rates of eggshell contamination at the onset of lay could be attributed to increased *Salmonella* shedding in feces at that point [5, 16]. There was no linear correlation between *Salmonella* shedding in feces and egg shell contamination of infected birds and this is in agreement with earlier reports [32]. Of note, in this study *Salmonella* was not detected from egg internal contents.

The *Salmonella* Typhimurium IgG antibody titres increased after week 1 pi and peaked at week 6 pi. Birds were seropositive till the end of the trial at week 14 pi but the immune response did not result in complete clearance of *Salmonella* spp. It is also important to note that the antibody response contributes to the clearance of extracellular bacteria, intracellular bacteria can persist in the host thus cell mediated immune response is essential for clearance of *Salmonella* Typhimurium (reviewed in [33]). Overall decreased IgG antibody response in multi-serovar infection group could perhaps be due to the competitive and immunoprotective mechanism between both *Salmonella* strains. However, the absence of an infection treatment with only *Salmonella* Mbandaka in this study limits this conclusion.

In the multi-serovar group, a low MPN was obtained at week 6 yet qPCR results revealed similar loads of both *Salmonella* Typhimurium and *Salmonella* Mbandaka. The discrepancy may be due to the detection of both live and dead bacteria using PCR method. However it is unclear why that has happened specifically at week 6 pi.

Laying hens mounted immune response to invasive strain of *Salmonella* Typhimurium DT9 without inducing clinical signs. Variation in qPCR and MPN results could be attributed to the sensitivity of the tests used. Several factors such as heterogeneous distribution of the pathogen in sample, number of stressed cells, sample matrix, enrichment time and enrichment media can influence the accuracy of quantitation [34].

In *Salmonella* Typhimurium infected group there were increased levels of FCM concentrations, antibody titres and bacterial shedding (as detected by MPN method) at week 6 pi (onset of lay) which supports the theory that the presence of stress hormones can stimulate *Salmonella* growth and enhance bacterial colonisation in the intestine [35]. However present data suggests that this theory may not apply when host is infected with multiple *Salmonella* serovars. Concentration of corticosterone levels in sera can increase or decrease the antibody response [36]. In this study the high corticosterone levels did not suppress the humoral immune response against *Salmonella* Typhimurium.

Stress can stimulate the recrudescence of bacteria from internal organs resulting in high bacterial load in feces [37]. Our findings indicated that *Salmonella* Typhimurium persisted in internal organs despite high levels of circulating specific IgG antibody. Previous studies reported *Salmonella* Typhimurium clearance from liver and other internal organs due to Th-1 dominated responses and high levels of interferon-γ expression at around 14–28 days pi [38]. Some studies reported low frequency of *Salmonella* Enteritidis in liver and other internal organs for up to 22 weeks pi [39]. It has also been suggested that age at exposure did not affect recovery of *Salmonella* Typhimurium from liver [40]. Our observations could not be compared with previous reports because such studies were performed using broilers for short period of time. It could be hypothesised that persistence of *Salmonella* Typhimurium in internal organs including liver could be due to the timing of challenge (prior to lay in this case). Sexual maturity can induce immunosuppression by altering cellular and humoral immune response [33]. This could ultimately cause bacteria to avoid clearance and dominate host leading to a recrudescence of infection. However further studies are required to confirm this hypothesis. It is interesting to note that in mixed infection group, only *Salmonella* Mbandaka was detected from liver.

Previous literature stated that intestinal persistence of *Salmonella* Typhimurium in chickens was longer when birds were challenged at day old compared to day 7 and that older birds are considerably more resistant to salmonellae than are young chicks [41, 42]. Our study indicated that infection of adult birds (14 weeks old in this study) can also result in continued harbouring of the *Salmonella* Typhimurium and intermittent faecal shedding. This shedding can be associated with the stress event such as onset of lay. However interplay between stress, immune response and *Salmonella* Typhimurium shedding in single or mixed infection group at the onset of lay is more complex to understand.

To conclude, *Salmonella* Typhimurium DT9 persistently infected hens causing intermittent bacterial shedding in faeces. At the onset of lay shedding of *Salmonella* Typhimurium was affected in mixed infection group. Increased immune response did not result in clearance of *Salmonella spp* (except for *Salmonella* Typhimurium at week 6 pi). There was no correlation between FCM and *Salmonella* shedding. This long term *Salmonella* Typhimurium infection model provided useful insights on the continued persistence and or recrudescence of *Salmonella* Typhimurium, although further investigation is necessary to understand the immunobiology of long term and systemic *Salmonella* Typhimurium infection.

Competing interests
The authors declare that they have no competing interests.

Authors' contributions
PS, VP, AM and KC designed the experiments and were involved with preparation of this manuscript. PS, VP, AM and KC conducted the layer hen trial. PS performed all sampling and microbiological processing. TM performed corticosterone extractions from fecal samples. PS and TM conducted FCM experiments. TM and KC performed qPCR. All authors read and approved the final manuscript.

Acknowledgements
We thank Associate Professor Milton McAllister, Dr. Vaibhav Gole and Dr. Rebecca Forder for their assistance with this study.

Funding
This research work was supported by Australian Egg Corporation Limited (AECL) Australia. Mr. Pardeep Sharma is a recipient of an International Postgraduate Research Scholarship from the University of Adelaide Australia.

References
1. Moffatt CR, Musto J, Pingault N, Miller M, Stafford R, Gregory J, Polkinghorne BG, Kirk MD (2016) *Salmonella* Typhimurium and outbreaks of egg-associated disease in Australia, 2001 to 2011. Foodborne Pathog Dis 13:379–385
2. Threlfall E, Wain J, Peters T, Lane C, De Pinna E, Little C, Wales A, Davies R (2014) Egg-borne infections of humans with salmonella: not only an *S. Enteritidis* problem. World Poultr Sci J 70:15–26
3. Chousalkar KK, Sexton M, McWhorter A, Hewson K, Martin G, Shadbolt C, Goldsmith P (2015) *Salmonella* Typhimurium in the Australian egg industry: multidisciplinary approach to addressing the public health challenge and future directions. Crit Rev Food Sci Nutr. doi:10.1080/10408398.2015.1113928
4. Williams A, Davies A, Wilson J, Marsh P, Leach S, Humphrey T (1998) Contamination of the contents of intact eggs by *Salmonella* Typhimurium DT104. Vet Rec 143:562–563
5. Okamura M, Sonobe M, Obara S, Kubo T, Nagai T, Noguchi M, Takehara K, Nakamura M (2010) Potential egg contamination by *Salmonella* enterica serovar Typhimurium definitive type 104 following experimental infection of pullets at the onset of lay. Poult Sci 89:1629–1634
6. Okamura M, Miyamoto T, Kamijima Y, Tani H, Sasai K, Baba E (2001) Differences in abilities to colonize reproductive organs and to contaminate eggs in intravaginally inoculated hens and in vitro adherences to vaginal explants between *Salmonella* Enteritidis and other *Salmonella* serovars. Avian Dis 45:962–971
7. Leach SA, Williams A, Davies AC, Wilson J, Marsh PD, Humphrey TJ (1999) Aerosol route enhances the contamination of intact eggs and muscle of experimentally infected laying hens by *Salmonella* Typhimurium DT104. FEMS Microbiol Lett 171:203–207
8. Borsoi A, Quinteiro-Filho WM, Calefi AS, Piantino Ferreira AJ, Astolfi-Ferreira CS, Florio JC, Palermo-Neto J (2015) Effects of cold stress and *Salmonella* Heidelberg infection on bacterial load and immunity of chickens. Avian Pathol 44:490–497
9. Quinteiro-Filho WM, Rodrigues M, Ribeiro A, Ferraz-de-Paula V, Pinheiro M, Sa L, Ferreira A, Palermo-Neto J (2012) Acute heat stress impairs performance parameters and induces mild intestinal enteritis in broiler chickens: role of acute hypothalamic-pituitary-adrenal axis activation. J Anim Sci 90:1986–1994
10. Holt PS (1993) Effect of induced molting on the susceptibility of White Leghorn hens to a *Salmonella* Enteritidis infection. Avian Dis 37:412–417
11. Nakamura M, Nagamine N, Takahashi T, Suzuki S, Kijima M, Tamura Y, Sato S (1994) Horizontal transmission of *Salmonella* Enteritidis and effect of stress on shedding in laying hens. Avian Dis 38:282–288
12. Shini S, Kaiser P, Shini A, Bryden WL (2008) Biological response of chickens (*Gallus gallus domesticus*) induced by corticosterone and a bacterial endotoxin. Comp Biochem Physiol B: Biochem Mol Biol 149:324–333
13. Mashaly M, Hendricks G, Kalama M, Gehad A, Abbas A, Patterson P (2004) Effect of heat stress on production parameters and immune responses of commercial laying hens. Poult Sci 83:889–894
14. Quinteiro-Filho W, Gomes A, Pinheiro M, Ribeiro A, Ferraz-de-Paula V, Astolfi-Ferreira C, Ferreira A, Palermo-Neto J (2012) Heat stress impairs performance and induces intestinal inflammation in broiler chickens infected with *Salmonella* Enteritidis. Avian Pathol 41:421–427
15. Gole VC, Torok V, Sexton M, Caraguel CG, Chousalkar KK (2014) Association between indoor environmental contamination by *Salmonella* enterica and contamination of eggs on layer farms. J Clin Microbiol 52:3250–3258
16. Gole VC, Caraguel CG, Sexton M, Fowler C, Chousalkar KK (2014) Shedding of *Salmonella* in single age caged commercial layer flock at an early stage of lay. Int J Food Microbiol 189:61–66
17. Pulido-Landínez M, Sanchez-Ingunza R, Guard J, Nascimento V (2013) Assignment of serotype to *Salmonella* enterica isolates obtained from poultry and their environment in Southern Brazil. Lett Appl Microbiol 57:288–294
18. Chousalkar K, Gole V, Caraguel C, Rault JL (2016) Chasing *Salmonella* Typhimurium in free range egg production system. Vet Microbiol 192:67–72
19. Glass K, Fearnley E, Hocking H, Raupach J, Veitch M, Ford L, Kirk MD (2016) Bayesian source attribution of salmonellosis in South Australia. Risk Anal 36:561–570
20. Doyle EM (2013) White paper on human illness caused by *Salmonella* from all food and non-food vectors. Update 2013 in: FRI Food Safety Reviews (Ed), Madison, pp 1-45
21. Guard J, Sanchez-Ingunza R, Shah DH, Rothrock MJ, Gast RK, Jones DR (2015) Recovery of *Salmonella* enterica serovar Enteritidis from hens initially infected with serovar Kentucky. Food Chem 189:86–92
22. Pulido-Landínez M, Sanchez-Ingunza R, Guard J, do Nascimento VP (2013) Presence of *Salmonella* Enteritidis and *Salmonella* Gallinarum in commercial laying hens diagnosed with fowl typhoid disease in Colombia. Avian Dis 58:165–170
23. Pande VV, Devon RL, Sharma P, McWhorter AR, Chousalkar KK (2016) Study of *Salmonella* Typhimurium infection in laying hens. Front Microbiol 7:203
24. USDA, U.S. Department of agriculture, food safety and inspection services (2008) most probable number procedure and tables. In: Microbiology Laboratory Guidebook. https://www.fsis.usda.gov/wps/wcm/

connect/8872ec11-d6a3-4fcf-86df-4d87e57780f5/MLG-Appendix-2. pdf?MOD=AJPERES. Accessed 14 Jan 2015

25. Pande VV, Gole VC, McWhorter AR, Abraham S, Chousalkar KK (2015) Antimicrobial resistance of non-typhoidal *Salmonella* isolates from egg layer flocks and egg shells. Int J Food Microbiol 203:23–26

26. Akiba M, Kusumoto M, Iwata T (2011) Rapid identification of *Salmonella* enterica serovars, Typhimurium, Choleraesuis, Infantis, Hadar, Enteritidis, Dublin and Gallinarum, by multiplex PCR. J Microbiol Methods 85:9–15

27. Gole V, Chousalkar K, Roberts J (2012) Prevalence of antibodies to *Mycoplasma synoviae* in laying hens and possible effects on egg shell quality. Prev Vet Med 106:75–78

28. Greiner M, Sohr D, Gobel P (1995) A modified ROC analysis for the selection of cut-off values and the definition of intermediate results of serodiagnostic tests. J Immunol Methods 185:123–132

29. Dehnhard M, Schreer A, Krone O, Jewgenow K, Krause M, Grossmann R (2003) Measurement of plasma corticosterone and fecal glucocorticoid metabolites in the chicken (*Gallus domesticus*), the great cormorant (*Phalacrocorax carbo*), and the goshawk (*Accipiter gentilis*). Gen Comp Endocrinol 131:345–352

30. Rettenbacher S, Mostl E, Hackl R, Ghareeb K, Palme R (2004) Measurement of corticosterone metabolites in chicken droppings. Br Poult Sci 45:704–711

31. Shini S, Huff G, Shini A, Kaiser P (2010) Understanding stress-induced immunosuppression: exploration of cytokine and chemokine gene profiles in chicken peripheral leukocytes. Poult Sci 89:841–851

32. Gast RK, Guard-Bouldin J, Holt PS (2005) The relationship between the duration of fecal shedding and the production of contaminated eggs by laying hens infected with strains of *Salmonella* Enteritidis and *Salmonella* Heidelberg. Avian Dis 49:382–386

33. Chappell L, Kaiser P, Barrow P, Jones MA, Johnston C, Wigley P (2009) The immunobiology of avian systemic salmonellosis. Vet Immunol Immunopathol 128:53–59

34. Malorny B, Lofstrom C, Wagner M, Kramer N, Hoorfar J (2008) Enumeration of *Salmonella* bacteria in food and feed samples by real-time PCR for quantitative microbial risk assessment. Appl Environ Microbiol 74:1299–1304

35. Verbrugghe E, Dhaenens M, Leyman B, Boyen F, Shearer N, Van Parys A, Haesendonck R, Bert W, Favoreel H, Deforce D, Thompson A, Haesebrouck F, Pasmans F (2016) Host stress drives *Salmonella* recrudescence. Sci Rep 6:20849

36. Campos-Rodriguez R, Kormanovski A, Stephano AQ, Abarca-Rojano E, Berczi I, Ventura-Juarez J, Drago-Serrano ME (2012) The central nervous system modulates the immune response to Salmonella. In: Kumar Yashwant (ed) Salmonella—a diversified superbug. Intech Open Access Publisher, Croatia, pp 375–398

37. Rostagno M, Wesley I, Trampel D, Hurd H (2006) *Salmonella* prevalence in market-age turkeys on-farm and at slaughter. Poult Sci 85:1838–1842

38. Beal RK, Powers C, Wigley P, Barrow PA, Smith AL (2004) Temporal dynamics of the cellular, humoral and cytokine responses in chickens during primary and secondary infection with *Salmonella* enterica serovar Typhimurium. Avian Pathol 33:25–33

39. Gast RK, Beard CW (1990) Isolation of *Salmonella* enteritidis from internal organs of experimentally infected hens. Avian Dis 34:991–993

40. Gast RK, Beard CW (1989) Age-related changes in the persistence and pathogenicity of *Salmonella* Typhimurium in chicks. Poult Sci 68:1454–1460

41. Groves PJ, Sharpe SM, Muir WI, Pavic A, Cox JM (2016) Live and inactivated vaccine regimens against caecal *Salmonella* Typhimurium colonisation in laying hens. Aust Vet J 94:387–393

42. Gast RK (2008) Paratyphoid infections. In: Saif Y (Ed) Diseases of Poultry, 12th edn. Blackwell, Ames, pp 636–655

16

Impact of diversity of *Mycoplasma hyopneumoniae* strains on lung lesions in slaughter pigs

Annelies Michiels[1][*] ⓘ, Katleen Vranckx[2], Sofie Piepers[1], Rubén Del Pozo Sacristán[1], Ioannis Arsenakis[1], Filip Boyen[3], Freddy Haesebrouck[3] and Dominiek Maes[1]

Abstract

The importance of diversity of *Mycoplasma hyopneumoniae* (*M. hyopneumoniae*) strains is not yet fully known. This study investigated the genetic diversity of *M. hyopneumoniae* strains in ten pig herds, and assessed associations between the presence of different strains of *M. hyopneumoniae* and lung lesions at slaughter. Within each herd, three batches of slaughter pigs were investigated. At slaughter, from each batch, 20 post mortem bronchoalveolar lavage fluid samples were collected for multiple locus variable-number tandem repeat analysis (MLVA), and lung lesions (*Mycoplasma*-like lesions, fissures) were examined. Multivariable analyses including potential risk factors for respiratory disease were performed to assess associations between the number of different strains per batch (three categories: one strain, two–six strains, ≥seven strains), and the lung lesions as outcome variables. In total, 135 different *M. hyopneumoniae* strains were found. The mean (min.–max.) number of different strains per batch were 7 (1–13). Batches with two–six strains or more than six strains had more severe *Mycoplasma*-like lesions ($P = 0.064$ and $P = 0.012$, respectively), a higher prevalence of pneumonia [odds ratio (OR): 1.30, $P = 0.33$ and OR: 2.08, $P = 0.012$, respectively], and fissures (OR = 1.35, $P = 0.094$ and OR = 1.70, $P = 0.007$, respectively) compared to batches with only one strain. In conclusion, many different *M. hyopneumoniae* strains were found, and batches of slaughter pigs with different *M. hyopneumoniae* strains had a higher prevalence and severity of *Mycoplasma*-like lung lesions at slaughter, implying that reducing the number of different strains may lead to less lung lesions at slaughter and better respiratory health of the pigs.

Introduction

Mycoplasma hyopneumoniae (*M. hyopneumoniae*) is the causative agent of enzootic pneumonia, and infections occur in all countries with an intensive pig production [1]. Infections with *M. hyopneumoniae* cause tremendous economic losses, either directly or indirectly, by increasing the susceptibility of infected animals to other respiratory pathogens [2].

Mycoplasmas have small genomes (580–1300 kb) [3, 4], and genetic diversity might be one solution to adapt to the adverse environment of the host [5, 6]. Many regions in the genome of *M. hyopneumoniae* related to adherence in the host contain variable number of tandem repeats (VNTRs). These regions are prone to recombination events and slipped strand mispairing, which can possibly lead to expression of a different sized protein [7]. Multiple locus variable number of tandem repeat analysis (MLVA) has been used successfully to genetically characterize *M. hyopneumoniae* isolates [8–12]. This technique has a high discriminatory power, and can be applied directly to clinical samples without the necessity to grow the bacterium, which is very fastidious in the case of *M. hyopneumoniae* [9].

Previous studies have shown that there is a high diversity of *M. hyopneumoniae* field isolates, especially between strains from different herds [10]. Other studies including a limited number of herds not practising

*Correspondence: Annelies.Michiels@UGent.be
[1] Department of Reproduction, Obstetrics and Herd Health, Unit Porcine Health Management, Faculty of Veterinary Medicine, Ghent University, Salisburylaan 133, 9820 Merelbeke, Belgium
Full list of author information is available at the end of the article

vaccination against *M. hyopneumoniae*, showed that in some herds, only one strain was detected, whereas different strains were found in other herds, even in the same pig [9, 12]. The importance of genetic diversity of *M. hyopneumoniae* strains however is not fully known. A possible link between the presence of multiple simultaneous or subsequent infections with different *M. hyopneumoniae* strains and the presence and severity of lung lesions has been suggested [9, 10, 13], but no systematic study has been conducted to answer this question. If the presence of different *M. hyopneumoniae* strains is associated with more clinical disease and/or lung lesions, then measures decreasing the diversity of strains may be helpful to control respiratory problems in pig herds.

The aim of this study was to investigate the presence of different *M. hyopneumoniae* strains in consecutive batches of slaughter pigs from different herds, to type the strains using MLVA and to investigate associations between the occurrence of multiple strains of *M. hyopneumoniae* and the prevalence and severity of lung lesions.

Materials and methods
Study population
A list of herds ($n = 56$) complying with following criteria: closed herd or closed production system, herd with at least 100 breeding sows and vaccination of piglets against *M. hyopneumoniae* was provided by one of the largest slaughter houses in Belgium (Covalis). The list of these farms was randomized (Excel 2010, Microsoft Corp., Redmond, WA, USA) and the farmers were contacted in order of appearance on the randomized list until ten herds willing to participate to the study were obtained. Descriptive data of the ten study herds are presented in Table 1. Different potential risk factors for respiratory disease were collected from these herds during a herd visit by the first author. During the visit, a questionnaire was completed, the stables were visited and the fattening pigs inspected. The potential risk factors in the questionnaire were based on previous studies [14] and pertained to biosecurity, management, housing and vaccination status (Table 2).

Sampling at the slaughterhouse and lung lesion scoring
Three different batches of fattening pigs per herd were evaluated at the slaughterhouse during a time span of one to three months. All visits were performed from November 2012 until April 2013. From each batch, 20 randomly selected blood samples were collected at exsanguination, and from 20 other randomly selected pigs, the lungs were collected. For practical reasons, only the left half of the lung was taken. The blood samples and lungs were transported to the laboratory of Bacteriology of the Faculty of

Veterinary Medicine, Ghent University immediately after the slaughterhouse visit.

Additionally, as many lungs as possible of each batch (min. 50) were evaluated for lung lesions. The lungs that were sampled were not included in the lung lesion scoring. The lungs were scored for presence of pneumonia and severity of *Mycoplasma*-like lesions using the method described by Morrison et al. [15]. *Mycoplasma*-like lesions were defined as macroscopic greyish to purplish consolidated pneumonia areas, generally located on the cranio-ventral parts of the lung lobes. The lungs were also evaluated for the presence of fissures and pleurisy. Fissures were defined as areas of collapsed alveoli adjoining alveolar emphysema (recovery lesions) [16], while pleurisy was defined as fibrotic adherences between the parietal and visceral membranes of the pleural cavity [17]. No approval of the ethical committee of Ghent University was necessary, as the pigs were destined for slaughter.

Nested polymerase chain reaction (NPCR)
Upon arrival in the laboratory, the lung halves were flushed with 20 mL phosphate buffered saline (PBS, 8 g/L NaCl, 0.34 g/L KH_2PO4, 1.21 g/L K_2HPO_4, pH 7.3). The recovered fluid was centrifuged at 2000 g during 30 min to obtain the remaining pellet by carefully removing the supernatant. The pellet was resuspended in 1 mL of PBS and 200 µL of the resuspension was used to perform the DNA extraction using the DNeasy blood and tissue kit (Qiagen, Belgium) according to the instructions in the protocol manual. *Mycoplasma hyopneumoniae*-DNA was detected with a two steps nested polymerase chain reaction (nPCR) [18]. The nPCR products were analyzed by gel electrophoresis on a 1.5% agarose gel in Tris–Borate–EDTA (TBE)-buffer and stained with GelRed™ (Biotium. Inc., CA, USA) with visualization under UV illumination.

Multiple locus variable-number tandem repeat analysis (MLVA)
All nPCR positive samples were submitted to a multiplex PCR as previously described [9]. Briefly, loci h1, h5 repeat 2, p97 repeat 1 and p146 repeat 3 were amplified in a multiplex reaction with a mastercycler epgradient S (Eppendorf, Hamburg, Germany) in a final volume of 20 µL containing 1× PCR buffer [20 mM Tris–HCl (pH 8.4), 50 mM KCl], 3 mM $MgCl_2$, 0.2 mM deoxynucleotide triphosphate, 0.75 U of Platinum® *Taq* DNA Polymerase (Invitrogen, Merelbeke, Belgium), 0.1 µM of each primer and finally 2 µL of template DNA. Ten cycles (30″94 °C; 30″63 °C; 1′15″69 °C) in which the annealing temperature was incrementally decreased with 1 °C per cycle were performed. Next, forty cycles (30″94 °C; 30″53 °C;

Table 1 Description of the ten study herds (A–J) enrolled in the study

Herd	A	B	C	D	E	F	G	H	I	J
Number of sows	170	200	250	200	150	250	200	250	150	125
Sows breed	LW (50%) + ELR (25%) + FLR (25%)	Topigs	ELR (50%) + FLR (50%)	Danbred (70%) + Hypor	Topigs	Topigs	Danbred	Rattlerow-Seghers	Hypor (90%) + Danbred (10%)	Hypor
Batch production system for sows	3-week	3-week	4-week	3-week	Day system	1-week	4-week	1-week	4-week	4-week
Stocking density nursery (m²/animal)	>0.30	<0.30	<0.30	>0.30	<0.30	>0.30	<0.30	>0.30	>0.30	<0.30
Stocking density fatteners (m²/animal)	>0.70	>0.7	0.65–0.70	0.65–0.7	0.7	<0.65	0.65–0.70	0.65–0.70	0.65–0.70	0.65
Purchase of gilts (occasions per year)	No	Yes (5)	No	Yes (4)	Yes (4)	No	No	Yes (8)	Yes every month[a]	Yes (5)
Duration of quarantine period for gilts	n.a.	9 week	n.a.	8 week	4 week	n.a.	n.a.	No	4 week	6 week
Mycoplasma hyopneumoniae vaccination gilts	No	Yes	No	Yes	No	No	No	No	Yes	No
Age (days) at vaccination of piglets against M. hyopneumoniae	8 and 26	21	14	7	14	7	35	3–8 and 28	18	21
Other vaccinations in piglets	No	PCV-2 (21)	No	PRRSv (18)	PCV-2 (14)	No	PCV-2 (35)	No	PCV-2 (18)	No
Age at weaning (days of age)	26	26	21	23	25	24	19	28	20–21	21
Clinical signs of M. hyopneumoniae	No	No	No	Yes	Yes	No	No	No	No	No
Coughing score for fattening pigs provided by the farmer (0–10)	3	2	0	7	4	2	3	0	1	0

LW: large white, ELR: English land race, FLR: French land race, n.a.: not applicable, PCV-2: porcine circovirus type 2, PRRSv: porcine reproductive and respiratory syndrome virus.
[a] Schedule of purchasing gilts has been accelerated with transition to Danbred.

Table 2 Potential risk factors for respiratory disease that were collected from the ten herds

Continuous variables	
Times per year farmer is purchasing gilts	"X" times per year that the farmer purchased gilts
Number of herds surrounding the herd in a perimeter of <5 km	calculated with Lambert coordinates and the Pythagoras theorem
Number of sows present on the herd	Measure for the size of the herd
Production system for the sows	0: no week system, 1, 2, 3, 4-week system
Coughing score given by the farmer	(0–10) fatteners
Categorical variables	
Purchase of gilts	1 = yes, 0 = no
Purchase of gilts always from the same supplier	1 = yes, 0 = no
Quarantine period for gilts	1 = yes, 0 = no
Herd located close to a highway (<5 km)	1 = yes, 0 = no
Herd located near a slaughter house (<5 km)	1 = yes, 0 = no
Distance herd to the public road (<100 or >100 m)	1 (<100 m), 2 (>100 m)
Sow breed	0: Topigs, 1: LW + ELR + FLR, ELR + FLR, Danbred + hypor, Danbred, RA-SE, Hypor
Dynamic or stable groups for pregnant sows	Stable (0) or dynamic (1) group sows
AIAO farrowing unit	1 = yes, 0 = no
AIAO nursery unit	1 = yes, 0 = no
AIAO fattening unit	1 = yes, 0 = no
Stocking density nursery	$1 < 0.30\ m^2/pig$; $2 >$ or $= 0.30\ m^2/pig$
Cross fostering during first week of life piglets	0 = no, 1 < 10%, 2 ≥10%
Cross fostering after first week of life piglets	0 = no, 1 < 10%, 2 ≥ 10%
Stocking density fattening unit	$1 ≥ 0.70\ m^2/pig$, $2 = 0.70–0.65\ m^2/pig$, $3 < 0.65\ m^2/pig$
Cleaning and disinfection farrowing unit	1 = yes, 0 = no
Cleaning and disinfection nursery	1 = yes, 0 = no
Cleaning and disinfection fattening unit	1 = yes, 0 = no, 2 = only cleaned not disinfected
Stand empty period farrowing unit	1 = yes, 2 = not always, 0 = no
Stand empty period nursery unit	1 = yes, 2 = not always, 0 = no
Stand empty period fattening unit	1 = yes, 2 = not always, 0 = no
Gilts vaccinated against *M. hyopneumoniae*	1 = yes, 0 = no
Clinical signs of *M. hyopneumoniae* in grower-finishers	1 = yes, 0 = no

LW + ELR + FLR: large white, English landrace, French landrace, ELR + FLR: English landrace, French landrace, RA-SE: Rattlerow-Seghers.

1'15"69 °C) and a final extension step of 5 min at 69 °C followed.

The PCR-products were diluted 1:10 with high performance liquid chromatography filtered water (HPLC–H_2O). Amplicons were kept at 4 °C for a maximum of 48 h. A volume of 165 µL Hi-Di formamide (one run, 16 samples) (Applied Biosystems, Halle, Belgium) or a multitude of 165 µL for multiple runs was pipetted in an 1.5 µL Eppendorf (Eppendorf Belgium N.V.-S.A, Rotselaar, Belgium) and 1.5 µL of 600 LIZ standard (Applied Biosystems, Halle, Belgium) was added. 10 µL of this mixture was added to 1 µL of sample (PCR-product). Samples were denatured at 95 °C for 5 min, cooled on ice and electrophoresis was applied on the ABI 3130xl genetic analyzer (Applied Biosystems) for 16 samples at 15 kV during 14 000 s at 65 °C or for more than 16 samples on the ABI 3730xl (Applied Biosystems) at 15 kV during 14 000 s at 70 °C.

The resulting electropherogram files were imported into BioNumerics version 7.5 (Applied Maths, Sint-Martens-Latem, Belgium). After normalization, the VNTR numbers were calculated automatically from the detected peaks. A minimal spanning tree was constructed with the Prims' algorithm using the multistate categorical coefficient. Only samples for which all four loci were detected, were included in the tree. A weight factor was assigned to each locus according to its' allelic variation in the obtained dataset with the highest weight assigned to the locus with the lowest variation. Following weights were assigned to each locus: 2, 3, 3 and 6 to p146, h1, h5, and p97, respectively. A strain was defined as a unique MLVA-type, e.g. if the combination of repeat numbers was unique. Clonal complexes were defined when strains differed in no more than one locus, with the exception of the most stable locus p97. The Hunter-Gaston discriminatory index was calculated for the complete dataset, as well as for each herd [19].

Serology

The sera of the blood samples (20 per batch) were tested for presence of antibodies against *M. hyopneumoniae* using a blocking ELISA (IDEIA™ *Mycoplasma hyopneumoniae* EIA kit, Oxoid Limited, Hampshire, UK). Sera with optical density (OD) <50% of the average value of the OD-buffercontrol were considered to be positive (ELISA *M. hyopneumoniae* positive samples). All values above or equal to 65% of the average value of the OD-buffercontrol were classified as negative. All doubtful samples equal to 50% and less than 65% of the average value of the OD-buffercontrol were considered to be negative as well.

Eight of the 20 samples from each batch were also tested for presence of antibodies against porcine reproductive and respiratory syndrome virus (PRRSv) (Herd-Check PRRS X3, IDEXX, Liebefeld-Bern, Switzerland) and subtypes H1N1, H1N2 and H3N2 of swine influenza virus (SIV) (standard haemagglutination-inhibition test).

Statistical analyses

Different statistical models were used to assess the associations between the number of strains on the one hand and the presence and severity of lung lesions on the other hand. The number of different strains found in each batch of pigs was categorized as follows: category 1 (CAT 1): one *M. hyopneumoniae* strain per batch, category 2 (CAT 2): two to six different strains per batch, and category 3 (CAT 3): ≥seven different strains per batch. The category one strain per batch was used as reference; the classification in category 2 and 3 was made to obtain the same number of strains in these categories.

The number of strains per batch was considered as explanatory variable in the models. As lung lesions may not only be caused by infection with *M. hyopneumoniae* and/or determined by the number of strains, the effect of the different potential risk factors for respiratory disease (Table 2) was also taken into account in the models. A forward selection procedure was used during the model building, and risk factors with a *P* value >0.15 were removed. Remaining risk factors (with *P* value <0.15) were tested for collinearity. Correlations were assessed using Pearson's (continuous variables) or Spearman rank (categorical variables) correlation, and in case two variables were highly correlated ($|r| > 0.6$), the most significant factor was retained. In the final model, only risk factors with a *P* value <0.05 were retained. Confounding factors were identified when the regression coefficient (β) of another risk factor deviated more than 25% or 0.1 when $\beta < 0.4$ when removing the factor from the model. Such factors were excluded, but mentioned below each model. In total, four separate multivariable models were tested. The outcome variables for the different models were: severity of *Mycoplasma*-like lesions, likelihood of

pneumonia lesions, fissures and pleurisy. Ln-transformation of the severity of the *Mycoplasma*-like lesions was performed to normalize the data. In all models, herd and lung were included as a random effect and batch was included as fixed effect.

A linear mixed regression model (MLwiN 2.26 [20]) was used to assess the influence of category of number of strains on the severity of the *Mycoplasma*-like lesions in each batch. The assumptions of normality and homogeneity of variance of the final model were tested by examining normal probability plots of residuals and plots of residuals versus predicted values. No patterns indicating heteroscedasticity were present. The multilevel linear regression model may be represented mathematically as: $Y_{ij} = \beta_0 + \beta_1 \text{category } 2_{ij} + \beta_2 \text{category } 3_{ij} + \text{batch}2_{ij} + \text{batch}3_{ij} + \varepsilon_{ij}$, where Y_{ij} is the continuous outcome variable (severity of *Mycoplasma*-like lesions), βs are the model coefficients, category is the fixed effect of the category of different number of strains, batch is the fixed effect of batch 1–3, herd is the random effect of herd i ($i = 1$–10), j refers to the jth lung in the ith herd and ε_{ij} is the random error term, assumed to be normally distributed with mean 0 and variance σ^2.

Logistic mixed regression models using 1st order marginal quasi-likelihood algorithms were used to assess the influence of strain category on the likelihood of pneumonia, fissures and pleurisy (MLwiN 2.26—Centre for Multilevel Modeling, Bristol, UK [20]). The fit of the models was evaluated by inspection of the lung standardized residuals plotted against the normal scores and the lung level predicted values. The Hosmer–Lemeshow goodness-of-fit measure was calculated for the explanatory variable models using SAS 9.3 (PROC LOGISTIC, SAS Institute Inc., NC, USA). The results were represented as odds ratio (OR) with the 95% confidence interval calculated around these odds ratios. The multilevel logistic regression model may be represented mathematically as: $g(Y_{ij}) = \beta_0 + \beta_1 \text{category } 2_{ij} + \beta_2 \text{category } 3_{ij} + \text{batch}2_{ij} + \text{batch}3_{ij} + \varepsilon_{ij}$, where (g) refers to the logit link function, Y_{ij} is the probability of the outcome variable on the logit scale (likelihood of pneumonia, fissures and pleurisy), β_s are the model coefficients, category is the fixed effect of category of number of strains, batch is the fixed effect of batch 1–3, herd is the random effect of herd i ($i = 1$ to 10), j refers to the jth lung in the ith herd and ε_{ij} is the random error term, assumed to be normally distributed with mean 0 and variance σ^2.

Results

Descriptive results of the nPCR, MLVA, lung lesions and serology

Nested PCR

From the 600 bronchoalveolar fluid samples, 495 (82.5%) tested positive using nPCR for *M. hyopneumoniae*. The

Table 3 Descriptive results in the three category groups: prevalence of nPCR positive results, average number of different strains, severity of *Mycoplasma*-like lesions ±SD, prevalence pneumonia, fissures and pleurisy expressed in percentages

	Category			Overall
	1	2	3	
nPCR results	42.5	79.6	91.1	82.5
Average number of different strains	1	4	9	7
Severity of *Mycoplasma*-like lesions ± SD	0.78 ± 2.4	3.97 ± 10.7	5.54 ± 12.7	4.59 ± 11.7
Prevalence of pneumonia	11.8	23.2	29.7	25.9
Prevalence of fissures	29.2	41.4	42.3	41.3
Prevalence of pleurisy	10.2	21.2	29.1	24.6

Severity of *Mycoplasma*-like lesions: minimum 0% and maximum 100% of the lung surface affected with pneumonia.

1 = batches with only one strain detected, 2 = batches with 2–6 different strain and 3 = batches with ≥7 strains detected, SD: standard deviation, *n*: number, nPCR results: nested polymerase chain reaction: percentage of positive animals for *M. hyopneumoniae*-DNA detected in the bronchoalveolar lavage fluid.

average percentage of positive samples in each category (Table 3) per batch were: CAT 1: 42.5%, CAT 2: 79.6% and CAT 3: 91.1%. In all batches of each herd, nPCR positive samples were detected. The descriptive nPCR results for each herd and for each batch per herd separately are shown in Table 4.

Multiple locus variable number tandem repeat analysis (MLVA)

Samples that were positive using nPCR were submitted to MLVA. In the entire dataset, 135 different *M. hyopneumoniae* strains were found (Figure 1). The Hunter-Gaston discriminatory index for the complete dataset and for each herd separately is presented in Table 5.

The average number of different strains per batch was 7 (min 1; max 13). The total number of strains and the number of different strains per batch are presented in Table 4.

The average number of different strains per batch in CAT 1, 2 and 3 were 1, 4 and 9, respectively (Table 3).

The most prominent strain was strain 2, with 24 detections in the whole data set of all herds. This strain was detected in herds C, I and J. Strain 113 was the second most prominent strain and was found in herd A and D for a total of 20 times. Strain 135 was only detected 5 times in the dataset, however in herd D, H and I. Hundred and ten strains out of 135 were only detected 5 times or less and 60 out of 135 strains were only detected once. Strain 2, 42, 45, 59, 61, 77, 78, 109 and 117 were found in each of the three sampling periods in herds C, F, F, E, E, H, H and A respectively. In herds B, D, G, I, J no strains were found circulating throughout all three sampling periods. In all herds, strains were identified that were detected in at least two out of three sampling periods, except for herd B. Most returning strains per batch were found in two consecutive sampling points. Five strains were found in the

first and the third sampling point only: strain 2, 19, 21, 99 and 113 in respectively herd I, E, E, G and A. In a lot of lungs (102), two and a few lungs (6) three different strains were detected (Table 4). In herds B and J, no samples with two different strains were obtained. In two lungs of herd F, three different strains were found. In herds A, C, E, and G, always in the second batch, one sample with detection of three strains was found. In herds B, D, H, I and J no samples with three strains were detected.

Lung lesions

In total, 3820 lungs were evaluated at the slaughter line. The average (min.–max.) number of lungs scored per herd and per batch were 382 (200–494) and 127 (54–186), respectively. The average severity of *Mycoplasma*-like lesions in CAT 1, 2 and 3 were 0.78 ± 2.4%, 3.97 ± 10.7 and 5.54 ± 12.7. The average prevalence of pneumonia was 11.8, 23.2 and 29.7% in CAT 1, CAT 2 and CAT 3, respectively. The average prevalence of fissures was 29.2, 41.4 and 42.3% in CAT 1, CAT 2 and CAT 3, respectively. The average prevalence of pleurisy in CAT 1, CAT 2 and CAT 3 was 10.2, 21.2 and 29.1%, respectively (Table 3). The severity scores of *Mycoplasma*-like lesions, and the prevalence of pneumonia, fissures and pleurisy of each herd and each batch are shown in Table 6.

Serology

The serological results for *M. hyopneumoniae*, PRRSv and H1N1, H1N2, H3N2 swine influenza viruses of each herd and each batch per herd are shown in Table 7.

Associations between diversity of *M. hyopneumoniae* strains and lung lesions

The results of the final multivariable models are shown in Table 8. The severity of *Mycoplasma*-like lesions and the prevalence of pneumonia were higher in batches of CAT

Table 4 Descriptive results of the strain data of ten herds and the three batches (1–3) within each herd: prevalence of nPCR (n = 600) positive results, number of different *M. hyopneumoniae* strains, total number of *M. hyopneumoniae* strains and number of bronchoalveolar lavage fluid samples obtained with detection of double or triple different strains

Herd	A	B	C	D	E	F	G	H	I	J	Total
nPCR	88 (53/60)	63 (38/60)	87 (52/60)	80 (48/60)	95 (57/60)	83 (50/60)	98 (59/60)	100 (60/60)	63 (38/60)	66 (40/60)	83 (495/600)
1	100 (20/20)	55 (11/20)	85 (17/20)	95 (19/20)	100 (20/20)	95 (19/20)	95 (19/20)	100 (20/20)	15 (3/20)	5 (1/20)	75 (149/200)
2	65 (13/20)	55 (11/20)	90 (18/20)	90 (18/20)	85 (17/20)	90 (18/20)	100 (20/20)	100 (20/20)	90 (18/20)	95 (19/20)	86 (172/200)
3	100 (20/20)	80 (16/20)	85 (17/20)	55 (11/20)	100 (20/20)	65 (13/20)	100 (20/20)	100 (20/20)	85 (17/20)	100 (19/20)	87 (174/200)
Number of different strains	16	6	10	19	18	23	14	15	12	7	135
1	9	2	5	8	11	13	6	10	2	1	65
2	9	3	6	9	8	11	9	6	8	4	71
3	7	1	3	6	10	7	4	5	3	3	49
Number of strains	67	11	66	49	94	46	69	53	23	18	496
1	25	5	15	18	32	17	21	20	2	1	156
2	19	4	30	21	29	20	26	19	15	8	191
3	23	2	21	10	33	9	22	14	6	9	149
BALF double strains	16	0	15	4	36	11	13	6	1	0	102
1	6	0	1	0	12	5	4	3	0	0	31
2	5	0	10	3	10	4	5	2	1	0	40
3	5	0	4	1	14	2	4	1	0	0	31
BALF triple strains	1	0	1	0	1	2	1	0	0	0	6
1	0	0	0	0	0	0	0	0	0	0	0
2	1	0	1	0	1	2	1	0	0	0	6
3	0	0	0	0	0	0	0	0	0	0	0

Where applicable the prevalence data are followed by the number of positive samples (nPCR)/total number of samples (nPCR) between brackets.

nPCR: nested polymerase chain reaction, BALF: bronchoalveolar lavage fluid, 1, 2, 3: respectively 1st, 2nd and 3rd batch of each herd.

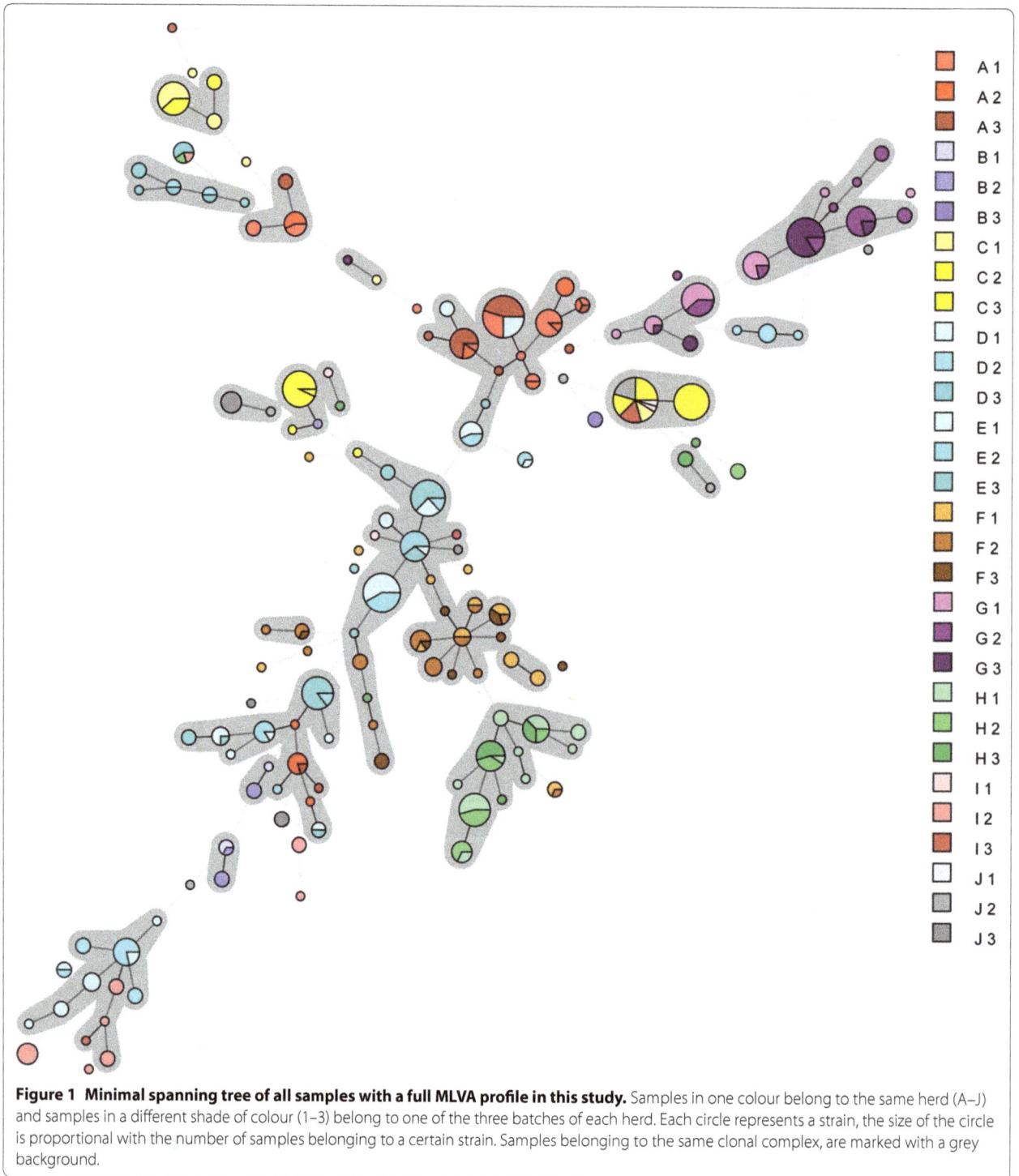

Figure 1 Minimal spanning tree of all samples with a full MLVA profile in this study. Samples in one colour belong to the same herd (A–J) and samples in a different shade of colour (1–3) belong to one of the three batches of each herd. Each circle represents a strain, the size of the circle is proportional with the number of samples belonging to a certain strain. Samples belonging to the same clonal complex, are marked with a grey background.

2 than in batches of CAT 1 and significantly higher in batches of CAT 3 than in batches of CAT 1 ($P = 0.064$ for CAT 2 to CAT and $P = 0.012$ for CAT 3 to CAT 1 and OR: 1.30; $P = 0.33$ for CAT 2 to CAT 1 and OR: 2.08; $P = 0.012$ for CAT 3 to CAT 1, respectively for the severity of *Mycoplasma*-like lesions and the prevalence of pneumonia).

In batches of CAT 2 and 3, there was a higher prevalence of fissures than in batches of CAT 1: CAT 2 to CAT 1: OR = 1.35; $P = 0.094$ and CAT 3 to CAT 1: OR = 1.70; $P = 0.007$).

Batches belonging to CAT 2 and 3 showed a lower prevalence of pleurisy (overall $P < 0.001$, CAT 2- CAT 1:

Table 5 The Hunter-Gaston discriminatory index was calculated for the complete dataset, for each VNTR, as well as for each of the 10 herds (A–J)

	Hunter-Gaston discriminatory index									
Herd	A	B	C	D	E	F	G	H	I	J
	89.7	89.1	82.0	93.8	89.1	95.7	85.8	88.2	92.3	85.2
VNTR	h1	h5	p146	p97	Total					
	88.0	88.5	90.8	77.5	98.4					

h1, h5, p146, p97: four VNTRs in the genome of *M. hyopneumoniae* of which the length of the amplified fragments were measured.

Total: the Hunter-Gaston DI calculated for the entire dataset.

$OR = 0.35$; $P < 0.001$ and CAT 3 to CAT 1: $OR = 0.34$; $P < 0.001$).

Discussion

The present study revealed that, using MLVA, many different *M. hyopneumoniae* strains are present in slaughter pigs from different pig herds and batches within a herd. The results also showed that prevalence and severity of pneumonia lesions at slaughter were significantly higher in batches where more different *M. hyopneumoniae* strains were found.

The ten selected study herds can be considered as representative for other pig herds, as the housing, feeding and management practices are quite similar to most Belgian and West-European herds. Also the prevalence of lung lesions (pneumonia 26%, fissures 41%, and pleurisy 25%) was similar to the results of previous studies [21]. The fact that three different batches of pigs were investigated within a herd, allowed to account for possible variations over time within a herd.

The minimal spanning tree (MST) visualizes the phylogenetic relationship of the analysed strains. In comparison with previous work [12], the MST in the present study had a wide distribution, confirming the high diversity of the *M. hyopneumoniae* strains. A weighing factor was assigned to each locus according to its abundancy in the dataset. This allowed to take into account the importance of variation of less abundant loci. To the author's knowledge this is the first time this approach is used for analysing the diversity of an organism. The Hunter-Gaston discriminatory index (98.4 when all four VNTRs are combined), confirmed that MLVA is a suitable and discriminatory technique to investigate genetic differences in *M. hyopneumoniae* [9]. The high variation in strains is also illustrated by the large number of different strains found at batch and even at animal level: in 102 pigs, two different strains were found, and in six pigs, three different strains were present. In theory more than three strains at animal level can be present and detected if multiple peaks in the electropherograms of each VNTR can be distinguished. In practice the MLVA-technique, has

some limitations: the detection limit is 100 organisms/ μL in bronchoalveolar lavage fluid and multiple strains can be detected if the differences in concentration are less than tenfold. Therefore, it cannot be excluded that only the dominant strains in the herd were detected [9]. Although it is known from previous studies that pigs may be infected with more than one strain [9, 11, 12], the results of the present study in vaccinated herds document a higher diversity of *M. hyopneumoniae* strains than shown by previous authors [6, 22–24]. The results also suggest that vaccination of piglets against *M. hyopneumoniae* does not lead to an important decrease in the diversity of *M. hyopneumoniae* strains in slaughter pigs. Some of the measures that might influence introduction of new strains in the farm might be purchasing and quarantine policy, swine density in the area, pig transport, all-in/all-out management and animal flow. It is not known whether contamination of the sampled pigs' lungs had occurred through the scalding water. Marois et al. showed that although *M. hyopneumoniae* was detected in the scalding water, the lungs of SPF pigs remained negative by nested PCR [25].

The prevalence and severity of pneumonia lesions at slaughter were significantly higher in batches where more different *M. hyopneumoniae* strains were found, illustrating for the first time the importance of strain diversity at batch level. The severity of *Mycoplasma*-like lesions, the prevalence of pneumonia and the prevalence of fissures was significantly higher in batches of CAT 3 compared to CAT 1, and numeric differences were obtained when batches of CAT 2 were compared to CAT 1. The effect of batch was significant in all models, indicating that there is quite some variation between successive batches in a herd. It also indicates the importance of investigating more batches from each herd.

The exact explanation why more different *M. hyopneumoniae* strains at batch level may lead to more pneumonia lesions is not known. Some strains have been shown to be more virulent than others [26], and infection with a low virulent strain did not protect against subsequent infection with a highly virulent strain [13]. On

Table 6 Descriptive results of lung lesions in the ten herds (A–J) and the three batches (1, 2, 3) within each herd: severity of *Mycoplasma*-like lesions (*n* = 3605), prevalence of pneumoniae (*n* = 3605), fissures (*n* = 3605) and pleurisy (*n* = 3820)

Herd	A	B	C	D	E	F	G	H	I	J	Overall
Mycoplasma-like lesions	7.2 ± 12.6	0.6 ± 1.9	4.8 ± 11.5	1.8 ± 5.1	10.2 ± 17.3	2.7 ± 9.0	7.8 ± 14.4	3.9 ± 10.8	4.0 ± 11.6	2.3 ± 7.7	4.6 ± 11.6
1	7.3 ± 12.2	0.6 ± 1.9	1.7 ± 3.4	2.1 ± 4.2	5.9 ± 10.1	0.4 ± 1.4	6.4 ± 12.8	6.7 ± 13.8	2.1 ± 10.3	1.2 ± 2.9	3.6 ± 9.3
2	8.3 ± 12.7	0.6 ± 1.9	4.1 ± 9.2	1.3 ± 4.7	10.9 ± 17.9	0.9 ± 5.7	6.7 ± 14.0	2.1 ± 7.6	1.4 ± 6.0	0.1 ± 0.9	3.6 ± 10.5
3	6.3 ± 13.0	0.5 ± 1.9	8.6 ± 16.7	1.8 ± 5.9	13.2 ± 20.5	6.6 ± 13.3	10.4 ± 15.9	2.5 ± 9.1	7.9 ± 15.2	4.9 ± 11.5	6.4 ± 14.0
Pneumonia %	42 (83/197)	9 (29/310)	30 (69/229)	19 (81/432)	45 (205/455)	17 (70/422)	41 (179/433)	22 (91/407)	19 (71/382)	16 (54/338)	26 (932/3605)
1	41	10	22	26	42	7	38	37	11	17	26
2	48	10	30	13	45	4	35	16	7	2	20
3	38	8	38	17	48	37	51	12	35	28	32
Fissures %	46 (90/197)	32 (99/310)	34 (78/229)	38 (164/432)	48 (217/455)	37 (155/422)	39 (170/433)	52 (213/407)	51 (194/382)	32 (107/338)	41 (1487/3605)
1	29	31	50	48	28	22	31	34	38	25	33
2	33	33	17	32	54	30	44	66	46	33	41
3	71	32	42	34	59	57	42	57	63	34	49
Pleurisy %	15 (30/200)	8 (25/319)	29 (73/250)	35 (162/461)	37 (185/494)	27 (119/445)	16 (71/454)	33 (149/445)	29 (120/411)	2 (6/341)	25 (940/3820)
1	1	2	7	39	38	21	16	25	32	3	21
2	26	7	45	35	37	28	20	34	27	2	27
3	20	15	26	32	37	32	11	43	30	1	26

Where applicable the prevalence data are followed by the number of positive results (prevalence lung lesions)/total number of lungs scored (lung lesions) between brackets.

Mycoplasma-like lesions: minimum 0% and maximum 100% of the lung surface affected with pneumonia.

Number of lungs scored for severity of *Mycoplasma*-like lesions, prevalence of pneumonia and fissures: 3605 (because of severe pleurisy in some lungs it was not possible to evaluate all lungs entirely).

Number of lungs scored for prevalence of pleurisy: 3820.

SD: standard deviation, *n*: number, 1, 2, 3: respectively 1st, 2nd and 3rd batch of each herd.

Table 7 Seroprevalence of *M. hyopneumoniae*, PRRSV, swine influenza subtypes H1N1, H1N2 and H3N2 in the ten herds (A–J)

Herd	A	B	C	D	E	F	G	H	I	J	Overall
ELISA *M. hyopneumoniae* n = 600	85 (51/60)	33 (20/60)	90 (54/60)	77 (46/60)	100 (60/60)	98 (59/60)	97 (58/60)	87 (52/60)	20 (12/60)	48 (29/60)	74 (441/600)
ELISA PRRSv n = 240	100 (24/24)	96 (23/24)	96 (23/24)	100 (24/24)	100 (24/24)	100 (24/24)	100 (24/24)	100 (24/24)	100 (24/24)	100 (24/24)	99 (238/240)
HI influenza H1N1 n = 240	88 (21/54)	100 (24/24)	100 (24/24)	100 (24/24)	79 (19/24)	92 (22/24)	100 (24/24)	100 (24/24)	100 (24/24)	100 (24/24)	96 (230/240)
HI influenza H1N2 n = 240	96 (23/24)	100 (24/24)	100 (24/24)	100 (24/24)	100 (24/24)	100 (24/24)	100 (24/24)	100 (24/24)	100 (24/24)	100 (24/24)	100 (239/240)
HI influenza H3N2 n = 240	54 (13/24)	71 (17/24)	67 (16/24)	42 (10/24)	75 (18/24)	71 (17/24)	54 (13/24)	21 (5/24)	54 (13/24)	79 (19/24)	59 (141/240)

Seroprevalence data are followed with number of positive samples/total number of samples between brackets.

n: number, PRRSv: porcine reproductive, HI: hemagglutination inhibition titers, SIV: swine influenza virus.

Table 8 Results of the four final multivariable models, with severity of *Mycoplasma*-like lesions, prevalence of pneumonia, fissures and pleurisy as outcome variables

	β	SE	OR	CI$_{min}$	CI$_{max}$	P
Severity of *Mycoplasma*-like lesions						
Intercept	−2.85	0.18	–	–	–	
CAT						0.027
CAT 2	0.35	0.19	–	–	–	0.064
CAT 3	0.51	0.20	–	–	–	0.012
Batch						<0.001
Batch 2	0.16	0.07	–	–	–	0.027
Batch 3	0.38	0.07	–	–	–	0.0021
Distance to public road[a]						0.0015
<100						
>100	0.24	0.08	–	–	–	0.0015
Stand empty farrowing unit[b]						<0.001
No						
Yes	−0.31	0.08	–	–	–	<0.001
Not always	0.03	0.09	–	–	–	0.70
Likelihood of pneumonia						
Intercept	−2.24	0.34	0.11	0.05	0.21	
CAT						<0.001
CAT 2	0.26	0.27	1.30	0.77	2.19	0.33
CAT 3	0.73	0.29	2.08	1.18	3.68	0.012
Batch						<0.001
Batch 2	−0.45	0.11	0.64	0.52	0.78	<0.001
Batch 3	0.42	0.10	1.53	1.25	1.86	<0.001
Number of herds surrounding the trial herd in a perimeter <5 km	0.01	0.00	1.01	1.01	1.01	<0.001
Vaccination gilts *M. hyopneumoniae*[b]						<0.001
No						
Yes	−0.99	0.23	0.37	0.24	0.58	<0.001
Likelihood of fissures						
Intercept	−0.94	0.20	0.39	0.26	0.58	
CAT						0.008
CAT 2	0.30	0.18	1.35	0.95	1.93	0.094
CAT 3	0.53	0.20	1.70	1.15	2.50	0.007
Batch						<0.001
Batch 2	0.29	0.09	1.34	1.12	1.59	0.001
Batch 3	0.74	0.09	2.09	1.75	2.48	<0.001
Distance to public road[a]						0.009
<100						
>100	0.26	0.10	1.30	1.07	1.58	0.009
Stand empty farrowing unit[b]						<0.001
Yes	−0.40	0.10	0.67	0.55	0.82	<0.001
Not always	−0.76	0.14	0.47	0.36	0.61	< 0.001

Table 8 continued

	β	SE	OR	CI$_{min}$	CI$_{max}$	P
Likelihood of pleurisy						
Intercept	0.25	0.72	1.29	0.32	5.25	
CAT						<0.001
CAT 2	−1.06	0.27	0.35	0.21	0.59	<0.001
CAT 3	−1.07	0.30	0.34	0.19	0.62	<0.001
Batch						0.002
Batch 2	0.35	0.10	1.41	1.16	1.72	<0.001
Batch 3	0.25	0.11	1.29	1.04	1.59	0.021
Cross fostering piglets during first week of life[b]						0.002
No						
<10%	−0.32	0.71	0.73	0.18	2.91	0.67
>10%	−1.96	0.77	0.14	0.03	0.64	0.040

Clinical signs *M. hyopneumoniae* with intensity cross fostering confounded. For severity of *Mycoplasma*-like lesions, a linear model was used. For the other outcome variables, a logistic model was used. For category (CAT), CAT 1 was the reference, for Batch, Batch 1 was the reference.

OR: odds ratio, CI: confidence interval, SE: standard error, *P*: *P* value, batch 1, 2, 3: referring to respectively the first, second and third sampling point in each herd, CAT (category) 1 (one *M. hyopneumoniae* strain per batch per herd), CAT 2: category 2 (two to six strains per batch per herd), CAT 3: category 3 (≥seven strains per batch per herd).

[a] <100 m is reference category.

[b] No is reference category.

the contrary, clinical symptoms and lesions were more severe in case of dual infection. It is therefore possible that also at batch level, the presence of many different *M. hyopneumoniae* strains may lead to more (severe) pneumonia lesions. Further research to explain the mechanisms is necessary. Charlebois et al. did not find a significant association between the number of different *M. hyopneumoniae* strains and severity of lung lesions in slaughter pigs [10].

To account for infection pressure possibly influencing the lung lesion data, rather than the number of different strains, all models were run with nPCR results included in the model. Only in the pneumonia model, the factor nPCR needed to be retained, but the overall conclusions for each model, including the pneumonia model remained the same (data not shown). Apart from *M. hyopneumoniae*, also other respiratory pathogens may be involved in pneumonia lesions [27]. Almost all pigs tested for swine influenza and PRRS virus were positive, and therefore, it is unlikely that these pathogens have biased the results. As lung lesions are multifactorial, the effect of potential non-infectious risk factors was taken into account in the multivariable models [14, 28, 29]. This allowed to investigate the effect of strain diversity in batches, apart from the effect of these risk factors. As the aim of the study was mainly to assess the importance of strain diversity, the other significant risk factors in the final models will only be discussed briefly.

The severity of *Mycoplasma*-like lesions was higher in batches from herds located further away from a public road (more than 100 versus less than 100 m), and when a stand-empty period in the farrowing unit was not practiced. The same two variables were also significant in the model for prevalence of fissures. One would expect that severity of lesions and prevalence of fissures to be higher in herds located closer to the public road, as this has been shown to be a risk factor for infection with *M. hyopneumoniae* [30]. One explanation could be that herds located further away from the public road are smaller herds with a lower biosecurity [31]. Also, all herds were located quite close to a public road in the present study. Not practicing a stand-empty period can be considered as one aspect of poor hygiene and biosecurity, which has been shown as a risk factor for respiratory disease [29].

The prevalence of pneumonia lesions was higher in case more other pig herds surrounded the herd, and when breeding gilts were not vaccinated against *M. hyopneumoniae*. Pig herd density in the region has been shown to be a risk factor for introduction of *M. hyopneumoniae* in the herd or for increased seroprevalence of *M. hyopneumoniae* [14, 32]. Purchasing gilts compared to no purchase was a risk factor for higher seroprevalence of *M. hyopneumoniae* in slaughter pigs [32]. Younger sows are more likely to transmit the infection to their piglets [33] and vaccination of breeding sows may lead to a lower infection level in weaned pigs [34] and to a lower prevalence of pneumonia in slaughter pigs [35].

Pleurisy was also measured in the study, as it is a common and economically important lesion. Experimental *M. hyopneumoniae* infection does however not lead to pleurisy lesions. Under field conditions, positive associations have been found between *M. hyopneumoniae* infection and pleurisy lesions [21], although the results are not consistent [36]. In the present study, although the descriptive values showed a higher prevalence of pleurisy when comparing CAT 2 and CAT 3 with CAT 1, the final models resulted in a higher number of different *M. hyopneumoniae* strains being associated with a lower prevalence of pleurisy, though the effect was small. A high intensity of mixing and cross-fostering pigs (>10%) compared to no cross-fostering of piglets was associated with a lower prevalence of pleurisy. This might be explained by the fact that cross-fostering may lead to a better colostrum intake by the piglets, resulting in better performance and health during their lifetime [37, 38].

MLVA testing on bronchoalveolar lavage fluid showed a high diversity of *M. hyopneumoniae* strains in slaughter pigs from herds vaccinated against *M. hyopneumoniae*. *Mycoplasma*-like lesions were more severe and the prevalence of pneumonia and fissures were higher when more different *M. hyopneumoniae* strains were present in a group of pigs. These results imply that inter- and intra-herd biosecurity measures decreasing the introduction of new *M. hyopneumoniae* strains, may lead to less (severe) pneumonia lesions in slaughter pigs.

Abbreviations

M. hyopneumoniae: Mycoplasma hyopneumoniae; MLVA: multiple locus variable-number tandem repeat analysis; VNTRs: variable number of tandem repeats; PBS: phosphate buffered saline; nPCR: nested polymerase chain reaction; TBE: tris–borate–EDTA; OD: optical density; PRRSv: porcine reproductive and respiratory syndrome virus; SIV: swine influenza virus; CAT: category; OR: odds ratio.

Competing interests

The authors declare that they have no competing interests.

Authors' contributions

AM designed the study protocol, selected and visited the farms and collected the questionnaires, visited the slaughter houses, performed the laboratory analysis, performed the statistical analysis, interpreted the data and wrote the manuscript. KV performed the analysis of the electropherograms and reviewed the manuscript. SP designed the statistical models and reviewed the manuscript. RDPS assisted with the slaughter house visits, reviewed the study protocol and the manuscript. IA reviewed the manuscript. FB, FH and DM reviewed the study protocol and the manuscript. All authors read and approved the final manuscript.

Acknowledgements

The authors want to thank the farmers for their cooperation and the slaughter houses Covameat and Comeco involved in the trial, especially Tine Delhaye, Trees Parmentier, Patrick Deceuninck, Benny Lammertyn and Christiaan Geldhof.

Funding

The study was financially supported by Pfizer A.H./Zoetis under the project name of "Effect of the diversity of Mycoplasma hyopneumoniae strains". The role of the funding body was merely financial for purchasing of materials and the analysis of the data. They did not have any role in the collection, interpretation, analysis and writing of the data.

Author details

[1] Department of Reproduction, Obstetrics and Herd Health, Unit Porcine Health Management, Faculty of Veterinary Medicine, Ghent University, Salisburylaan 133, 9820 Merelbeke, Belgium. [2] Applied Maths, Sint-Martens-Latem, Belgium. [3] Department of Pathology, Bacteriology and Avian Diseases, Faculty of Veterinary Medicine, Ghent University, Salisburylaan 133, 9820 Merelbeke, Belgium.

References

1. Thacker EL (2004) Diagnosis of *Mycoplasma hyopneumoniae*. J Swine Health Prod 12:252–254
2. Thacker E (2006) Mycoplasmal diseases. In: Zimmerman JJ, D'Allaire S, Taylor DJ (eds) Diseases of swine. Blacwell Publishing Ltd, Oxford
3. Minion FC, Lefkowitz EJ, Madsen ML, Cleary BJ, Swartzell SM, Mahairas GG (2004) The genome sequence of *Mycoplasma hyopneumoniae* strain 232, the agent of swine mycoplasmosis. J Bacteriol 186:7123–7133

4. Hutchison CA, Montague MG (2002) Mycoplasmas and the minimal genome concept. In: Razin S, Herrmann R (eds) Molecular biology and pathogenicity of mycoplasmas. Kluwer Academic/Plenum Publishers, New York

5. Madsen ML, Oneal MJ, Gardner SW, Strait EL, Nettleton D, Thacker EL, Minion FC (2007) Array-based genomic comparative hybridization analysis of field strains of Mycoplasma hyopneumoniae. J Bacteriol 189:7977–7982

6. Vranckx K, Haesebrouck F, Maes D, Pasmans F (2012) Mycoplasma hyopneumoniae diversity in pigs. Ph.D. Thesis, Ghent University, Department of Pathology, Bacteriology and Poultry Diseases, Faculty of Veterinary Medicine

7. Torres-Cruz J, van der Woude MW (2003) Slipped-strand mispairing can function as a phase variation mechanism in Escherichia coli. J Bacteriol 185:6990–6994

8. Dos Santos LF, Sreevatsan S, Torremorell M, Moreira MAS, Sibila M, Pieters M (2015) Genotype distribution of Mycoplasma hyopneumoniae in swine herds from different geographical regions. Vet Microbiol 175:374–381

9. Vranckx K, Maes D, Calus D, Villarreal I, Pasmans F, Haesebrouck F (2011) Multiple locus variable number of tandem repeats analysis is a suitable tool for the differentiation of Mycoplasma hyopneumoniae strains without cultivation. J Clin Microbiol 49:2020–2023

10. Charlebois A, Marois-Créhan C, Hélie P, Gagnon CA, Gottschalk M, Archambault M (2014) Genetic diversity of Mycoplasma hyopneumoniae isolates of abattoir pigs. Vet Microbiol 168:348–356

11. Nathues H, Beilage EG, Lothar Kreienbrock L, Rosengarten R, Spergser J (2011) RAPD and VNTR analyses demonstrate genotypic heterogeneity of Mycoplasma hyopneumoniae isolates from pigs housed in a regionwith high pig density. Vet Microbiol 152:338–345

12. Vranckx K, Maes D, Del Pozo Sacristán R, Pasmans F, Haesebrouck F (2011) A longitudinal study of the diversity and dynamics of Mycoplasma hyopneumoniae infections in pig herds. Vet Microbiol 156:315–321

13. Villarreal I, Maes D, Meyns T, Gebruers F, Calus D, Pasmans F, Haesebrouck F (2009) Infection with a low virulent Mycoplasma hyopneumoniae isolate does not protect piglets against subsequent infection with a highly virulent M. hyopneumoniae isolate. Vaccine 27:1875–1879

14. Villarreal I (2010) Epidemiology of Mycoplasma hyopneumoniae infections and effect of control measures. Ph.D. Thesis, Ghent University, Department of Reproduction, Obstetrics and Herd Health, Faculty of Veterinary Medicine

15. Morrison RB, Hilley HD, Leman AD (1985) Comparison of methods for assessing the prevalence and extent of pneumonia in market weight swine. Can Vet J 26:381–384

16. Kobish M, Blanchard B, Le Potier MF (1993) Mycoplasma hyopneumoniae infection in pigs: duration of the disease and resistance to reinfection. Vet Res 24:67–77

17. Michiels A, Piepers S, Ulens T, Van Ransbeeck N, Del Pozo Sacristán R, Sierens A, Haesebrouck F, Demeyer P, Maes D (2015) Impact of particulate matter and ammonia on average daily weight gain, mortality and lung lesions in pigs. Prev Vet Med 121:99–107

18. Stärk KDC, Nicolet J, Frey J (1998) Detection of Mycoplasma hyopneumoniae by air sampling with a nested PCR assay. Appl Environ Microbiol 64:543–548

19. Hunter PR, Gaston M (1988) Numerical index of the discriminatory ability of typing systems: an application of Simpson's index of diversity. J Clin Microbiol 26:2465–2466

20. Rasbash J, Charlton C, Browne WJ, Healy M, Cameron B (2012) MLwiN Version 2.26. University of Bristol, Centre for Multilevel Modelling

21. Meyns T, Van Steelant J, Rolly E, Dewulf J, Haesebrouck F, Maes D (2011) A cross-sectional study of risk factors associated with pulmonary lesions in pigs at slaughter. Vet J 187:388–392

22. Calus D (2010) Phenotypic characterization of Mycoplasma hyopneumoniae isolates of different virulence. Ph.D. Thesis, Ghent University, Departement of Pathology, Bacteriology and Poultry Diseases, Faculty of Veterinary Medicine

23. Mayor D, Zeeh F, Frey J, Kuhnert P (2007) Diversity of Mycoplasma hyopneumoniae in pig farms revealed by direct molecular typing of clinical material. Vet Res 38:391–398

24. Nathues H (2011) Influence of Mycoplasma hyopneumoniae strain variation, environmental factors and co-infections on enzootic pneumonia in pigs. Ph.D. Thesis, University of Hannover, Field Station for Epidemiology, Bakum

25. Marois C, Cariolet R, Morvan H, Kobisch M (2008) Transmission of pathogenic respiratory bacteria to specific pathogen free pigs at slaughter. Vet Microbiol 129:325–332

26. Vicca J, Stakenborg T, Maes D, Butaye P, Peeters J, de Kruif A, Haesebrouck F (2003) Evaluation of virulence of Mycoplasma hyopneumoniae field isolates. Vet Microbiol 97(97):177–190

27. Sibila M, Pieters M, Molitor T, Maes D, Haesebrouck F, Segalés J (2009) Current perspectives on the diagnosis and epidemiology of Mycoplasma hyopneumoniae infection. Vet J 181:221–231

28. Del Pozo Sacristán R (2014) Treatment and control of Mycoplasma hyopneumoniae infections. Ph.D. Thesis, Ghent University, Department of Reproduction, Obstetrics and Herd Health, Faculty of Veterinary Medicine

29. Stärk KDC (2000) Epidemiological investigation of the influence of environmental risk factors on respiratory diseases in swine—a literature review. Vet J 159:37–56

30. Stärk KDC, Keller H, Eggenberger E (1992) Risk factors for the reinfection of specific pathogen-free pig breeding herds with enzootic pneumonia. Vet Rec 23:532–535

31. Amass F, Clark LK (1999) Biosecurity considerations for pork production units. Swine Health Prod 7:217–228

32. Maes D, Deluyker H, Verdonck M, Castryck F, Miry C, Vrijens B, de Kruif A (2000) Herd factors associated with the seroprevalences of four major respiratory pathogens in slaughter pigs from farrow-to-finish pig herds. Vet Res 31:313–327

33. Fano E, Pijoan C, Dee S, Torremorell M (2006) Assessment of the effect of sow parity on the prevalence of Mycoplasma hyopneumoniae in piglets at weaning IPVS, 19th edn. Denmark, Copenhagen

34. Ruiz AR, Utrera V, Pijoan C (2003) Effect of Mycoplasma hyopneumoniae sow vaccination on piglet colonization at weaning. J Swine Health Prod 11:131–135

35. Sibila M, Bernal R, Torrents D, Riera P, Llopart D, Calsamiglia M, Segalés J (2008) Effect of sow vaccination against Mycoplasma hyopneumoniae on sow and piglet colonization and seroconversion, and pig lung lesions at slaughter. Vet Microbiol 127:165–170

36. Fraile L, Alegre A, López-Jiménez R, Nofrarías M, Segalés J (2010) Risk factors associated with pleuritis and cranio-ventral pulmonary consolidation in slaughter-aged pigs. Vet J 184:326–333

37. Quesnel H (2011) Colostrum production by sows: variability of colostrum yield and immunoglobulin G concentrations. Animal 5:1546–1553

38. Declerck I, Dewulf J, Sarrazin S, Maes D (2016) Long-term effects of colostrum intake in piglet mortality and performance. J Anim Sci 94:1633–1643

Permissions

All chapters in this book were first published in VR, by BioMed Central; hereby published with permission under the Creative Commons Attribution License or equivalent. Every chapter published in this book has been scrutinized by our experts. Their significance has been extensively debated. The topics covered herein carry significant findings which will fuel the growth of the discipline. They may even be implemented as practical applications or may be referred to as a beginning point for another development.

The contributors of this book come from diverse backgrounds, making this book a truly international effort. This book will bring forth new frontiers with its revolutionizing research information and detailed analysis of the nascent developments around the world.

We would like to thank all the contributing authors for lending their expertise to make the book truly unique. They have played a crucial role in the development of this book. Without their invaluable contributions this book wouldn't have been possible. They have made vital efforts to compile up to date information on the varied aspects of this subject to make this book a valuable addition to the collection of many professionals and students.

This book was conceptualized with the vision of imparting up-to-date information and advanced data in this field. To ensure the same, a matchless editorial board was set up. Every individual on the board went through rigorous rounds of assessment to prove their worth. After which they invested a large part of their time researching and compiling the most relevant data for our readers.

The editorial board has been involved in producing this book since its inception. They have spent rigorous hours researching and exploring the diverse topics which have resulted in the successful publishing of this book. They have passed on their knowledge of decades through this book. To expedite this challenging task, the publisher supported the team at every step. A small team of assistant editors was also appointed to further simplify the editing procedure and attain best results for the readers.

Apart from the editorial board, the designing team has also invested a significant amount of their time in understanding the subject and creating the most relevant covers. They scrutinized every image to scout for the most suitable representation of the subject and create an appropriate cover for the book.

The publishing team has been an ardent support to the editorial, designing and production team. Their endless efforts to recruit the best for this project, has resulted in the accomplishment of this book. They are a veteran in the field of academics and their pool of knowledge is as vast as their experience in printing. Their expertise and guidance has proved useful at every step. Their uncompromising quality standards have made this book an exceptional effort. Their encouragement from time to time has been an inspiration for everyone.

The publisher and the editorial board hope that this book will prove to be a valuable piece of knowledge for researchers, students, practitioners and scholars across the globe.

List of Contributors

Lukas Schwarz, Bettina Wöchtl and Andrea Ladinig
Department for Farm Animals and Veterinary Public Health, University Clinic for Swine, University of Veterinary Medicine Vienna, Veterinaerplatz 1, 1210 Vienna, Austria

Christiane Riedel, Leonie J. Sinn, Till Rümenapf and Benjamin Lamp
Department of Pathobiology, Institute of Virology, University of Veterinary Medicine Vienna, Veterinaerplatz 1, 1210 Vienna, Austria

Sandra Högler, Nora Dinhopl, Barbara Rebel-Bauder and Herbert Weissenböck
Department of Pathobiology, Institute of Pathology and Forensic Veterinary Medicine, University of Veterinary Medicine Vienna, Veterinaerplatz 1, 1210 Vienna, Austria

Thomas Voglmayr
Traunkreis Vet Clinic, Großendorf 3, 4551 Ried im Traunkreis, Austria

Sean R. Wattegedera, Yvonne Pang, David Frew, Tom N. McNeilly and Colin J. McInnes
Moredun Research Institute, International Research Centre, Pentlands Science Park, Bush Loan, Penicuik, Scotland EH26 0PZ, UK

Yolanda Corripio-Miyar and Gary Entrican
Moredun Research Institute, International Research Centre, Pentlands Science Park, Bush Loan, Penicuik, Scotland EH26 0PZ, UK
The Roslin Institute and Royal (Dick) School of Veterinary Studies, The University of Edinburgh, Easter Bush, Midlothian, Scotland EH25 9RG, UK

Javier Palarea-Albaladejo
Biomathematics and Statistics Scotland, JCMB, The King's Buildings, Peter Guthrie Tait Road, Edinburgh, Scotland EH9 3FD, UK

Jayne C. Hope and Elizabeth J. Glass
The Roslin Institute and Royal (Dick) School of Veterinary Studies, The University of Edinburgh, Easter Bush, Midlothian, Scotland EH25 9RG, UK

Katharina Sobotta, Katharina Bonkowski, Elisabeth Liebler-Tenorio and Christian Menge
Institute of Molecular Pathogenesis, Friedrich-Loeffler-Institut (FLI), Naumburger Strasse 96a, 07743 Jena, Germany

Pierre Germon and Pascal Rainard
ISP, INRA, Université Tours, UMR 1282, 37380 Nouzilly, France

Nina Hambruch and Christiane Pfarrer
Department of Anatomy, University of Veterinary Medicine Hannover, Bischofsholer Damm 15, 30173 Hannover, Germany

Ilse D. Jacobsen
Research Group Microbial Immunology, Leibniz Institute for Natural Product Research and Infection Biology/Hans Knoell Institute, Beutenbergstrasse 11a, 07745 Jena, Germany

Caroline S. Corbett, Jeroen De Buck, Karin Orsel and Herman W. Barkema
Department of Production Animal Health, Faculty of Veterinary Medicine, University of Calgary, Calgary, AB, Canada

Lenka Kavanová
Veterinary Research Institute, Hudcova 296/70, 62100 Brno, Czech Republic
Institute of Experimental Biology, Faculty of Science, Masaryk University, Kotlářská 267/2, 61137 Brno, Czech Republic

Katarína Matiašková
Veterinary Research Institute, Hudcova 296/70, 62100 Brno, Czech Republic
University of Veterinary and Pharmaceutical Sciences Brno, Palackého třída 1946/1, 612 42 Brno, Czech Republic

Lenka Levá, Hana Štěpánová, Kateřina Nedbalcová, Ján Matiašovic, Martin Faldyna and Jiří Salát
Veterinary Research Institute, Hudcova 296/70, 62100 Brno, Czech Republic

Zehui Liu, Yangkun Liu, Yuanyuan Zhang, Yajuan Yang, Jingjing Ren, Xiaoying Zhang and Enqi Du
College of Veterinary Medicine, Northwest A&F University, Yangling, Shaanxi 712100, People's Republic of China

Jitka Mucksová, Jiří Kalina, Barbora Benešová and Pavel Trefil
BIOPHARM, Research Institute of Biopharmacy and Veterinary Drugs, Jílové U Prahy, Czech Republic

Jiří Plachý and Jiří Hejnar
Institute of Molecular Genetics, Academy of Sciences of the Czech Republic, Prague, Czech Republic

Ondřej Staněk
Institute of Microbiology, Academy of Sciences of the Czech Republic, Prague, Czech Republic

Viktor Ahlberg, Bernt Hjertner, Stina Hellman and Caroline Fossum
Department of Biomedical Sciences and Veterinary Public Health, Swedish University of Agricultural Sciences, SLU, Uppsala, Sweden

Per Wallgren
National Veterinary Institute, SVA, Uppsala, Sweden

Karin Lövgren Bengtsson
Novavax AB, Uppsala, Sweden

Zuzana Sekelova, Hana Stepanova, Ondrej Polansky, Karolina Varmuzova, Marcela Faldynova, Ivan Rychlik and Lenka Vlasatikova
Veterinary Research Institute, Hudcova 70, 621 00 Brno, Czech Republic

Radek Fedr
Department of Cytokinetics, Institute of Biophysics of the CAS, Kralovopolska 135, 612 65 Brno, Czech Republic

Center of Biomolecular and Cellular Engineering, International, Clinical Research Center, St. Anne's University Hospital Brno, Pekarska 53, 656 91 Brno, Czech Republic

D. J. Begg, A. C. Purdie, K. de Silva, N. K. Dhand, K. M. Plain and R. J. Whittington
Farm Animal and Veterinary Public Health, Sydney School of Veterinary Science and School of Life and Environmental Sciences, Faculty of Science, The University of Sydney, 425 Werombi Rd, Camden, NSW 2570, Australia

C. De Witte, B. Flahou, I. Bosschem, R. Ducatelle and F. Haesebrouck
Department of Pathology, Bacteriology and Avian Diseases, Faculty of Veterinary Medicine, Ghent University, Merelbeke, Belgium

B. Devriendt
Department of Virology, Parasitology, Immunology, Faculty of Veterinary Medicine, Ghent University, Merelbeke, Belgium

A. Smet
Laboratory of Experimental Medicine and Pediatrics, Faculty of Medicine and Health Sciences, Antwerp University, Antwerp, Belgium

Mary J. Pantin-Jackwood, Mar Costa-Hurtado, Kateri Bertran, Eric DeJesus, Diane Smith and David E. Swayne
Exotic and Emerging Avian Viral Diseases Research Unit, Southeast Poultry Research Laboratory, U.S. National Poultry Research Center, Agricultural Research Service, U.S. Department of Agriculture, 934 College Station Rd, Athens, GA 30605, USA

Han Zheng, Xiaotong Qiu and Jianguo Xu
State Key Laboratory for Infectious Disease Prevention and Control, Collaborative Innovation Center for Diagnosis and Treatment of Infectious Diseases, National Institute for Communicable Disease Control and Prevention, Chinese Center for Disease Control and Prevention, Changping, Beijing, China

David Roy, Mariela Segura and Marcelo Gottschalk
Faculty of Veterinary Medicine, Swine and Poultry Infectious Diseases Research Center, University of Montreal, Quebec, Canada

Pengchen Du
Institute of Infectious Diseases, Beijing Ditan Hospital, Capital Medical University, Beijing Key Laboratory of Emerging Infectious Diseases, Beijing, People's Republic of China

Elena L. Sassu, Andrea Ladinig, Christian Knecht, Heiko Stein and Isabel Hennig-Pauka
University Clinic for Swine, Department of Farm Animals and Veterinary Public Health, University of Veterinary Medicine, Vienna, Austria

Stephanie C. Talker, Maria Stadler and Wilhelm Gerner
Institute of Immunology, Department of Pathobiology, University of Veterinary Medicine Vienna, Vienna, Austria

Janna Frömbling, Joachim Spergser and Monika Ehling-Schulz
Functional Microbiology, Institute of Microbiology, Department of Pathobiology, University of Veterinary Medicine Vienna, Vienna, Austria

Barbara Richter
Institute of Pathology and Forensic Veterinary Medicine, Department of Pathobiology, University of Veterinary Medicine Vienna, Vienna, Austria

Robert Graage
Division of Swine Medicine, Department of Farm Animals, University of Zurich, Vetsuisse Faculty, Zurich, Switzerland

Pardeep Sharma, Vivek V. Pande, Talia S. Moyle, Andrea R. McWhorter and Kapil K. Chousalkar
School of Animal and Veterinary Sciences, The University of Adelaide, Roseworthy, SA 5173, Australia

Annelies Michiels, Sofie Piepers, Rubén Del Pozo Sacristán, Ioannis Arsenakis and Dominiek Maes
Department of Reproduction, Obstetrics and Herd Health, Unit Porcine Health Management, Faculty of Veterinary Medicine, Ghent University, Salisburylaan 133, 9820 Merelbeke, Belgium

Katleen Vranckx
Applied Maths, Sint-Martens-Latem, Belgium

Filip Boyen and Freddy Haesebrouck
Department of Pathology, Bacteriology and Avian Diseases, Faculty of Veterinary Medicine, Ghent University, Salisburylaan 133, 9820 Merelbeke, Belgium

Index

www.ingramcontent.com/pod-product-compliance
Lightning Source LLC
Chambersburg PA
CBHW082041190326
41458CB00010B/3430